BEST PRACTICES IN TEACHING NURSING

National League for Nursing

BEST PRACTICES IN TEACHING NURSING

Edited by:

Joanne Noone, PhD, RN, CNE, FAAN, ANEF

Paula Gubrud, EdD, RN, CHSE, FAAN, ANEF

. Wolters Kluwer

Philadelphia · Baltimore · New York · London
Buenos Aires · Hong Kong · Sydney · Tokyo

Vice President, Nursing Segment: Julie K. Stegman
Director, Nursing Education and Practice Content: Jamie Blum
Senior Development Editor: Meredith L. Brittain
Marketing Manager: Greta Swanson
Editorial Assistant: Sara Thul
Manager, Graphic Arts and Design: Steve Druding
Art Director: Jennifer Clements
Production Project Manager: Catherine Ott
Manufacturing Coordinator: Margie Orzech
Prepress Vendor: Aptara, Inc.

Noone, J., & Gubrud, P. (2024). *Best practices in teaching nursing*. National League for Nursing.

9 8 7 6 5 4 3 2 1

Printed in the United States of America

Library of Congress Cataloging-in-Publication Data available upon request.
978-1-9752-3220-7

shop.LWW.com   www.NLN.org

About the Editors

Joanne Noone, PhD, RN, CNE, FAAN, ANEF, is an AB Youmans Spaulding Distinguished Professor and Director of the Master's in Nursing Education Program at the Oregon Health & Science University School of Nursing. Dr. Noone has over three decades of experience teaching nursing in associate degree and baccalaureate programs; RN to BS completion programs; as well as master's and doctoral programs. She currently teaches in the Master's in Nursing Education program at OHSU in which three of the courses she teaches are certified by Quality Matters, meeting national standards for best practices in online education. Dr. Noone received her PhD in nursing from the University of Hawaii in 2003. She has been certified since 2009 as an academic nurse educator by the National League for Nursing (NLN) and was inducted as a fellow into the NLN Academy of Nursing Education in 2017 and into the American Academy of Nursing in 2018. Dr. Noone's contributions to nursing education aim to promote health equity through learning activities to prepare nurses to care for diverse populations and an educational strategy to improve nursing workforce diversity. She developed a model for undergraduate nursing programs to improve workforce diversity focused on recruitment, enrollment, retention, and graduation strategies. This has had an impact on the improved representation of underrepresented minority graduates in associated nursing programs.

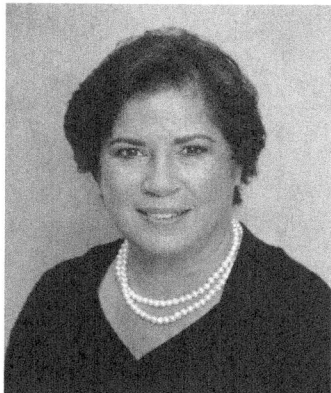

Paula Gubrud, EdD, RN, CHSE, FAAN, ANEF, is an Associate Professor Emeritus from Oregon Health & Science University School of Nursing. Dr. Gubrud has over 30 years of experience in nursing and health professions education. She received her EdD in post-secondary education in 2008 from Portland State University, an MS in community health nursing from Oregon Health & Science University in 1993, and a BS in nursing from Walla Walla University in 1980. Dr. Gubrud is one of the architects of the Oregon Consortium of Nursing Education (OCNE) and served as the co-director of the partnership for over 10 years. Her nursing education experience expands multiple levels of nursing education from LPN to graduate programs. Dr. Gubrud is a national and international speaker and consultant for colleges, universities, and health systems providing faculty development courses and curricular integration expertise focused on clinical education and simulation-based

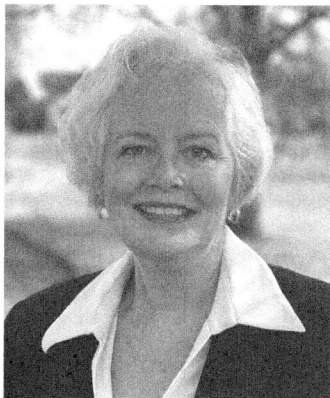

learning experiences. She led the initiative in creating the OCNE Clinical Education Model. The model integrates the science of learning and is designed to facilitate clinical learning designed to align with competency-based curriculum. Dr. Gubrud has authored a medical-surgical textbook, numerous book chapters, and articles on simulation and clinical education. Her research interests are focused on applying clinical learning and simulation-based learning experiences to facilitate development of clinical reasoning.

About the Contributors

Gail Armstrong, PhD, DNP, RN, ACNS-BC, CNE, FAAN, is a professor and faculty development coordinator at the University of Colorado College of Nursing. Known as a strong educator, Gail's two-decade career in higher education has included teaching and curricular development in prelicensure, master's degree, and DNP programs. Gail's clinical practice began at the bedside as a medical-surgical nurse, then as an adult clinical nurse specialist, and more recently, was focused in the area of quality and safety. Gail's academic and practice career has focused on teaching health professionals how to integrate health care systems improvement into their practice. Gail's scholarly work includes developing strategies for early and sustained integration of the IOM/NAM competencies into prelicensure curricula, which challenged decades-old models of curricular progression. Gail is the primary author of Leadership and Systems Improvement for the DNP, a 2020 text that offers leadership and systems improvement content for DNP nursing clinical leaders.

Holly Fiock, MSEd, is a senior instructional design manager and adjunct professor at Purdue University in West Lafayette, Indiana. With over a decade of teaching experience in various programs, she specializes in online learning, curriculum development, and instructional design. Ms. Fiock has published and presented extensively in the field of online learning, with a specific focus on utilizing the Community of Inquiry framework in online learning environments. Her contributions have been recognized through prestigious awards, including the UPCEA's Outstanding Service in Postsecondary Instructional Design award, D2L Excellence Award, and Association for Educational Communications and Technology's Outstanding Research and Theory Division Sponsored Accepted Student Proposal Award.

Susan Gross Forneris, PhD, RN, CNE, CHSE-A, FAAN, is currently the associate dean and professor for academic programs at the University of Minnesota. Dr. Forneris has been a nurse educator for over 25 years. As a former director for innovation in education excellence at the National League for Nursing, she traveled globally working closely with many nursing education influencers to prepare faculty in teaching and learning best practices with emphasis in simulation. She is instrumental in the design and implementation of faculty development courses focused on the science of teaching and learning, curriculum and instructional design, simulation foundations, debriefing, and learner evaluation. Her research and publications focus on the development and use of reflective teaching strategies to enhance critical thinking. She co-authored the publications *Critical Conversations: The NLN Guide for Teaching Thinking* and *Critical Conversations: From Monologue to Dialogue*. Recognized nationally and internationally for her expertise and leadership driving programs on faculty preparation to teach, she was inducted as a fellow in the American Academy of Nursing in 2018.

Ashley E. Franklin, PhD, RN, CNE, CHSE-A, is an associate professor and the Rankin Endowed Professor at Texas Christian University in Fort Worth, Texas, where she teaches primarily in simulation and coordinates simulation faculty onboarding. Dr. Franklin has expertise in faculty development, curriculum development and evaluation, experiential learning, and mentoring. She is president-elect of the International Nursing Association for Clinical Simulation and Learning, and she received the American Association of College of Nursing's Scholarship of Teaching and Learning Excellence Award in 2019. Dr. Franklin facilitates simulation with prelicensure nursing students in dedicated simulation courses and has taught simulation pedagogy graduate courses. Her program of research centers on nurses' simulation behavioral performance and factors that underpin behavior. Dr. Franklin's research has been supported by Sigma Theta Tau International, the National League for Nursing, the National Network of Libraries of Medicine, and the US Army Research Institute.

Heather Hawk, DNP, RN, CCRN-K, CNE, is an assistant professor of clinical nursing at Oregon Health and Science University, where she teaches in the RN baccalaureate completion program. Her clinical expertise is in pediatric critical care. As an NLN-certified nurse educator and participant in OHSU's Education Scholars Program, Heather is passionate about creating learning environments that allow nursing students to excel. She is particularly interested in how human connection can support learning and resilience. Heather is active in the National League for Nursing, Sigma Theta Tau, and Quality Matters, and serves as co-chair of the curriculum committee for the Oregon Consortium of Nursing Education.

Jeremy Hutson, MSN, RN, began teaching prelicensure nursing at Clackamas Community College in Portland, Oregon in 2018. His roles included theory instructor, clinical instructor, and simulation instructor. Jeremy has participated in multiple-patient simulation research focusing on learner behaviors and pre-briefing methods. Jeremy is currently pursuing his PhD in Health Sciences-Nursing at Texas Christian University with a focus on simulation education.

Seiko Izumi, PhD, RN, FPCN, is an associate professor at Oregon Health & Science University School of Nursing in Portland, Oregon. She has over 20 years of experience teaching in the BSN, MSN, and doctoral (DNP and PhD) programs in both the US and Japan. Dr. Izumi has expertise in program evaluation, learning theories, and interprofessional education. Her areas of interest include palliative care, health system research, interprofessional collaboration, and professional ethics. She has over 100 publications and presented nationally and internationally. She is a recipient of the Excellence in Teaching Award, a Sojourns Palliative Leadership Scholar, a Fellow in Palliative Care Nursing, and a Fellow in Western Academy of Nursing, and is recognized as a nurse leader in the palliative care field.

Kathie Lasater, EdD, RN, FAAN, ANEF, is a professor emerita at Oregon Health & Science University, where she taught all levels of nursing students for 19 years. As an educationalist, Dr. Lasater was deeply engaged in a major statewide curriculum development project, spanning several years, and has consulted on other curricular development and revision projects. As a nursing education researcher, Dr. Lasater is best known as the creator of the Lasater Clinical Judgment Rubric, which describes a trajectory of clinical judgment development and is also used as an assessment tool. The rubric has been translated or is in the process of translation into 19 languages. Her primary clinical focus lies in population and community health. In 2018, Dr. Lasater was a Fulbright Research Scholar at Edinburgh Napier University, where she currently serves as a visiting professor, helping to lay the groundwork for a deepening emphasis on social determinants of health and the care of populations. In addition to being a frequent speaker, she is also an assistant editor for *Nurse Education Today*.

Glenise McKenzie, PhD, MN, RN, is an associate professor of nursing at Oregon Health & Science University where she has been a faculty member since 2006 and director of the Bachelor's Completion Online Program for 8 years. She has experience in various teaching delivery methods, with a content focus on communication, mental health, gerontology, ethics, and leadership. Dr. McKenzie has worked as a nurse in the areas of gerontology and psychiatry for over 30 years. Her scholarship in teaching and learning has focused on inquiry-based strategies for addressing and minimizing the stigma surrounding individuals with mental health disorders and, most recently, on enhancing collaborative learning in online courses and improving student engagement online. Dr. McKenzie is a leader in the implementation of Quality Matters (QM), a peer-review process for best practices, in online learning at OHSU.

Teri A. Murray, PhD, PHNA-BC, RN, FAAN, ANEF, is a professor and dean emerita at Saint Louis University School of Nursing. She serves as their inaugural chief diversity and inclusion officer. She is the project director for her third Department of Health and Human Services, Health Resource and Service Administration, Nursing Workforce Diversity Grant. Dr. Murray works tirelessly to advance diversity in nursing education and the nursing workforce. In addition, she has served on the AACN Board of Directors and on the HRSA National Advisory Committee for Nurse Education and Practice. She has held positions as a national adviser to the Robert Wood Johnson Foundation New Careers in Nursing program, president and board member of the Missouri State Board of Nursing, and Missouri delegate to the National Council of State Boards of Nursing. Her research and policy interests are focused on the social determinants of health and the interplay in the social environment, the political environment, and health outcomes.

Rana Halabi Najjar, PhD, RN, CPNP (she, her, هي), is an associate professor at Oregon Health & Science University, teaching in the undergraduate and graduate programs in the School of Nursing for the last 12 years. Dr. Najjar's research and scholarship focus on bias, discrimination, and equitable and inclusive practices in health care education. She is a 2022 AACN Diversity Institute Leadership Fellow and has served on the Western Institute of Nursing Diversity Equity and Inclusion committee since its inception. Dr. Najjar has developed an online platform to engage educators interested in trauma-informed education practices (TIEP) and is leading a collaborative effort at OHSU to design, implement, and evaluate faculty/staff training on TIEP. She has published manuscripts and presented at regional, national, and international conferences with the goal of raising awareness of the impact of inequities on learning and building a community of trauma-informed educators.

Ann Nielsen, PhD, RN, is an associate professor of clinical nursing emerita at Oregon Health & Science University in Portland, Oregon, where she taught in the Bachelor of Science in Nursing and Masters in Nursing Education programs, as well as directed the Undergraduate Nursing Program. Her clinical experience is in neonatal, perinatal, pediatric, and community nursing practice. Dr. Nielsen's scholarship interests are the development of clinical judgment and reasoning, effective clinical education using concept-based learning and reflection, and transition to practice. She has done research, published, and presented on a wide range of nursing education topics.

Barbara J. Patterson, PhD, RN, FAAN, ANEF, is a distinguished professor and director of the PhD program in the School of Nursing and associate dean for scholarship and inquiry at Widener University in Chester, Pennsylvania. She is also the Distinguished Scholar in the NLN/Chamberlain Center for Advancing the Science of Nursing Education. She has chaired over 50 PhD dissertations, many investigating nursing education topics. Dr. Patterson has presented and published extensively on nursing education, specifically in the areas of evidence-based teaching, veterans' academic transitions, and leadership in nursing education. Her passion is in the generation and translation of evidence for nursing education practice. She has served as faculty and mentor for novice nurse educators in the Nurse Faculty Leadership Academies of Sigma focusing on leadership development. Dr. Patterson serves as staff of NLN's Research in Nursing Education Grants Program reviewing nursing education research grants. She is the editor-in-chief for Nursing Education Perspectives.

Kathleen Poindexter, PhD, RN, CNE, ANEF, is an associate professor and interim associate dean of academic affairs and faculty development at MSU College of Nursing (CON) as well as chair of the National League for Nursing. In addition, she is the director of the College Teaching in Nursing Certificate Program, CON teaching assistant program, and faculty mentoring program. She provides faculty consultations on teaching to support student learning outcomes, including teaching in online environments, and scholarship of teaching and learning (SOTL) projects. Dr. Poindexter is involved beyond the discipline of nursing as a member of the Interprofessional Education Strategic Planning and Development Committee in collaboration with the College of Osteopathic Medicine and multiple regional community colleges. Dr. Poindexter is board-certified in nursing education and is a fellow in the Academy of Nurse Educators. Dr. Poindexter has over 30 years of academic experience and leadership in curricular and program development.

Christine Tanner, PhD, RN (ret), FAAN, ANEF, is a professor emerita at the Oregon Health & Science University School of Nursing and a national leader in nursing education innovation and scholarship. Dr. Tanner served as editor-in-chief for the *Journal of Nursing Education* from 1991 to 2012. Her program of research, spanning four decades, focused on the development of expertise in clinical judgment and the impact of different education models on the development of skill in clinical judgment. She has published scores of books and journal articles on the topic, as well as presented numerous workshops, lectures, and keynote addresses both in the United States and internationally. Dr. Tanner was one of the leads in the development of the innovative Oregon Consortium for Nursing Education competency-based curriculum and the adoption of research-based pedagogies.

Heather C. Voss, PhD, RN, is an associate professor at Oregon Health & Science University where she has taught in the BSN, accelerated BSN, and MSN programs for 17 years. Her clinical experience consists of population/community health as RN and FNP. Dr. Voss has expertise in faculty development, curriculum development, implementation, evaluation, community-academic partnering, and service-learning. Dr. Voss is a 2018 NLN Jonas Scholar.

Foreword

In 2012, the National League for Nursing published *Best Practices in Teaching and Learning in Nursing Education,* which translated advances in the science of learning to nursing pedagogies. The book followed on the heels of the landmark Carnegie Nursing Education Study, which highlighted the fact that teaching a practice discipline across the three apprenticeships—professional knowledge base, skilled know-how and clinical reasoning, and ethical comportment—is necessary to teach the neophyte how to think, act, and perform with integrity (Benner et al., 2010). Since then, the National Council of State Boards of Nursing has further emphasized the importance of clinical reasoning through its development of the Next-Generation NCLEX (NGN), administered for the first time in April 2023.

This book, which updates and expands on the earlier *Best Practices in Teaching Nursing,* comes at an important juncture in nursing education. Accreditation standards and changes in the licensure exam have prompted new outcomes in prelicensure education, with a new emphasis on clinical judgment and clinical practice in a variety of roles across the health-illness continuum. Educators are faced with designing curricula that include an ever-expanding amount of content to be mastered and used in the practice of nursing. Nursing education researchers have intensified efforts to understand clinical reasoning and to test pedagogical approaches that will foster skill development in clinical judgment. We have developed a clearer understanding of the relationship between clinical judgment and patient safety (Billings, 2019). There continue to be reports of new graduates' poor performance in clinical reasoning (Kavanagh & Szweda, 2017; Kavanagh & Shapnack, 2021), raising the possibility that the amount of content covered in prelicensure nursing programs is inversely related to the ability to apply this content in clinical reasoning. Historically, NCLEX pass rates were a required minimum indicator of program quality, which consistently contributed to the faculty's sense of responsibility for assuring high pass rates; the result has been faculty's press to "cover" increasing amounts of content.

CLINICAL REASONING AND DEEP LEARNING

The focus on clinical reasoning in the NGN is likely to produce very different results in educational practices. We now understand that content coverage through fast-paced, PowerPoint-laden lectures is certain to defeat the goal of competence in clinical reasoning. Development of skill in clinical judgment requires effective education in the professional knowledge base, distilled for relevance and taught contextually based, as it will be used in practice. Thus, in order to teach skill in clinical reasoning, faculty must commit to focusing on deep understanding of the discipline's most important concepts, the interrelationship among key concepts, and their expression in clinical practice (Bransford et al., 2000).

Deep learning often involves sophisticated insights and abilities, and it is essential for nursing practice in increasingly complex situations. To teach for deep understanding, we must use pedagogies that actively engage the learner in solving problems about authentic clinical situations. To contextualize complex concepts, one can simulate clinical practice in the classroom, through strategies such as case-based instruction. This in turn necessarily requires a reduction in the amount of content covered in traditional fire-hose approaches and employs new ways of engaging the learner in using their new knowledge as they make clinical judgments.

BOOK ORGANIZATION AND KEY THEMES

Best Practices in Teaching Nursing describes advances in nursing pedagogies that support development of a deep understanding of nursing's most important concepts and, hence, skill in clinical judgment.

Section 1: Introduction

Section 1 sets a foundation for the book. Chapter 1 describes the evolution of nursing education in response to the Carnegie Study's call for radical transformation. Chapter 2 analyzes what it means to teach in a practice discipline, reminding readers of the importance of teaching across the three apprenticeships, and highlighting some of the discipline's most important concepts.

Turning to advances in the science of learning, Chapter 3 summarizes current thought about how people learn, the importance of contextualized learning, and practices that promote integration and connection across concepts—in other words, how to facilitate the deep learning required for clinical reasoning. This chapter will interest both seasoned faculty and those new to teaching. An old adage about college teachers in general, and nursing faculty in particular, is that we teach as we were taught. But educational literature appearing at the turn of this century radically changed our views on the effectiveness of that approach. The Scholarship of Teaching and Learning, a movement advanced by the American Association of Higher Education and continued through the Carnegie Foundation for the Advancement of Teaching, brought financial support and faculty development to foster pedagogical inquiry. New advances in the science of learning led to a major critical and integrative review of the many sciences seeking to understand how people learn, and experts have extracted pedagogical implications for K-12 learning and beyond (Bransford et al., 2000; Wiggins & McTighe, 2005). Institutions of higher learning now invest in faculty development (particularly around instructional design), use of new technologies for distance education, and (in the health professions) use of high-fidelity simulation.

Chapter 4 explores the continuing need for nursing faculty development, highlighting the skills needed in the faculty role and in clinical and classroom teaching.

Section 2: Best Teaching Practices

Section 2 describes specific pedagogies that will promote deep learning, integration of clinical and classroom teaching, and situated practice in clinical reasoning.

Chapter 5 explores how faculty-student interactions can promote equity and belonging; it also examines the use of trauma-informed teaching principles and strategies for recognizing and addressing microaggressions in the classroom and clinical learning environments. Chapter 6 explores diverse learner engagement in meaningful learning experiences. Chapter 7 describes intentional course design, which promotes the alignment of learning outcomes, methods of assessment, and design of learning activities. This chapter unpacks the meaning of significant (or deep) learning and the type of activities suitable for different kinds of learning. Chapter 8 discusses the flipped classroom, which is a way to provide content through reading and/or brief lectures prior to engaging students in classroom learning activities. The described activities are well suited for the practice of clinical reasoning, such as unfolding cases, and this chapter provides specific guidelines for facilitating discussion. Chapter 9 extends this discussion to intentional design of online learning activities. Each of these chapters should help the reader in the design of courses and learning activities that will engage the learner in clinical reasoning.

Traditional clinical education in acute care settings, in which the student takes responsibility for the care of one or two patients, was first introduced to nursing education in the mid-1930s. Chapter 10 describes models of clinical education that made their appearance two decades ago including dedicated education units; this chapter also explains the intentional design of clinical learning activities that support concept learning and clinical reasoning. Chapter 11 explains the use of concept-based learning activities, which have been demonstrated to deepen learning and improve performance in clinical judgment. Chapter 12 describes best practices in high-fidelity simulation, an approach that has greatly augmented the teaching of clinical reasoning, as well as other competencies such as interprofessional collaboration, interpersonal communication, and leadership. Lastly, Chapter 13 discusses the best practices for creating service-learning clinical experiences that can benefit both learners and clinical partners.

Section 3: Assessment of Learning

The last decade has marshaled a new era of racial reckoning in the United States, recognizing the extent of systemic racism, the impact on health disparities, and the need to create learning environments that are welcoming to a diverse student body. These themes are echoed throughout Sections 2 and 3 of this book. Addressing themes of equity and justice, Chapter 14 explores equitable grading practices, examining issues of high-stakes testing and other grading practices that often have a negative impact on learning. Chapters 15 and 16 discuss best practices in creating the assessment tools commonly used in nursing education: test items and rubrics.

Chapter 17 describes the effect of implicit bias on clinical reasoning and explains that this bias may be responsive to anti-bias training, citing Ochs's (2023) argument that because of the impact of structural racism on health outcomes, nursing education must incorporate anti-racist teaching. Chapter 17 also provides an overview of Tanner's updated model of clinical judgment, recommending that readers review the original model's description (Tanner, 2006) as a companion to this chapter. Skillful clinical judgment is dependent on a highly interrelated network of knowledge, both conceptual and gained from experience. This deep store of knowledge allows recognition of potential problems as well as the selection and interpretation of relevant clinical data to determine appropriate courses of action. The chapter emphasizes the practice of engaging the student in clinical reasoning through conversations about particular clinical situations, using the clinical judgment model as a framework for the conversation. This kind of situated coaching, over several varied clinical situations, encourages students to deepen their knowledge and use it to interpret and respond to clinical situations. Chapter 18 explores ethical and legal considerations in assessment, including methods to reduce bias and the concept of justice in assessment.

CONCLUSION

The science of learning continues to evolve and influence best practices in teaching. This text provides critical information to nurse educators who may not have had formal preparation in teaching as well as experienced nurse educators needing an update on current best practices. Faculty are encouraged to develop a practice of periodically reviewing journals that focus on pedagogical practices, such as *Nursing Education Perspectives, Journal of Nursing Education*, and *Nurse Educator*. We must evolve ways to keep the nursing curriculum and our pedagogical practices alive, changing with advances in nursing practice and pedagogical science. This text provides a strong foundation for engaging in dynamic pedagogical practices.

Christine Tanner, PhD, RN (ret), FAAN, ANEF
Professor Emerita
Oregon Health & Science University
Portland, Oregon

References

Benner, P., Sutphen, M., Leonard, V., & Day, L. (2010). *Educating Nurses: A Call for Radical Transformation*. John Wiley & Sons.

Billings, D. M. (2019). Teaching nurses to make clinical judgments that ensure patient safety. *Journal of Continuing Education in Nursing, 50*(7), 300–302. https://doi.org/10.3928/00220124-20190612-04

Bransford, J. D., Brown, A. L., & Cocking, R. R. (2000). *How people learn: Brain, mind, experience, and school: Expanded Edition.* The National Academies Press. https://doi.org/10.17226/9853

Kavanagh, J. M., & Sharpnack, P. A. (2021). Crisis in competency: A defining moment in nursing education. *Online Journal of Issues in Nursing, 26*(1). https://doi.org/10.3912/OJIN.Vol26No01Man02

Kavanagh, J., & Szweda, C. (2017). A crisis in competency: The strategic and ethical imperative to assessing new graduate nurses' clinical reasoning. *Nursing Education Perspectives, 38*(2), 57–62. https://doi.org/10.1097/01.NEP.0000000000000112

Ochs, J. H. (2023). Addressing health disparities by addressing structural racism and implicit bias in nursing education. *Nurse Education Today, 121*(105670), 105670. https://doi.org/10.1016/j.nedt.2022.105670

Tanner, C. A. (2006). Thinking like a Nurse: A research-based model of clinical judgment in nursing. *Journal of Nursing Education, 45*(6), 204–211. https://doi.org/10.3928/01484834-20060601-04

Wiggins, G., & McTighe, J. (2005). *Understanding by design* (2nd edition). Prentice-Hall.

Preface

The purpose of this book is to provide up-to-date information on best practices in teaching nursing education based on learning science. Written by expert nurse educators, the text presents salient information and emphasizes practical application focused on teaching and assessing learners to provide excellent educational experiences. This text is a valuable resource for graduate students readying themselves for a teaching practice, expert clinicians and researchers transitioning to an academic career, as well as experienced nurse educators needing an update on best practices. Current and best practices provided are grounded within nursing as a practice profession and incorporate the science of learning. This book is also written with an equity lens to promote educating diverse learners, and all chapters integrate concepts as well as teaching and learning activities that focus on addressing the social determinants of health (SDOH). The text expands teaching and learning activities beyond acute care and incorporates concepts needed to design instruction related to population-based care, care coordination, and interprofessional education. This approach supports the recommendations of both the *IOM Report on the Future of Nursing: Leading Change, Advancing Health* and *The Future of Nursing 2020–2030: Charting a Path to Achieve Health Equity* to facilitate the education of diverse learners.

This book provides information critical for nurse educators to fulfill their role in teaching in the classroom and in a variety of clinical settings. It highlights foundational elements nurse educators need to know to design and assess learning activities. It emphasizes the most relevant knowledge and skills informed by learning science that a nurse educator needs to provide instruction, and each chapter introduces important pedagogical concepts and the most salient information needed to teach best practices. Section 1 contains introductory chapters that focus on important elements in a practice-based educational program, current evidence in the science of learning, and how nurse educators can best prepare to teach. The chapters in Section 2 delve into best teaching practices, including providing information on frameworks to structure learning and how to create inclusive learning environments. This section presents best practices in the design of learning activities and assessments to align with outcomes. Best teaching practices for classroom, online, and clinical learning follow, with particular emphasis on concept-based, simulation, and service-learning. The book concludes with Section 3, which contains a full discussion on assessment, focusing on equitable assessment, item-writing, the design of rubrics, assessing clinical judgment, and ethical-legal considerations in assessment.

In 2010, the NLN published a monograph titled *Best Practices in Teaching and Learning in Nursing Education*, coauthored by faculty from Oregon Health & Science University School of Nursing. This book revisits the topic with updated information and extends the discussion into a chaptered text. We are grateful to the National League for Nursing for collaborating with us to produce this updated information, and we are thankful for the expert educators who joined us on this journey to share their wisdom, knowledge, and expertise. We are honored for the opportunity to share best practices in teaching in nursing education and are confident the information in this text is valuable to you and will support your journey as a nurse educator.

Editors: *Joanne Noone, PhD, RN, CNE, FAAN, ANEF*
Paula Gubrud, EdD, RN, CHSE, FAAN, ANEF

Contents

List of Figures, Tables, and Boxes

LIST OF BOXES

1

Introduction

1

Educating Nurses: Where We've Been and Where We're Going

Kathleen Poindexter, PhD, RN, CNE, ANEF
Joanne Noone, PhD, RN, CNE, FAAN, ANEF
Paula Gubrud, EdD, RN, CHSE, FAAN, ANEF

CHAPTER OVERVIEW

This chapter introduces a brief history of nursing education and summarizes historical past influences that continue to influence nursing education. Recent and future trends from national surveys and reports and practice changes in the professional arena are emphasized. The impact of technology on nursing education is reviewed.

EVOLUTION OF NURSING EDUCATION

Nurses are the largest group of health care workers around the globe, sometimes the only workers, to support global health care needs. According to the *State of the World's Nursing 2020*, approximately 28 million, or 59% of the global health care workforce, are nurses (WHO, 2020). Globally, 19.3 million are professional nurses, 6 million are associate professional nurses, and the remainder were not classified in the report. Despite these numbers, predictions indicate a total of 36 million nurses will be required to provide adequate care around the globe by 2030. The report calls on governments to increase support for nursing education including recruitment of faculty, development of infrastructures, technology, and student resources.

The COVID-19 pandemic reinforced the need for a well-educated health care workforce to build a resilient international health care system. Globally, the World Bank has invested over $5 billion to support nursing education in more than 50 countries to improve the training of qualified nurses (Tanaka & Miyamoto, 2022). While the nursing scope of practice, licensure, and educational requirements vary extensively around the globe, there is universal recognition of the value of education to ensure a qualified, sustainable, nursing workforce.

The evolution of nursing education is a direct reflection of historical events, social movements, values, and public health priorities with a long legacy of responding to the health care needs of society. Nursing and nursing education continue to evolve since their early roots in the mid-1800s, to a unique profession grounded in the art of caring and compassion, framed by a foundation of nursing science. A reflection of the profession's growth and social influence will illuminate the roots of nursing education and practices as they exist today in the U.S.

EARLY NURSING AND THE BIRTH OF NURSING EDUCATION

In early human societies, individuals were appointed as caregivers and the practices and customs developed to promote healing, facilitate comfort, and support death were passed down through mentoring and oral traditions (Enges, 2018). Nurses or healers formed themselves into organized groups during the emergence of Christianity. Early hospitals were created by members of religious communities, nuns, and monks who devoted their lives to caring for the sick (Enges, 2018). Patients cared for in early hospitals throughout Europe were typically poor and destitute and did not have family who could care for them at home. The Protestant Reformation resulted in the closure of many monasteries and convents. Consequently, caring for the sick occurred in almshouses and public hospitals, and women—often from a lower-class underprivileged background—were recruited to provide care, often lacking any knowledge of nursing care (Enges, 2018). During the early 19th century, social reformers recruited religious women often referred to as deaconesses to staff hospitals (Enges, 2018). Deaconesses received some instruction in nursing ministrations but also spent significant time in religious instruction and prayer (Enges, 2018). The deaconess training programs set the stage for the establishment of formal nursing education initiated by Florence Nightingale (Enges, 2018).

Historians credit Florence Nightingale as the founder of modern nursing based on her work in a field hospital during the Crimean War (1853–1856). Her work brought attention to public health; the use of data to improve practice; and principles of hygiene, sanitation, ventilation, and infection control measures to improve health outcomes (Selanders, 2023). She began her educational preparation as a nurse at the Institute of St. Vincent de Paul in Alexandria, Egypt, and completed three months of training at a Protestant community hospital in Kaiserwerth, Germany, to be considered a trained nurse. In 1854, Ms. Nightingale was appointed as superintendent of the English General Hospitals in Turkey and 37 of her nurses were sent to provide care for soldiers wounded in the Crimean War. These early roots of training nurses to provide care established the groundwork for what was to become organized nursing education as we know it today.

In 1859, Florence Nightingale published *Notes on Nursing: What it is and what it is not* (Nightingale, 1860), the first document to outline principles of nursing care that formed the foundation for early nursing education programs. Nightingale went on to establish the first fully organized training program for nurses, *The Nightingale Home and Training School for Nurses* in 1860 (Nutting & Dock, 1907–1912). Her programs differed from earlier models of nursing education because the curriculum included a combination of classroom learning with an emphasis on clinical training. However, the programs were designed using an apprenticeship model of nursing education. This model served as a standard for nursing programs around the world for over 100 years.

Origins of Nursing Education in the United States

The need for nursing education in the U.S. gained importance during the Civil War (1861–1865). Thousands of patriotic women challenged social norms that prioritized women's work at home by serving as nurses. Despite the challenging work and dedicated care provided by these nurses, the majority lacked any formal training or experience. Similar to the conditions noted by Nightingale during the Crimean War, more soldiers were said to have died from unsanitary conditions, poor hygiene, and infection than from enemy fire. As a result of the Civil War, society recognized the value and need for trained nurses. The success of the Nightingale School of Nursing encouraged social reformers and some physicians in the U.S. to promulgate the idea that safe and quality nursing care resulted when nurses received formal education (Enges, 2018).

Physician support for formal education of nurses was minimal during the early establishment of nurse training programs as many believed nurses only needed basic training (Enges, 2018). Despite this opposition, committees of laywomen opened three more nurse training programs in 1873 (Enges, 2018). See Table 1.1 for a list of the first nurse training programs in the U.S.

Emergence of Hospitals

After the Civil War, cities in the U.S. experienced rapid growth due to the migration of rural citizens to urban areas and the rapid influx of European immigration. Crowded living conditions fostered the spread of disease and new arrivals to the cities frequently did not have family members available to provide care in times of illness. The only option was to obtain care in municipal almshouses, which evolved into public hospitals. Because the Civil War had changed the perceptions of the value of formal education for those caring for the sick, the development of training schools for nurses was endorsed (Enges, 2018). The late 1800s was a momentous time as formalized nursing education developed. Social norms evolved to recognize the value and worth of educated nurses as a notable and respectable profession triggered by the ravages of wars in Europe and the U.S.

By the end of the 1800s, the number of nursing programs in the country was estimated to be greater than six hundred (Anderson, 1981). Most of the schools were either closely aligned or owned by a hospital system. Pupils were primarily young, single, women of stature, and teaching was overseen by physicians. The type of educational process that persisted consisted of two to three years of training with a strong emphasis on students supplying clinical care, and less time spent on didactic or classroom education. A diploma was awarded to those pupils who successfully completed the program making them eligible to pursue jobs as trained nurses. These apprenticeship programs remained the predominant model of education for over one hundred years, with nursing students, primarily educated by physicians, providing the majority of patient care in exchange for training.

THE INFLUENCE OF WAR ON NURSING EDUCATION

Declaration of war has played a significant driving force behind the development of training programs for students in the provision of nursing care. The Spanish-American War (1898)

TABLE 1.1

Early Nurse Training Programs in the United States

Training Program	Historical Impact
New England Hospital for Women and Children—Opened 1872	Directed by Dr. Susan Dimock Recruited women between the ages of 21–31 with good reputation, character, and disposition Admitted for a 2-week probationary period prior to formal admission Placed significant importance on the training of nurses Considered the value of nurses to be equal to that of physicians Sixteen-month curriculum included practical study, medical, surgical, maternity, and night nursing (Davis, 1991)
The New York Training School at Bellevue Hospital—Opened 1873	Opened by Dr. W. Gill Wylie with a letter of recommendation from Florence Nightingale Lectures provided by physicians on anatomy, physiology, and hygiene Incorporated strict rules of hygiene and cleanliness GP Putman and Sons published a Manual of Nursing prepared for the Training School of Nurses in 1887 (Bellevue Hospital, 1887) Credited with establishing the first nursing alumni association of trained nurses in 1889
Connecticut Training School—Opened 1873	Offered a two-year curriculum beginning with lectures taught primarily by physicians Students spent majority of the first year working on the wards, then transitioned to private-duty nursing Developed a manual for nursing caring for families in the home titled "*A hand-book of nursing for family and general use*" (Connecticut Training School, 1879)
Boston Training School at Massachusetts General Hospital—Opened 1873	One year of training offered to women between ages 25–35 years in good health and of moral character Didactic training consisted of: ➤ Care of the environment ➤ Patient hygiene ➤ Dressings ➤ Medication administration Treatments under the direction of the physician and nursing supervisor Pupils signed an agreement to remain in school for the first year of training and a second year to work as paid nurses After completing the second year, pupils received a diploma (Boston Training School for Nurses)

was the first to accept only trained nurses to serve as members of the military (Kalisch, 1975). The number of available male nurses was inadequate to provide the required care for diseases such as typhoid, malaria, and yellow fever, so the military reluctantly contracted with fifteen hundred nurses to provide additional care (Army Nurse Corp Association, 2023). The Naval Appropriations Bill in 1908 authorized the establishment of the Navy Nurse Corp, allowing the first females to serve in the Navy (Naval History and Heritage Commission, 2017).

World War I

World War I saw a rapid increase in women applying to nursing programs and an increased demand for nurses. The Army Nurse Corps, founded in 1901, was significantly under-staffed with a little more than 4,000 nurses. Out of the total 80,000–90,000 nurses in the U.S. during WWI, slightly more than 16,000 were in active service with the Red Cross or the Army and Navy Nurse Corps. In response, the Vassar Training Camp (1918) for Nurses was created to address the need for nurses to serve. The camp accepted only women who held a college degree and agreed to complete a three-month intensive training program in the sciences for entrance into nursing schools (National Council of Defense & American Red Cross, 1918). Women completed an additional two years of nursing education by attending one of thirty-five select nursing schools. The historic significance of the Vassar Training Camps represents the early movement of nursing education into university settings.

World War II

World War II once again required a significant increase in nurses and civilian hospitals were in danger of closing due to short staffing. Congress responded by passing the "Bolton Act" authorizing the U.S. Nurse Cadet Corps (CNC) (1943) a program to prepare nurses as quickly as possible. In order to remain competitive and serve as a partnering school, nursing programs were forced to increase enrollments, shorten the curriculum, demonstrate program standards in alignment with the National League for Nursing Education (NLNE), and partner with hospitals to arrange clinical training (Petry, 1943). The Bolton Act has a significant ongoing influence on nursing education by establishing mandated standards for nursing education programs and eliminating school policies that discriminated against students' gender, marital status, ethnicity, or race (Enges, 2018).

ORGANIZATION OF NURSING AS A PROFESSION

The early beginnings of hospital-based nursing education were a mixture of basic train-ing followed by student provision of nursing care. Hospital labor costs to deliver nursing care by students were minimal, leaving many trained nurses unemployed unless they were promoted to hospital supervisors or provided home care to families with greater wealth. Nurses began to organize and move toward assuming responsibility for stand-ardizing education. As nursing care became more complex, patients were no longer sat-isfied with the level of care delivered by students. This transition required an increase in the number of trained nurses to meet the complex care needs of hospitalized patients. Nursing schools eventually increased oversight by state boards, provided greater struc-ture to subjects taught, and reduced student responsibility for delivering patient care.

Isabelle Hampton Robb, founding supervisor for the Johns Hopkins Hospital, led the promotion of standards for nursing education (Moody, 1938). She organized nursing sessions during the *International Congress of Charities, Corrections, and Philanthropy* (Chicago's World Fair), in Chicago in 1893. Ms. Hampton urged superintendents to establish standards for nursing education, called for expanding nursing education to three years, reduce training to eight-hour days, and set admission dates during established times of the year (Moody, 1938). She proclaimed hospitals have a responsibility to provide education for nursing students and founded nursing's first *Society of Superintendents of Training Schools for Nurses* to organize nursing education and practice. The initial goals of the organization were to increase minimum nursing education entrance standards, improve the living and working conditions for pupils, and increase opportunities for postgraduate nurses adding education for specialized areas of practice. In 1893, Isabell Hampton Robb published *Hampton's Nursing: Its Principles and Practice for Hospital and Private Use* and the first nursing ethics text, *Nursing Ethics: For Hospital and Private Use* (Hampton Robb, 2013). Her text outlined a two-year nursing education curriculum including lesson content and clinical rotations (Moody, 1938). Hampton played a significant role in nursing and nursing education, moving nursing toward a professional stage.

Isabel Hampton Robb, Lavinia Lloyd Dock, and Mary Adelaide Nutting are considered the modern architects of nursing education (Poslusny, p. 64). Isabel Hampton Robb work set the foundation for the development of The *American Society of Superintendents of Training Schools for Nurses*, (later known as the National League for Nursing Education) followed by *the Associated Alumnae of Trained Nurse*s (later known as the American Nurses Association) and then organized the *American Journal of Nursing* (Poslusny, 1989). See Table 1.2 for details.

In 1920, the Rockefeller Foundation funded a study of nursing education in the U.S. appointing Annie Goodrich, Adelaide Nutting, and Lillian Wald as members of the committee. The committee studied over seventy nursing programs and published their findings in the Goldmark report, *Nursing and Nursing Education in the United States.* The conclusions in the report called for nursing education reform, such as moving programs to universities and away from hospital-based diploma education, establishing national accreditation standards, placing a stronger emphasis on education over service, and requiring faculty to hold advanced degrees (Goldmark, 1923).

In response to the Goldmark report, groups of prominent investors provided financial support to transition nursing education to university-based academic centers for learning. Universities such as Yale, Case Western Reserve, Vanderbilt, and the University of Chicago received generous endowments to support the advancement of nursing education. Yale School of Nursing was the first autonomous university-based nursing program with a Dean of Nursing (Yale, 2019).

DEVELOPMENT OF THREE MODELS OF NURSING EDUCATION
Diploma Nursing Education

During the first half of the 20th century, diploma programs flourished and evolved into the solution for staffing hospitals with a student workforce. The NLNE, the forerunner of today's National League for Nursing, attempted to redesign diploma nursing education

TABLE 1.2

Early Architects of Nursing Education in the United States

Nurse	Role
Isabel Hampton Robb (1860–1910)	Superintendent of the Illinois Training School and the Johns Hopkins School for Nurses
	Set the foundation for the development of:
	▸ *The American Society of Training Schools for Nurses* (forerunner of the National League for Nursing)
	▸ The Associated Alumnae of Trained Nurses (forerunner of the ANA)
	▸ Organized the *American Journal of Nursing*
Lavinia Lloyd Dock (1858–1956)	Served as a lecturer, author, and activist
	Campaigned for women's suffrage and participated in antiwar protests
	Authored the first nursing pharmacology text and other texts on public health nursing
	Provided leadership for the *International Council of Nurses*
Mary Adelaide Nutting (1858–1948)	Succeeded Hampton as the Superintendent at Johns Hopkins School where she instituted a 3-year program of study
	Joined Teacher's College at Columbia University where she designed the school's postgraduate program
	The first nurse to become a university-ranked full professor of nursing education
	Led the development of the first department of nursing and health in a university
	Compiled a study on the *Educational Status of Nursing* published by the U.S. Bureau of Education

Adapted from Scheckel (2018).

to decrease the time students worked in the hospital wards and increase the time spent in clinical classroom coursework. By the middle of the century changes in health care and advances in medical and disease science and technology required nurses to have a solid foundation of science-based preparation. These changes created a decline in hospital-based diploma programs as nursing education began to occur predominately in colleges and universities.

Associate Degree Nursing

Associate degree nursing education began in response to a serious post-World War II nursing shortage. The NLNE initiated talks with community colleges and developed a strong interest in associate degree nursing programs to train nurses in a shorter time period than a baccalaureate degree while still committing to the goal of moving nursing education to institutions of higher education. In 1951, Mildred Montag proposed a technical nursing program that would be embedded in junior colleges. These early programs were a combination of nursing courses, laboratory experiences, and clinical rotations administered over a two-year period. The associate degree program meant more nurses could be trained in a shorter period, they were less expensive, applicant standards were more liberal, and nurses could enroll in an associate degree to baccalaureate completion program post-graduation. The associate degree in nursing provided opportunity for individuals with minimal access to baccalaureate nursing programs the chance to become registered nurses (Scheckel, 2018).

Public Health Nursing and Baccalaureate Education

By the end of the 19th century, public health nursing emerged as a setting where nurse graduates could find employment outside the hospital (Enges, 2018). District nursing originated in England through funding from wealthy philanthropists, so nurses could provide care to sick and poor persons in their homes. The model spread to the U.S. in the late 1800s, when two district health associations were developed in Boston and Philadelphia. Lillian Wald was an early district nurse who eventually founded the Henry Street Settlement House to provide nursing care to the immigrant population in New York City's lower east side. Eventually, a team of district nurses and social workers provided home nursing care and a variety of social services to New York's immigrant population (Enges, 2018). After several years of positive outcomes, Lillian Wald began sending nurses to schools in an attempt to reduce chronic absenteeism. The experiment was successful and school nurses became a mainstay in public education settings. Public health and school health nurse roles eventually evolved into a curriculum distinct from the baccalaureate-prepared nurse as diploma and associate degree programs focused solely on preparing graduates to practice as bedside nurses in hospitals and other inpatient settings (Enges, 2018).

Baccalaureate nursing education aligns with Florence Nightingale's original vision. Nightingale believed that nursing should occur outside of hospitals and should not mimic the medical model of training by avoiding apprenticeships where students receive minimal education in the principles of nursing care because they were providing long hours of service to the hospitals. However, the labor provisions hospitals enjoyed through diploma programs prevailed for decades, and arguments that nurses do not need to be overeducated stifled the development of baccalaureate nursing education in universities. The University of Minnesota established the first baccalaureate nursing program in the U.S. in 1909. The movement toward baccalaureate education for nurses in place of a diploma was slow and steady for the next half of the 20th century (Scheckel, 2018). The Brown Report published in 1948 declared nursing education belonged in higher education institutions and that curricula needed to integrate both liberal coursework and technical training to prepare graduates competent for professional practice (Scheckel, 2018). Baccalaureate education was increasingly differentiated from a diploma or associate degree by the 1960s. The baccalaureate curriculum emphasized liberal arts, intellectual skills, leadership, management, community and public health, and the role of the nurse as a health teacher (Scheckel, 2018). In 1965, the American Nurses Association (ANA) published a position paper declaring the baccalaureate degree should be the entry-level degree for nursing. However, multiple stakeholders were cautious about embracing the ANA position. Conflict over the appropriate degree for entry into practice continues to this day as all graduates from approved diploma, associate, and baccalaureate degree programs must pass the same licensing examination to practice as a registered nurse.

CURRENT CHALLENGES EMBEDDED IN NURSING HISTORY
Influence of Feminism in Nursing

As described earlier, nursing as a profession in the U.S. arose during the Civil War. Fowler (2017) describes the emergence of nursing as a "sponsored profession" (p. 2) because, to overcome the opposition to females in military hospitals, all clinical decisions were either made by or attributed to military physicians. As formal nursing education programs emerged, curricula and coursework were controlled by physicians. Physicians administered, dictated policy, and even owned many nursing education programs for the primary purpose of exploiting free labor provided by female students (Fowler, 2017). Nursing practice and education were founded among gender politics and patriarchal hierarchy. While change for nursing as an autonomous and equal profession in partnership with medicine has systematically and consistently progressed, there continue to be opportunities for improved collaborative practice.

Lingel et al. (2022) write "In the United States, feminists movements and nursing have shared a tumultuous relationship marked by both mutually beneficial collaborations and mutually destructive conflicts" (p. 1150). Nursing has often and still can be caught in the middle between the long history of the patriarchal hierarchy of medicine, as a once male-dominated profession, over nursing as a past and current female-dominated profession (Lingel et al., 2022). Despite the historical expectation of the subordination of nursing to medicine, nursing as a profession has fought tirelessly for its own agency and for social justice since the early years of the profession. Fowler (2017) posits nursing fought for the abolition of slavery, women's suffrage, child labor laws, welfare for factory workers, vaccination, human treatment for the mentally ill, access to birth control, and gender-specific education. The ANA provided an early endorsement of the Equal Rights Amendment, yet nearly 50 years later, the law has not been passed (Lingel et al., 2022). Fowler (2017) voices concerns that graduates from today's nursing schools are not exposed to women's history and nursing history which are intricately intertwined. Fowler argues realizing the influence of feminism on the profession's history and tradition of "… addressing social injustices affecting not only women and nurses, but all socially marginalized, vulnerable voiceless, or stigmatized persons or groups" (p. 4) is critical to the social ethics that guide the profession. Lingel et al. (2022) argue even after the ANA first joined the women's suffrage movement the need for feminist transformation within the profession persists and suggests that today's curriculum should address nursing and women's history.

Roots of Diversity and Exclusion in Nursing Education

A diverse nursing workforce is essential to delivering equitable access to quality health care and reduction of health disparities for the populations under their care. When students and faculty can interact with persons who reflect their own community and cultural background, overall learning, well-being, and health improve. Members from all types of backgrounds benefit when there is mutual trust, respect, and willingness to listen and learn from each other. A goal of nursing and nursing education is to the development of a caring and well-rounded diverse nursing workforce. A reflective view of the history of nursing education explains the lack of diversity that continues to persist within the profession. The past cannot be changed; however, a strong understanding of the historical practices that occurred and a commitment to developing and creating a strong, agile, diverse, and inclusive nursing workforce is required to achieve equitable access to education, career advancement, and, ultimately, healthy outcomes. Persons of color, various religions, gender, and race were commonly banned from participating in white-dominated nursing professional organizations and education programs, joining the military, or the right to receive access to health care with the exception of a few open and inclusive programs. See Table 1.3 for a brief list of significant early people and events promoting diversity in nursing history.

The early beginnings of the profession were primarily women, lacking inclusion of racial diversity or male presence (with the exception of physicians), a reflection of social norms and discriminatory practices at the time. While nursing education has evolved since the 1800s, a closer analysis of the first training programs and manuals supplies greater insight into the development of health care's hierarchical structure, apprenticeship training model, patient care trends, and education content. A review of the history of nursing education and the embedded influence of racism in the U.S. significantly contributed to a lack of diversity and inclusion across the nursing profession. Despite tremendous efforts of a few bold leaders, the roots of exclusion and these early patterns had an impact on the growth of the profession that remain visible today. It is important to recognize and honor those early leaders and organizations that pushed beyond social norms to celebrate humanity and respect. Nursing education continues to work toward removing barriers to accessing quality education programs, diversifying student applicants, and supporting inclusive learning environments to prepare a more diverse nursing workforce.

RECENT TRENDS IMPACTING NURSING EDUCATION

In the past ten to fifteen years, national reports on the future of nursing and national studies on nursing education have created recommendations that have influenced the current state of nursing education. Explosions in technology have influenced the landscape of nursing education, creating opportunities for online education and simulation to become integral components of nursing education today. Lastly, nursing professional drivers for patient safety and evidenced-based practice have emphasized inclusion of these concepts in nursing education curricula and support for baccalaureate-prepared nurses.

Carnegie National Nursing Education Study

In 2010, Benner and colleagues (Benner et al., 2010) published a report on the state of nursing education as part of a broader focus on preparation for professional practice supported by the Carnegie Foundation for the Advancement of Teaching. The researchers conducted national surveys and site visits to schools of nursing, directly observing classroom and clinical teaching. While the report concluded that nursing education had strengths in forming professional identity, ethical comportment, and clinical teaching, the researchers identified the need to better integrate classroom and clinical teaching and to use effective pedagogies to prepare safe and effective practitioners. They recommended

TABLE 1.3

Diversity and Inclusion: Significant People and Events

Person or Event	Description
Mary Mahoney	First African American educated nurse in the U.S.; completed training at the New England Hospital for Women and Children (Steptoe, 2010)
Spelman Seminary (1886)	An early nursing program opened for African American women in Atlanta, Georgia; classes were held in a church basement (Steptoe, 2010)
Daniel Williams	A Black surgeon inspired by Emma Reynolds who was denied admission to a nurse training program and founded the first Black-owned and operated hospital in the U.S.: Providence Hospital in Chicago, which became a 12-bed training hospital for African American nurses (Chicago History Museum, 2021)
Howard University	In 1892, opened a training school for African American nurses later known as Freemen's Hospital School of Nursing, which was established to provide care in Washington, DC for former slaves. Also established the Bachelor of Science in Nursing Degree (Minority Nurse, 2013)
Estelle Massey Riddle Osborne	First Black nurse to earn a master of science in nursing degree (Montgomery et al., 2021)
Elizabeth Lipford Kent	First Black nurse to earn a PhD in nursing (Montgomery et al., 2021)
Darius Mills	Opened a formal nurse training program for men at Bellevue Hospital (Bellevue School of Nursing, ND)
Pennsylvania Hospital School for Men	Opened in 1914 at the Department for Mental and Nervous Diseases
Leroy Craig	First male nurse to be the head of the school (School of Nursing for Men, ND)
Edward Lyon	First male nurse commissioned to serve in the U.S. Army Nurse Corps in 1955, overturning the 1901 policy of restricting men (Mulkey, 2023)
Joe Hogan	An African American nurse with an associate degree who applied to Mississippi University for Women to receive his bachelor's degree in nursing and was denied. In 1982, the U.S. Supreme Court ruled in favor of Hogan based on gender discrimination (Mulkey, 2023).
American Nurses Association (1948)	Removes barriers to nurses of color joining ANA
Luther Christman	Founder and dean of Rush University College of Nursing; was denied admission to two nursing schools because of his gender but was eventually accepted to the Pennsylvania Hospital School of Nursing. Luther established the American Assembly for Men in Nursing and was the first man inducted into the ANA Hall of Fame for his advocacy in nursing education (Mulkey, 2023).
Sage Memorial Hospital, School of Nursing	First to open its doors to admit Native American students into nursing programs as part of the Ganado mission located on the Navajo Indian Reservation (Trennert, 2003). The accredited school of nursing graduated its first Indian registered nurses in 1933. The school welcomed students of all backgrounds and cultures, graduating about 150 native women from over 50 tribes, until its doors closed in 1950 (Trennert, 2003).

a better focus on teaching for a sense of salience and situated cognition so that students do not learn decontextualized information but rather are able to apply the knowledge learned to solve complex health problems. In particular, Benner and colleagues (2010) recommended moving away from content-laden cataloging of information in classroom learning to more active learning strategies. They recommended a shift from solely focusing on critical thinking to a model emphasizing clinical reasoning, and multiple ways of thinking that includes critical thinking as one of many approaches used in clinical reasoning and decision making. Lastly, they recommended a focus on the development of professional formation, rather than a narrow focus on socialization and role-taking. The full set of recommendations can be found in Table 1.4.

These recommendations have profoundly influenced nursing education pedagogies and intersected with other national reports, such as the 2010 Future of Nursing Report. Many of these recommendations are presented as best practices in this book. Benner (2012) provides examples of how programs have contextualized the curriculum, implemented original approaches to clinical, and closed the theory-practice gap through better integration of classroom and clinical learning. Active learning strategies, through case studies and simulations, can assist in promoting the development of clinical reasoning (Benner, 2015).

One response to these recommendations was a movement during this time period to a concept-based curriculum which was perceived to address some of the problems with teaching methods identified in the Carnegie Study. A concept-based curriculum was proposed to assist with developing learners' connection across concepts and between classroom and clinical learning. Active learning strategies for teaching concepts were advocated, including team-based learning, to promote a more student-centered approach (Hardin & Richardson, 2012). Outcome evaluations of this curriculum method have been mixed with some studies demonstrating no difference in student outcomes compared to the previous curriculum (Duncan & Schulz, 2015; Repsha et al., 2020) and others noting positive outcomes with this curriculum change (Repsha et al., 2020). While this curricular approach is not described in this text, an evidence-based unique clinical experiential approach to helping students develop skill in pattern recognition across concepts is discussed by Ann Nielsen in Chapter 11, *Concept-Based Learning in the Clinical Learning Environment.*

The 2011 Future of Nursing Report

The Institute of Medicine's (IOM) landmark report on *The Future of Nursing: Leading Change, Advancing Health* had a major influence on the direction of nursing education calling for radical reform to train a diverse nursing workforce to deliver safe, quality care, across care environments (Institute of Medicine, 2011). The report recommended 80% of all nurses be prepared at the baccalaureate level and double the number of nurses prepared at the doctoral level by 2020. The report encouraged seamless academic progression to facilitate baccalaureate attainment and an improvement in the diversity of the nursing workforce. Additionally, they recommended that nursing education accrediting bodies identify key clinical performance competencies, setting the stage for the development of competency-based education, including interprofessional competencies, that is now being endorsed by both the American Association of Colleges of Nursing (AACN) (2021) and the National League for Nursing (NLN) (2023).

TABLE 1.4

Recommendations from the Carnegie National Nursing Education Study

Program Area	Recommendations
Entry and Pathways	1. Come to agreement about a set of clinically relevant prerequisites.
	2. Require the BSN for entry to practice.
	3. Develop local articulation programs to ensure a smooth, timely transition from the ADN to the BSN.
	4. Develop more ADN-to-MSN programs.
Student Population	5. Recruit a more diverse faculty and student body.
	6. Provide more financial aid, whether from public or private sources, for all students, at all levels.
The Student Experience	7. Introduce prenursing students to nursing early in their education.
	8. Broaden the clinical experience (to beyond acute care settings and increasing the variety and flexibility of placements).
	9. Preserve postclinical conferences and small patient care assignments.
	10. Develop pedagogies that keep students focused on the patient's experience.
	11. Vary the means of assessing student performance.
	12. Promote and support learning the skills of inquiry and research.
	13. Redesign the ethics curricula (to include every-day ethical concerns, relational care, and self-care).
	14. Support students in becoming agents of change.
Teaching	15. Fully support ongoing faculty development for all who educate student nurses.
	16. Include teacher education courses in master's and doctoral programs.
	17. Foster opportunities for educators to learn how to teach students to reflect on their practice.
	18. Support faculty in learning how to coach.
	19. Support educators in learning how to use narrative pedagogies.
	20. Provide faculty with resources to stay clinically current.
	21. Improve the work environment for staff nurses and support them in learning to teach.
	22. Address the faculty shortage.
Entry to Practice	23. Develop clinical residencies for all new graduates.
	24. Change the requirements for licensure (to require a master's degree within 10 years of licensure).
National Oversight	25. Require performance assessments for licensure.
	26. Cooperate on accreditation (for national nursing education accrediting boards).

In an effort to achieve these recommendations, the Future of Nursing Campaign for Action website was developed (Campaign for Action, n.d.a.) and houses data dashboards on the IOM 2011 recommendations. Additionally, a 2015 progress update (National Academies of Sciences, Engineering, and Medicine, 2016) and the 2020–2030 Future of Nursing Report, which will be discussed below, address the original recommendations from the 2011 report.

THE IMPACT OF TECHNOLOGY

The advent of technology has had multiple impacts on nursing education and the evolution of technological growth will continue to enhance and influence education as the impact of Virtual and Augmented Reality unfolds. Online education and simulation are two technological impacts that have greatly influenced nursing education. In Chapter 9, Glenise McKenzie and Heather Hawk clearly describe the growing number of online education courses and programs and how the transition to online and remote learning during the pandemic highlighted to nursing educators and students the need for formal development in faculty teaching in the online setting. The chapter clearly demonstrates the best practices and educator skills required for effective online design and delivery of instruction. Likewise, in Chapter 12, Ashley Franklin and Jeremy Hutson delineate the historical roots and development of simulation learning and seminal research studies that have led to established best practices in simulation and influenced nursing regulation of simulation in nursing education.

PROFESSIONAL INFLUENCES ON EDUCATION

Trends and evidence within the nursing profession have built upon the Carnegie Study and IOM recommendations calling for a baccalaureate-prepared workforce. These trends include an emphasis on patient safety and evidence-based practice.

Baccalaureate Workforce and Patient Outcomes

The evidence of the critical impact of a baccalaureate-prepared workforce on patient care outcomes continues to accumulate. The sentinel work by Aiken et al. (2003) on reduced surgical patient mortality associated with a baccalaureate-prepared workforce has been replicated in multiple studies and patient populations (O'Brien et al., 2018). Additional improved patient care outcomes associated with a baccalaureate-prepared workforce include lower complications, such as decubitus ulcer formation, deep vein thrombosis, and pulmonary embolism; lower failure to rescue rates, decreased length of stay (Blegen et al., 2022); and greater odds of survival to discharge from cardiac arrest (Harrison et al., 2019). Projections of moving to an 80% BSN workforce report that the economic savings to an institution are estimated at $5.6 million due to reduced length of stays and readmission rates even taking into account the additional cost of BSN salaries (Yakusheva et al., 2014). A recent 2021 study identified a potential reduction in patient mortality of 25% in comparing an 80% BSN workforce to a 30% workforce and found no difference in improved outcomes with variations in educational pathways for attainment of the baccalaureate degree (whether by initial licensure or an RN to BSN pathway) (Porat-Dahlerbruch et al., 2022).

Quality and Safety Education for Nurses

In Chapter 18 of this volume on *Ethical and Legal Considerations in Assessment*, Paula Gubrud discusses the Quality and Safety Education Initiative (QSEN) and competencies more fully. The QSEN website (QSEN, n.d.) identifies prelicensure and graduate competencies related to quality and safety and hosts a variety of learning strategies to incorporate into nursing curricula to assist in achieving these competencies. Djukic and colleagues (Djukic et al., 2019) have monitored nursing graduates by degree and their preparedness in quality and safety education compared at two time periods (2007–2008 and 2014–2015). They identified 16 topics as pertinent to quality and safety education. During the first time period, 2007–2008, BSN graduates reported better preparation in 5 of the 16 identified topics than associate degree graduates (ADN); in the second time period, 2014–2015, BSN graduates reported better preparation in 12 of 16 topics, more than doubling in the 8-year time period. The authors suggested closing this gap through either improving ADN curricula in meeting QSEN competencies, facilitating academic progression of ADN to BSN, or legislation requiring BSN preparation for entry into practice or within a specific time period.

Magnet Recognition Program

The Magnet Recognition Program® established by the American Nurses Credentialing Center (ANCC) certifies health care organizations for excellence in nursing services. As of January 2023, approximately 10% of U.S. hospitals have received this recognition (ANCC, n.d.) with the number and percentage of certified U.S. health care institutions growing over the past decade. Magnet recognition requires all nurse leaders in an applicant organization to have at least a baccalaureate degree and an institutionally established benchmark for a baccalaureate-prepared nursing workforce. A recent systematic review of 21 studies of Magnet institutions compared to non-Magnet found safer work environments, higher quality and more cost-effective care with lower rates of nursing shortages, burnout, job dissatisfaction and turnover, patient mortality, falls, hospital-acquired infections, and pressure ulcers in Magnet hospitals (Rodríguez-García et al., 2020).

In summary, the evidence continues to accumulate demonstrating the impact of a baccalaureate-prepared nursing workforce on health outcomes, with certain organizations moving to meet or exceed this recommendation of an 80% baccalaureate-prepared nursing workforce (Clifford & Jurado, 2018; Straka et al., 2019).

FUTURE DIRECTIONS IMPACTING NURSING EDUCATION

The Future of Nursing Report 2020–2030

The Future of Nursing 2020–2030 Report (National Academy of Sciences, 2021) promotes nurses' role in achieving health equity. This report has implications for nursing education in order to prepare a nursing workforce skilled in addressing health equity issues. It identifies a diverse nursing workforce as a key component of the nursing profession's contribution to achieving health equity. The report recommends eliminating practices within nursing education that contribute to racism and discrimination of students and

> ### BOX 1.1

Future of Nursing 2020–2030 Educational Recommendations

> ➤ A curriculum embedded in coursework and experiential learning that effectively prepares students to promote health equity, reduce health disparities, and improve the health and well-being of the population will build the capacity of the nursing workforce.
> ➤ Learning experiences that develop nursing students' understanding of health equity, social determinants of health, and population health and prepare them to incorporate that understanding into their professional practice include opportunities to:
>> ➤ learn cultural humility and recognize one's own implicit biases;
>> ➤ gain experience with interprofessional collaboration and multisector partnerships to enable them to address social needs comprehensively and drive structural improvements;
>> ➤ develop such technical competencies as the use of telehealth, digital health tools, and data analytics; and
>> ➤ gain substantive experience with delivering care in diverse community settings, such as public health departments, schools, libraries, workplaces, and neighborhood clinics.
> ➤ Successfully diversifying the nursing workforce will depend on holistic efforts to support and mentor/sponsor students and faculty from a wide range of backgrounds, including cultivating an inclusive environment; providing economic, social, professional, and academic supports; ensuring access to information on school quality; and minimizing inequities.

Reprinted with permission from National Academies of Sciences, Engineering, and Medicine (2021). *The Future of Nursing 2020–2030: Charting a Path to Achieve Health Equity.* The National Academies Press. https://doi.org/10.17226/25982

focusing on cultivating an inclusive learning environment. Hassmiller & Wakefield (2022) identify a priority area for undergraduate and graduate nursing programs to ensure integration of social determinants of health and population health concepts throughout the curriculum. Sumpter et al. (2022) identify four pillars to address to transform nursing education in response to this report: 1) reconciling the shortage of nurses with expertise in public health and health equity; 2) creating policies that include and promote the tenets of diversity, antiracism, and well-being; 3) designing curricular resources and activities that address contemporary issues; and, 4) creating and supporting an ethos that invites, retains, and graduates diverse students and facilitates a sense of belonging. The report holds specific recommendations for the addition of health equity concepts into the curriculum (see Box 1.1) and the Campaign for Action website has an Action Hub website (Campaign for Action, n.d.b.) to assist with implementing the recommendations for this report.

Competency-Based Education and Clinical Judgment

Both nursing education professional organizations, AACN (2021) and NLN (2023), have recently endorsed competency-based education (CBE) in an effort to promote and graduate practitioners who meet the expected knowledge, skills, and abilities for professional nursing practice. These recommendations have been driven in part by the data showing that new nurse graduates may be underprepared for their first nursing job (Kavanagh & Szweda, 2017); other influences, such as the National Council of State Boards of Nursing's movement to better assess competency in clinical decision-making on the NCLEX-RN

TABLE 1.5	
American Association of Colleges of Nurses Domains and Concepts for Nursing Practice	
Domains	**Concepts**
Knowledge for Nursing Practice	Clinical Judgment
Person-Centered Care	Communication
Population Health	Compassionate Care
Scholarship for Nursing Practice	Diversity, Equity, and Inclusion
Quality and Safety	Ethics
Interprofessional Partnerships	Evidence-Based Practice
Systems-Based Practice	Health Policy
Informatics and Health Care Technologies	Social Determinants of Health
Professionalism	
Personal, Professional, and Leadership Development	

Source: American Association of Colleges of Nurses (2021).

and the resultant need for nursing programs to incorporate a clinical judgment framework into curriculum and assessment (Dickison et al., 2019); and the growing body of evidence demonstrating the effectiveness of CBE (Lewis et al., 2022). Table 1.5 illustrates the domains and concepts developed by the AACN (2021), which has a framework of ten domains and eight core concepts with associated subcompetencies within each domain. The NLN has created a framework depicted in Table 1.6 that defines 5 concepts with related competencies (Forneris et al., 2022). Both frameworks clearly link to other identified national competencies such as QSEN and interprofessional competencies (Interprofessional Education Collaborative, 2016; QSEN, 2020).

Future trends in CBE include the need to develop nursing competencies related to the burgeoning practice of telehealth nursing. Beginning work has started to identify these competencies for nurses and advanced practice nurses. van Houwelingen et al. (2016) completed a Delphi study, identifying 14 entrustable professional activities (see Box 1.2) and 32 competencies for nurses related to telehealth. Rutledge et al. (2021) identified advanced practice competencies related to planning, preparing, providing, and performance evaluation in telehealth with subsequent leveling of competencies according to readiness to practice (Dzioba et al., 2022).

PROFESSIONAL INFLUENCES ON EDUCATION

Addressing Racism in Nursing

Societal forces in the U.S. and beyond have stimulated nursing practice and education to begin the journey of addressing racism in nursing. In 2021, the ANA, in conjunction

TABLE 1.6

National League for Nursing Concepts and Competencies

Concepts	Competencies
Clinical Knowledge	Knowledge of pathophysiology and patient condition Medication management Interpretation of provider orders Use of evidence-based practice Compliance with legal and regulatory requirements Use of quality improvement methodologies
Clinical Reasoning	Recognition of need for assistance Patient safety Decision-making based on interpretation of patient data Recognizing and responding to changes in patient status Ability to anticipate risk
Management of Responsibility	Ability to take initiative Organization and prioritization Delegation of tasks
Communication	Interprofessional team communication Patient/caregiver education Conflict resolution Patient advocacy Rapport with patients and caregivers
Professionalism	Ability to work as part of a team Accountability for professional practice

Source: Forneris, Tagliareni, & Allen, 2022.

with multiple other nursing organizations, instituted the National Commission to Address Racism in Nursing (ANA, n.d.). Since that time foundational reports and resources have illustrated the history and prevalence of racism in education and practice and offered resources and strategies for change. The report on racism in nursing education discusses the historical roots of racism in nursing education and how it can continue to be perpetuated in pedagogy, access, climate and culture, and progression (National Commission to Address Racism in Nursing, n.d.). Teri Murray, in Chapter 5 of this text offers specific strategies to create more inclusive learning environments.

Impact of the COVID-19 Pandemic

The full impact of the *COVID-19* pandemic on nursing practice and education remains to be seen. Although the pandemic demonstrated the positive impact of nursing's role in health care, there continues to be an impact on nurses' mental and physical health and

---

BOX 1.2

Entrustable Activities for Telehealth

➤ Supporting patients in the use of technology
➤ Training patients in the use of technology as a way to strengthen their social network
➤ Providing health promotion remotely
➤ Triaging incoming calls and alarms
➤ Analyzing and interpreting incoming data derived from (automatic) devices for self-measurement
➤ Monitoring body functions and lifestyle
➤ Providing psychosocial support
➤ Encouraging patients to undertake health promotion activities
➤ Instructing patients and family caregivers in self-care
➤ Assessing patient capacity to use telehealth
➤ Evaluating and adjusting the patient care plan
➤ Coordination of care with the use of telehealth technology
➤ Independent double-check of high-risk medication
➤ Guidance and peer consultation

Reprinted with permission from van Houwelingen, C. T., Moerman, A. H., Ettema, R. G., Kort, H. S., & Ten Cate, O. (2016). Competencies required for nursing telehealth activities: A Delphi-study. *Nurse education today, 39*, 50–62. https://doi.org/10.1016/j.nedt.2015.12.025.

intention to remain in the profession (Esposito, 2021). This has exacerbated nursing shortages. The impact of curriculum modifications necessary during the pandemic related to an inability to be on campuses or in clinical situations is still unfolding. A recent report of nursing graduates educated during the pandemic indicates concerns about delivering safe patient care, being advocates, and having a long-term commitment to the profession (Djukic et al., 2023). Resources to support nurses' and nursing students' physical and emotional health and work environment are needed more than ever to sustain a healthy workforce.

CHAPTER SUMMARY

Nursing, as it has since its inception, continues to push forward to define itself as a profession, remove barriers to progression, and create consistent standards for education and practice. There are ongoing calls to require higher levels of nursing education to provide increasingly complex health care across diverse populations, while simultaneously increasing nursing enrollment in institutions with limited educational capacity, a shortage of faculty, and clinical training facilities. Professional organizations continue to debate degree requirements for levels of practice and education, regulations requirements are inconsistent, and nurse program enrollments are in jeopardy as the profession experiences elevated levels of burnout and safety concerns. The profession is young in terms of identity and purpose and continues to make great strides in creating an autonomous and respected profession. Throughout the period of development, nursing has been continuously challenged by external variables such as wars, plagues, finance, and at times conflicting societal values that can redefine or interfere with the direction and goals set forth by the nurse leaders. Despite these ongoing challenges and debates, nursing continues to demonstrate resilience as a profession, remaining true to core values and committed to providing quality health care.

References

Aiken, L. H., Clarke, S. P., Cheung, R. B., Sloane, D. M., & Silber, J. H. (2003). Educational levels of hospital nurses and surgical patient mortality. *Journal of the American Medical Association*, *290*(12), 1617–1623. https://doi.org/10.1001/jama.290.12.1617

American Association of Colleges of Nursing. (2021). *The essentials: Core competencies for professional nursing education*. Retrieved from https://www.aacnnursing.org/Essentials

ANA. (n.d.). *National Commission to Address Racism in Nursing*. Retrieved from https://www.nursingworld.org/practice-policy/workforce/racism-in-nursing/national-commission-to-address-racism-in-nursing/

ANCC. (n.d.). *Find a Magnet organization*. Retrieved from https://www.nursingworld.org/organizational-programs/magnet/find-a-magnet-organization/

Anderson, N. (1981). The historical development of American nursing education. *Journal of Nursing Education*, *21*(1), 14–26.

Bellevue Hospital School of Nursing Alumnae Association Records, 1873–2010 (MC19), Bellevue Alumnae Center for Nursing History, Foundation of New York State Nurses, Guilderland, NY. https://www.cfnny.org/archives/bellevue-hospital-school-of-nursing-alumnae-association-records/

Benner, P. (2012). Educating nurses: a call for radical transformation-how far have we come? *The Journal of Nursing Education*, *51*(4), 183–184. https://doi.org/10.3928/01484834-20120402-01

Benner, P. (2015). Curricular and pedagogical implications for the Carnegie Study, educating nurses: a call for radical transformation. *Asian Nursing Research*, *9*(1), 1–6. https://doi.org/10.1016/j.anr.2015.02.001

Benner, P., Sutphen, M., Leonard, V., & Day, L. (2010). *Educating nurses: A call for radical transformation*. Jossey-Bass.

Blegen, M. A., Goode, C. J., Park, S. H., Vaughn, T., & Spetz, J. (2013). Baccalaureate education in nursing and patient outcomes. *The Journal of Nursing Administration, 43*(2), 89–94. https://doi.org/10.1097/NNA.0b013e31827f2028

Campaign for Action. (n.d.a.) *Our story and timeline*. Retrieved from https://campaignforaction.org/about/our-story/

Campaign for Action. (n.d.b.). *Action Hub Future of Nursing 2030*. Retrieved from https://campaignforaction.org/resources/future-of-nursing-2030-action-hub/

Chicago History Museum (2021). The black nurses of Providence Hospital. The Black Nurses of Provident Hospital–Chicago History Museum.

Clifford, M. E., & Jurado, L.-F. M. (2018). The Impact of an All BSN Workforce Policy. *Journal of Nursing Practice Applications & Reviews of Research*, *8*(2), 60–67.

Davis, A. (1991). America's first school of nursing: the New England Hospital for Women and Children. *Journal of Nursing Education*, *30*(4), 158–161. https://doi.org/10.3928/0148-4834-19910401-06

Dickison, P., Haerling, K. A., & Lasater, K. (2019). Integrating the National Council of State Boards of Nursing Clinical Judgment Model Into Nursing Educational Frameworks. *The Journal of Nursing Education*, *58*(2), 72–78. https://doi.org/10.3928/01484834-20190122-03

Djukic, M., Padhye, N., Ke, Z., Yu, E., McVey, C., Manuel, W., Short, Y., Pine, R., & Caligone, S. (2023). Associations between the COVID-19 Pandemic and New Nurses' Transition to Practice Outcomes: A Multisite, Longitudinal Study. *Journal of Nursing Regulation*, *14*(1), 42–49. https://doi.org/10.1016/S2155-8256(23)00067-4

Djukic, M., Stimpfel, A. W., & Kovner, C. (2019). Bachelor's Degree Nurse Graduates

Report Better Quality and Safety Educational Preparedness than Associate Degree Graduates. *Joint Commission Journal on Quality and Patient Safety*, *45*(3), 180–186. https://doi.org/10.1016/j.jcjq.2018.08.008

Duncan, K., & Schulz, P. S. (2015). Impact of Change to a Concept-Based Baccalaureate Nursing Curriculum on Student and Program Outcomes. *Journal of Nursing Education*, *54*, S16–S20. https://doi.org/10.3928/01484834-20150218-07

Dzioba, C., LaManna, J., Perry, C. K., Toerber-Clark, J., Boehning, A., O'Rourke, J., & Rutledge, C. (2022). Telehealth Competencies: Leveled for Continuous Advanced Practice Nurse Development. *Nurse Educator*, *47*(5), 293–297. https://doi.org/10.1097/NNE.0000000000001196

Enges, K. J. (2018). History of nursing. In G. Roux, & J. A. Halstead (Eds.), *Issues and trends in nursing* (2nd ed., pp. 3–29). Jones & Barlett Learning LCC.

Esposito, L. (2021). Pandemic's impact on the nursing profession. *Us News & World Report*. Retrieved from https://health.usnews.com/health-care/patient-advice/articles/pandemics-impact-on-the-nursing-profession

Forneris, S. G., Tagliareni, M. E., & Allen, B. (2022). Accelerating to Practice: Defining a Competency-Based Curriculum Framework for Nursing Education Part 1. *Nursing Education Perspectives*, *43*(6), 363–368. https://doi.org/10.1097/01.NEP.0000000000000954

Fowler, M. D. (2017). Unladylike commotion: Early feminism and nursing's role in gender/trans dialogue. *Nursing Inquiry*, *24*, e12179. https://doi.org/10.1111/nin.12179

Goldmark, J. C.; Committee for the Study of Nursing Education. (1923). *Nursing and nursing education in the United States*. The Macmillan Company. Retrieved from https://books.google.com/books?id=0tR-AAAAIAAJ&pg=PA1#=onepage&q&f=false

Hampton Robb, I. (2013). Nursing Ethics: For hospital and private use. E. C. Koeckert Publisher.

Hardin, P. K., & Richardson, S. J. (2012). Teaching the concept curricula: theory and method. *The Journal of Nursing Education*, *51*(3), 155–159. https://doi.org/10.3928/01484834-20120127-01

Harrison, J. M., Aiken, L. H., Sloane, D. M., Brooks Carthon, J. M., Merchant, R. M., & Berg, R. A.; American Heart Association's Get With the Guidelines-Resuscitation, I. (2019). In hospitals with more nurses who have baccalaureate degrees, better outcomes for patients after cardiac arrest. *Health Affairs*, *38*(7), 1087–1094, https://doi.org/10.1377/hlthaff.2018.05064.

Hassmiller, S. B., & Wakefield, M. K. (2022). The Future of Nursing 2020–2030: Charting a path to achieve health equity. *Nursing Outlook*, *70*(6 Suppl 1), S1–S9. https://doi.org/10.1016/j.outlook.2022.05.013

Institute of Medicine. (2011). *The Future of Nursing: Leading Change, Advancing Health*. National Academies Press.

Interprofessional Education Collaborative. (2016). *Core Competencies for Interprofessional Collaborative Practice: 2016 Update*. Retrieved from https://ipec.memberclicks.net/assets/2016-Update.pdf

Kalisch, P. A. (1975). Heroines of '98: female Army nurses in the Spanish-American war. *Nursing Research*, *24*(6), 411–429.

Kavanagh, J. M., & Szweda, C. (2017). A crisis in competency: The strategic and ethical imperative to assessing new graduate nurses' clinical reasoning. *Nursing Education Perspectives*, *38*(2), 57–62. https://doi.org/10.1097/01.NEP.0000000000000112

Lewis, L. S., Rebeschi, L. M., & Hunt, E. (2022). Nursing Education Practice Update 2022: Competency-Based Education in Nursing. *SAGE Open Nursing*, *8*, 23779608221140774. https://doi.org/10.1177/23779608221140774

Lingel, J., Clark-Parsons, R., & Branciforte, K. (2022). More than handmaids: Nursing, labor activism and feminism. *Gender, Work and Organization*, *29*, 1149–1163. https://doi.org/10.1111.gwao.12816

Minority Nurse. (2013). *Preserving the history of black nurses*. Minority Nurse, Springer Publishing Company, Black and African-American Nurses, Magazine, Nursing

Associations. https://minoritynurse.com/preserving-the-history-of-black-nurses/

Montgomery, T., Bundy, J., Cofer, D., & Nicholls, E. (2021). Black Americans in nursing education. *American Nurse.* Black Americans in Nursing Education–what the future holds (myamericannurse.com)

Moody, S. (1938). Isabel Hampton Robb: Her Contribution to Nursing Education. *The American Journal of Nursing, 38*(10), 1121–1139. https://doi.org/10.2307/3413723

Mulkey, D. C. (2023). The History of Men in Nursing: Pioneers of the Profession. *Journal of Christian Nursing, 40*(2), 96–101. https://doi.org/10.1097/CNJ.0000000000001040

National Academies of Sciences, Engineering, and Medicine. (2016). *Assessing progress on the institute of medicine report the future of nursing.* The National Academies Press. https://doi.org/10.17226/21838

National Academies of Sciences, Engineering, and Medicine. (2021). *The Future of Nursing 2020–2030: Charting a path to achieve health equity.* The National Academies Press. https://doi.org/10.17226/25982

National Council of Defense & American Red Cross. (1918). *The training camp for nurses at Vassar College.* Poughkeepsie, New York.

National Commission to Address Racism in Nursing. (n.d.). How Does Racism in Nursing Show Up in the Education Space? Retrieved from https://www.nursingworld.org/~49b97e/globalassets/practiceandpolicy/workforce/commission-to-address-racism/3racismintheeducationspace.pdf

National League for Nursing. (2023). NLN vision statement: Integrating competency-based education in the nursing curriculum. Retrieved from https://www.nln.org/news/newsroomnln-position-documents/nln-vision-series

Naval History and Heritage Command. (2017). United States Navy Nurse Corps, World War 1. https://www.history.navy.mil/our-collections/artifacts/exhibits/uniform--navy-nurse-corps--world-war-i.html

Nightingale, F. (1860). *Notes on nursing: What it is and what it is not.* https://digital.library.upenn.edu/women/nightingale/nursing/nursing.html

O'Brien, D., Knowlton, M., & Whichello, R. (2018). Attention Health Care Leaders: Literature Review Deems Baccalaureate Nurses Improve Patient Outcomes. *Nursing Education Perspectives, 39*(4), E2–E6. https://doi.org/10.1097/01.NEP.0000000000000303

Petry, L. (1943). U. S. Cadet Nurse Corps: Established under the Bolton Act. *The American Journal of Nursing, 43*(8), 704–708. http://www.jstor.org/stable/3456272

Porat-Dahlerbruch, J., Aiken, L. H., Lasater, K. B., Sloane, D. M., & McHugh, M. D. (2022). Variations in nursing baccalaureate education and 30-day inpatient surgical mortality. *Nursing Outlook, 70*(2), 300–308. https://doi.org/10.1016/j.outlook.2021.09.009.

Poslusny, S. M. (1989). Feminist friendship: Isabel Hampton Robb, Lavinia Lloyd Dock, & Mary Adelaide Nutting. *Image Journal Nursing Scholarship. Summer, 21*(2), 63–68. https://doi.org/10.1111.j.1547-5069.1989.tb00099x

Quality and Safety Education for Nurses (QSEN). (n.d). http://qsen.org/.

Repsha, C. L., Quinn, B. L., & Peters, A. B. (2020). Implementing a Concept-Based Nursing Curriculum: A Review of the Literature. *Teaching & Learning in Nursing, 15*(1), 66–71. https://doi.org/10.1016/j.teln.2019.09.006

Rodríguez-García, M. C., Márquez-Hernández, V. V., Belmonte-García, T., Gutiérrez-Puertas, L., & Granados-Gámez, G. (2020). Original Research: How Magnet Hospital Status Affects Nurses, Patients, and Organizations: A Systematic Review. *The American Journal of Nursing, 120*(7), 28–38. https://doi.org/10.1097/01.NAJ.0000681648.48249.16

Rutledge, C. M., O'Rourke, J., Mason, A. M., Chike-Harris, K., Behnke, L., Melhado, L., Downes, L., & Gustin, T. (2021). Telehealth Competencies for Nursing Education and Practice: The Four P's of Telehealth. *Nurse Educator, 46*(5), 300–305. https://doi.org/10.1097/NNE.0000000000000988

Scheckel, M. (2018). Nursing education: Past, present and future. In G. Roux, & J. A. Halstead (Eds.), *Issues and Trends in Nursing* (2nd ed., pp. 3–29). Jones & Barlett Learning LCC.

School of Nursing for Men. (1914–1965). Historical timeline. History of Pennsylvania Hospital. https://www.uphs.upenn.edu/paharc/timeline/1901/tline26.html

Selanders, L. (2023). Florence Nightingale. Encyclopedia Britannica. https://www.britannica.com/biography/Florence-Nightingale

Steptoe, T. (2010). Spelman College (188-1). Blackpast. https://www.blackpast.org/african-american-history/spelman-college-1881/

Straka, K. L., Hupp, D. S., Ambrose, H. L., & Christy, L. (2019). Reaching beyond 80% BSN-prepared nurses: One organization's journey to success. *Nursing Management, 50*(5), 52–54. https://doi.org/10.1097/01.NUMA.0000557624.27437.25

Sumpter, D., Blodgett, N., Beard, K., & Howard, V. (2022). Transforming nursing education in response to the Future of Nursing 2020–2030 report. *Nursing Outlook, 70*(6S1), S20–S31. https://doi.org/10.1016/j.outlook.2022.02.00

Tanaka, N., & Miyamoto, K. (2022). The world needs more and better nurses. Published on education for global development. Worldbank.org. https://blogs.worldbank.org/education/world-needs-more-and-better-nurses-heres-how-education-sector-can-help

Trennert, R. A. (2003). Sage Memorial Hospital and the Nation's first all-Indian school of nursing. *The Journal of Arizona History, 44*(4), 353–374. http://www.jstor.org/stable/41696805

van Houwelingen, C. T., Moerman, A. H., Ettema, R. G., Kort, H. S., & Ten Cate, O. (2016). Competencies required for nursing telehealth activities: A Delphi-study. *Nurse Education Today, 39*, 50–62. https://doi.org/10.1016/j.nedt.2015.12.025

WHO. (2020). *State of the world's nursing 2020: Investing in education, jobs, and leadership.* World Health Organization. License: CC BY-NC-SA 3.0 IGO. https://www.who.int/publications/i/item/9789240003279

Yakusheva, O., Lindrooth, R., & Weiss, M. (2014). Economic evaluation of the 80% baccalaureate nurse workforce recommendation: A patient-level analysis. *Medical Care, 52*(10), 864–869.

Yale University Library Online Exhibitions. (2019–2022). 1870s–1933: Origins of the Yale School of Nursing. Yale School of Nursing: Better Health for All People—1870s–1933: Origins of the Yale School of Nursing—Yale School of Nursing: Better Health for All People—Yale University Library Online Exhibitions

2

Teaching in a Practice-Based Profession

Gail Armstrong, PhD, DNP, RN, ACNS-BC, CNE, FAAN

CHAPTER OVERVIEW

This chapter focuses on how teaching and learning are different in a practice-based program of study and the consideration of how practice standards impact teaching practice, course design, and evaluation. Standards significant for nurse educators include accreditation and regulatory requirements, as well as quintessential guiding practice concepts, such as patient safety. Topics addressed in this chapter include the dynamic nature of practice standards, how utilization of Benner's three apprenticeships model facilitates a holistic preparation for practice standards, the usefulness of referencing accreditation and practice standards in planning teaching/learning, and the necessity of continuously connecting classroom learning to clinical education.

TEACHING IN A PRACTICE PROFESSION

There are important differences in teaching in a practice profession, as compared to teaching in a discipline where graduates do not enter a practice. Prior to being granted full access to practice, clinical professionals must successfully complete rigorous academic and practical training (Shulman, 1998). As an educator in a practice profession, exemplary nurse educators teach knowledge, skills, and professional values as all are necessary for the provision of safe, high-quality patient care. Practice professions include clinical rotations, which ideally complement traditional didactic classes. Seasoned nurse educators are aware of the tension of teaching knowledge that must be applied in rapidly shifting nursing practice as a consistent element of teaching in a practice profession. Navigating this gap between education and practice is a core part of the work of nursing education. Effective nurse educators learn to navigate between nursing content, research, and practice, and thereby facilitate learners' ability to access, understand, appraise, apply, and support research in practice (Andiwatir & Betan, 2018). Table 2.1 offers five distinguishing characteristics of practice professions that influence educational standards within that profession.

TABLE 2.1

Characteristics of Practice Professions

Characteristic of Practice Professions	Explanation
Centrality of clients	Successful outcomes in clinical practice are co-produced by the practitioner and the client.
Knowledge demands	Safe practice is highly complex requiring general and specialized knowledge and skills as well as theoretical, practice, and technical knowledge.
Use of evidence and judgment in practice	Determining best practice requires knowing an individual client as well as knowing latest evidence-based practice.
Community and standards of practice	Clinical practice professions form a professional community that monitors quality, distributes knowledge, and creates standards of practice.
Education for clinical practice	Students in practice professions must learn to work effectively with clients, obtain a high degree of knowledge, understand how to use evidence and judgment in practice, and comprehend and value the standards in their profession.

Adapted from Alter, J., & Coggshall, J. G. (2009). Teaching as a clinical practice profession: Implications for teacher preparation and state policy. Issue brief. *National Comprehensive Center for Teacher Quality.*

THE DYNAMIC NATURE OF PRACTICE STANDARDS

Practicing nurses have a keen sense of the rapid infusion of new evidence continually affecting practice standards. Staying abreast of current nursing practice is vital for nursing programs to graduate nurses who are practice-ready. Few studies have quantified how quickly practice standards need to be updated. A 2001 study assessed the validity of 17 clinical practice guidelines published by the Agency for Healthcare Research and Quality (AHRQ). Analysis indicated that about half the guidelines were outdated in 5.8 years (Shekelle et al., 2001). Similar data were found in a 2007 study that examined how quickly systematic reviews go out of date. Shojania et al. (2007) found that the median duration that a systematic review remained current without needing to be updated was 5.5 years. This rapid cycle of new information entering health care creates a challenge for nurse educators in staying current with the content and practice standards that they teach.

A vital area of alignment is between dynamic practice standards and the content of the licensing exam to enter nursing. The National Council of State Boards of Nursing (NCSBN) serves as the regulatory guide for Boards of Nursing (BON) in all fifty states. NCSBN writes licensing exams taken by all levels of nurses (e.g., Registered Nurses, Licensed Practical Nurses, and Licensed Vocational Nurses). Because the US health care industry is rapidly changing, NCSBN conducts practice analysis studies every three years to ensure that the nursing licensing exams reflect current nursing practice.

Data from NCSBN's practice analysis studies drive evaluation of the content of the nursing licensure examination in assessing the licensing exam's alignment with practice (NCSBN, 2021). These NCSBN surveys track shifts in practice priorities. For example, the results of the 2021 survey identified the five most important knowledge areas for newly licensed RNs as airway management, client safety, basic life support, client assessment, and vital signs. These five areas were a shift from the 2017 survey data that identified the following knowledge areas as most important for newly licensed RNs: airway management, medication administration, vital signs, medication safety, and changes in client condition (NCSBN, 2021).

Across health professions education, evidence-based practice (EBP) offers key skills that health care professionals need to stay appraised of current practice, but this skill set is rarely well integrated where didactic teaching interfaces with clinical education models. A recent review of EBP in health professions education programs reveals that gaps exist between teaching current practice standards and facilitating the application of those standards in clinical rotations. Effective embedding of EBP throughout health professions curricula requires further development, with an emphasis on a real-world and more pragmatic approach (Lehane et al., 2019). Gaps identified by this research team include variables clustered around EBP curriculum considerations, the actual skills needed to effectively teach EBP, and engagement by interested parties in EBP education. Some recommendations include focusing on EBP as a core competency within a discipline's professional standards, increased emphasis on communication skills to facilitate shared decision-making, use of more dynamic assessment strategies that are context-specific, and a move towards scaffolding EBP learning across a program of study. This research team also highlights the necessity of identifying salient barriers and developing an expedient approach to overcoming identified barriers (Lehane, 2019).

PRACTICE-EDUCATION GAP

A commonly identified problem in nursing education is the inadvertent separate siloes between didactic knowledge and clinical education. The artificial separation between technical and scientific knowledge from practice and relational skills contradicts the reality that skill sets are intermingled in effective practice. A common definition of the practice-education gap (also called the theory-practice gap) is the distancing of theoretical knowledge from the practical dimension of nursing (Scully, 2011). The effect of this gap can be nurse graduates who are not ready for practice. Inadequately prepared new nurses may compromise patient safety (King et al., 2018). In resource-limited settings, this disparity can be more pronounced, with systemic elements exacerbating the separation. A 2019 international study discovered five causes contributing to the practice-education gap: system inadequacies; resource constraints; challenges of the clinical learning environment; clinical placement and supervision; and nurse faculty factors (Salifu et al., 2019). Encouraging nursing faculty to stay connected to the multifaceted demands of nursing practice through collaboration with clinical partners is an effective strategy for avoiding the practice-education gap.

During the Covid-19 pandemic, the practice-education gap was exacerbated by the temporary cessation of nursing clinical rotations and migration to increased utilization of online resources, virtual simulation, and artificial-intelligence teaching methodologies to bolster clinical education (Diaz et al., 2021). These interruptions in clinical education caused notable psychological distress for nursing students, impacting their sense of self-determination in transitioning into practice (Yang, 2022). Additionally, for students educated during the pandemic, the substitution of traditional clinical educational learning by skills laboratories, simulation, virtual simulation, or case studies has created doubt about their future role as new graduate nurses (Kang & Hwang, 2023).

Evidence-based resources are available for updated strategies to address the practice-education gap. In 2016 the American Association of Colleges of Nursing (AACN) published a robust report, *Advancing Healthcare Transformation*, which provided recommendations for strengthening academic-practice partnerships (AACN, 2016). Recommendations focused on addressing the historical gap between academic nursing and the dynamic changes in practice, missed opportunities for alignment between nursing education and practice, and the chronic problem of insufficient resources to address the practice-education gap (AACN, 2016). From this report, AACN offers valuable resources to address the practice-education gap including evidence-based Guiding Principles, an Implementation Tool Kit, and Exemplar Partnerships that have been recognized for their excellence (available at: https://www.aacnnursing.org/Academic-Practice-Partnerships).

BENNER'S THREE APPRENTICESHIPS MODEL

Utilization of an education model that closely links didactic and clinical learning can bridge the practice-education gap. To facilitate such blended learning, the nursing profession has a long history of an apprentice model for education. A recent close review of documentation of nursing apprenticeship models suggests that rigorous academic practice partnerships are necessary for effective, updated apprenticeships in nursing (Tesseyman et al., 2022). The complex practice demands on graduate nurses require that educators concurrently address teaching and learning not only at the intellectual level but also at the motor skills and values levels as well. Ideally, learners in nursing education programs experience concurrent development in all three areas. In the 2010 study, Educating Nurses, published by the Carnegie Foundation, Benner et al. (2010) introduce the three-apprenticeship model for nursing education. The value of this model is that it illuminates how nurses need continual development in knowledge development, clinical reasoning and skilled know-how, and ethical formation. Benner and colleagues differentiate their recommended apprenticeship model from historic nursing education apprenticeships where learners at diploma programs were mostly educated through on-the-job training. Benner's clarification of "higher apprenticeships" places an emphasis on identification of competence in learning over time, using a variety of pedagogies, with built-in processes for reflective practice. This updated definition of an apprenticeship emphasizes a multi-faceted approach to graduated learning in nursing, where apprenticeship captures the "experiential learning that requires interaction with a community of practice, situated coaching by teachers, and demonstration of aspects of complex practice that are not easily translated" (Benner et al., 2010, p. 24).

Benner updates the apprenticeship model through three apprenticeships for nursing education: (1) Acquiring and Using Knowledge and Science, (2) Using Clinical Reasoning and Skilled Know-How; and (3) Ethical Comportment and Formation. Knowledge of science is core to competent nursing practice. Nurses use knowledge from many fields. Subject matter expertise from various sciences (e.g., anatomy, physiology, pathophysiology, microbiology, chemistry, genetics, and pharmacology) is needed for patient care, interpretation of diagnostics, and staying current with practice. Making decisions in the context of the complexities of practice requires synthesis of knowledge and intellectual agility in being able to prioritize key concerns. Managing a patient's dynamic condition over time while utilizing various resources requires complex clinical reasoning skills. Integral to effective care are strong communication skills with patients, families, and the health care team. Effective clinical decisions require rapid interpretation of clinical indicators and synthesizing information from multiple sources. Lastly, ethics is interconnected to all aspects of nursing practice. Nurses need the skills of ethical decision-making, ethical reflection, and the ability to use moral resources in navigating complex care situations (Benner et al., 2010).

Through the interconnectedness of the three apprenticeships, Benner's model promotes integrative learning opportunities. Through the overlap across cognitive and clinical reasoning apprenticeships, learners have the opportunity to articulate and execute key aspects of competent care. Applying knowledge germane to a clinical situation encourages learners to discern relevant information and discern the salience of specific details. Supervised practice creates an opportunity where learners can share their thinking and learn from role-modeled clinical decision-making. The coaching inherent to supervised practice helps learners understand, reflect on, and articulate their emerging practice, especially in complex clinical situations. Guiding novice learners in recognizing priorities and demands embedded in clinical situations helps learners develop a sense of salience and determine the highest priority of care to attend to. The overlap across all three apprenticeships facilitates reflection on practice, as the teaching/learning goal is for learners to draw on all they learn in each apprenticeship and appropriately integrate their synthesized learning into practice (Benner et al., 2010).

Teaching across the three apprenticeships encourages nurse educators to consider holistic approaches to practice standards. An exemplar of using one's understanding of the three apprenticeships in teaching sexually transmitted diseases to prelicensure learners emphasizes an integrated learning design, where case studies, communication patterns, and learner self-awareness are interwoven to replicate the application of this knowledge and these clinical skills in actual nursing practice (Noone, 2009). A clinical simulation for prelicensure learners focusing on psychiatric mental health care addresses the three apprenticeships through baseline knowledge of chronic schizophrenia, an opportunity to interact with the patient and family (through high-fidelity simulation), and debriefing with expert clinician educators. Through attention to all three apprenticeships, the psychiatric mental health teaching team ensures the integration of information to address the demands of real practice (Crider & McNiesh, 2011). A nurse educator focusing on teaching end-of-life care created a meaningful and relevant learning experience for prelicensure learners by addressing the three apprenticeships. Knowledge acquisition focused on standards related to caring for dying patients, unfolding case studies, role playing, and volunteering as hospice volunteers facilitated clinical reasoning and application of knowledge in authentic *practice* situations, and moral reasoning was addressed through the reflective practice highlighted in class discussions and through reflection papers (Hold et al., 2014). Through attention to current practice standards and the three apprenticeships, nurse educators can effectively minimize the practice-education gap.

PROFESSIONAL ORGANIZATIONS

Resources from professional organizations can serve as a key source of information for nurse educators about updated practice standards. While there are a plethora of nursing professional organizations, most focus their priorities, work, and recommendations for a specific area of practice (e.g., American Psychiatric Nurse Association, Academy of Medical Surgical Nurses, Association of Perioperative Nurses, and Oncology Nursing Society). When teaching clinical content specific to a professional organization's clinical focus, it is prudent for nurse educators to review professional nursing organizations' white papers, position statements, or practice standards resources.

Valuable practice standard recommendations are also published by broader-based professional organizations. Patient safety is a primary focus in nursing practice and therefore a recurring priority in many nursing courses. Nurse educators can garner strong evidence-based guidelines for their teaching about patient safety from a variety of professional organizations.

The National Academy of Medicine

Consensus reports and workshop proceedings generated by the National Academy of Medicine (NAM) can be a rich resource for nurse educators. NAM is part of the National Academies of Sciences, Engineering, and Medicine. Until 2015, NAM was known as the Institute of Medicine (IOM). NAM's mission is to improve health for all by advancing science, accelerating health equity, and providing independent, authoritative, and trusted advice. NAM provides free resources as an evidence-based scientific advisor, functioning as a national academy with a global scope, with an emphasis on catalyzing action to lead collaborative and interdisciplinary work for a healthier future for all (NAM, n.d.). Table 2.2 lists recent NAM reports related to nursing that offer evidence-based guidelines for a variety of health care challenges, including URLs for downloads. NAM offers robust resources where a search on the NAM site can lead educators to a wealth of evidence-based resources. For example, using the prompt "health equity and social determinants of health" in the search bar on the NAM home page leads to a 2017 resource, *Perspectives on Health Equity and Social Determinants of Health* (Bogard, 2017). Along with the link to download the publication is a link to a free social media toolkit to enhance the teaching of this content.

With the release of *To Err is Human* in 2000, IOM was a key player in calling national attention to concerning data about poor patient safety outcomes. This important report was the first data-driven publication to examine patient safety outcomes from a systems perspective. The broad, national interest in it catalyzed tracking patient safety outcomes within health care systems. As more complete and accurate data about avoidable harm to patients in US health care systems became available, systematic improvements were recommended. From 2000 to 2006 IOM focused most of its resources on studying patient safety issues and publishing a series of ten reports to address these complex issues. This series of reports, *Crossing the Quality Chasm Series*, offered

TABLE 2.2

Examples of Recent National Academy of Medicine Reports Specific to Nursing

Year	Title	Type of Report
2022	The National Imperative to Improve Nursing Home Quality: Honoring Our Commitment to Residents, Families and Staff https://nap.nationalacademies.org/catalog/26526/the-national-imperative-to-improve-nursing-home-quality-honoring-our	Consensus study report
2022	Mechanisms for Organizational Behavior Change to Address the Needs of People Living with Alzheimer's Disease and Related Dementia https://nap.nationalacademies.org/catalog/26772/mechanisms-for-organizational-behavior-change-to-address-the-needs-of-people-living-with-alzheimers-disease-and-related-dementias	Proceedings
2021	The Future of Nursing 2020-2030: Charting a Path to Achieve Health Equity https://nap.nationalacademies.org/catalog/25982/the-future-of-nursing-2020-2030-charting-a-path-to	Consensus study report
2020	Understanding Nursing Home, Hospice, and Palliative Care for Individuals with Later-Stage Dementia: Proceedings of a Workshop—in Brief https://nap.nationalacademies.org/catalog/25902/understanding-nursing-home-hospice-and-palliative-care-for-individuals-with-later-stage-dementia	Proceedings
2016	Establishing an African Association for Health Professions Education and Research https://nap.nationalacademies.org/catalog/23485/establishing-an-african-association-for-health-professions-education-and-research	Proceedings
2016	Assessing Progress on the Institute of Medicine Report The Future of Nursing https://nap.nationalacademies.org/catalog/21838/assessing-progress-on-the-institute-of-medicine-report-the-future-of-nursing	Consensus study report
2015	Future Directions of Credentialing Research in Nursing https://nap.nationalacademies.org/catalog/18999/future-directions-of-credentialing-research-in-nursing-workshop-summary	Proceedings
2015	Empowering Women and Strengthening Health Systems and Services Through Investing in Nursing and Midwifery Enterprise: Lessons from Lower-Income Countries https://nap.nationalacademies.org/catalog/19005/empowering-women-and-strengthening-health-systems-and-services-through-investing-in-nursing-and-midwifery-enterprise	Proceedings

Source: https://nap.nationalacademies.org/search/?topic=288&term=nursing

TABLE 2.3	
Evidence-Based Toolkits Found on AHRQ's Patient Safety Network	
Title of Toolkit	**URL**
Getting Started with a Communication and Resolution Program Policy or Commitment Statement to Communication Resolution	https://psnet.ahrq.gov/issue/getting-started-communication-and-resolution-program-crp-policy-or-commitment-statement-cr
Toolkit to Improve Antibiotic Use in Ambulatory Care	https://psnet.ahrq.gov/issue/toolkit-improve-antibiotic-use-ambulatory-care
Calibrate Dx: A Resource to Improve Diagnostic Decisions	https://www.ahrq.gov/patient-safety/settings/multiple/calibrate-dx.html
How To Create a My Medicines List	https://psnet.ahrq.gov/issue/how-create-my-medicines-list
The Nursing Home Expert Panel's Falls Investigation Guide Toolkit: How-To-Guide	https://psnet.ahrq.gov/issue/nursing-home-expert-panels-falls-investigation-guide-toolkit-how-guide
Measure Dx: A Resource to Identify, Analyze and Learn from Diagnostic Safety Events	https://psnet.ahrq.gov/issue/measure-dx-resource-identify-analyze-and-learn-diagnostic-safety-events
Toolkit for Preventing CLABSI and CAUTI in ICUs	https://psnet.ahrq.gov/issue/toolkit-preventing-clabsi-and-cauti-icus
Safer Dx Checklist: 10 High Priority Practices for Diagnostic Excellence	https://psnet.ahrq.gov/issue/safer-dx-checklist-10-high-priority-practices-diagnostic-excellence
TeamSTEPPS® for Diagnosis Improvement	https://psnet.ahrq.gov/issue/teamsteppsr-diagnosis-improvement

Source: https://psnet.ahrq.gov/toolkits

evidence-based recommendations to policymakers and health care systems for systemic improvements to improve the quality and safety of patient care. Several reports in this series focused on nurses and nursing care.

AHRQ offers a plethora of resources for nursing educators to teach evidence-based patient safety, as well as updated research findings. A 2022 AHRQ study reveals the two-decade focus on patient safety outcomes has measurably improved patient outcomes for patients experiencing heart attack, heart failure, pneumonia patients, and major surgery (Eldridge et al., 2022). AHRQ's Patient Safety Network offers a wide variety of fact sheets, tool kits, measurement tools, and exemplary organization policies or guidelines for addressing patient safety. These resources can be found at: https://psnet.ahrq.gov/toolkits. Table 2.3 highlights some of the most useful tool kits for nursing educators found on AHRQ's Patient Safety Network website.

The National Quality Forum

Another example of a professional organization that offers quality measure guidelines for the improvement of health care is the National Quality Forum (NQF). Measures and standards developed by NQF serve as a critically important foundation for initiatives to enhance health care value, make patient care safer, and achieve better outcomes (NQF, n.d.). NQF works to advance the field of measurement science in health care by endorsing measures through a transparent endorsement process by experts. Currently, approximately 300 NQF-endorsed measures are used in health care systems (NQF, n.d.). NQF's primary website offers an abundance of resources specific to current standards in measuring improvement in health care.

REGULATORY AGENCIES

Regulatory agencies direct many aspects of nursing education programs and are a prolific resource for nurse educators to stay current with education and practice benchmarks. Their standards on educational programs in nursing can guide the development of relevant curricula and the structuring of clinical learning experiences. Regulatory agencies differ in several ways from professional organizations. Regulatory agencies offer a clear focus on protecting patient safety, and licensees are mandated to follow educational, licensing, and practice standards outlined by regulatory agencies. Table 2.4 spells out different structural, functional, and scope variances when considering the impact and roles of regulatory bodies and professional organizations.

State Boards of Nursing

State-level nursing regulatory bodies, State Boards of Nursing (BON), oversee the maintenance of education nursing education standards and licensing requirements with a primary focus on protection of the public. Literature focusing on contrast and comparison of BON regulations consistently find that there is a notable variation across the 50 BON in the United States. As early as Packard et al. (1994) found great disparity from state to state in both the content of nursing education programs and the processes required for acceptable nursing programs. As an example, a recent review of BON standards for nursing preceptors found that although some commonalities were noted (e.g., requirement of an RN license, a baccalaureate degree, and one to three years of experience), 11 states had no documented regulations. Many BON guidelines for preceptors lacked depth, specificity, and consistency (L'Ecuyer et al., 2018). Similarly, a 2014 examination of regulatory requirements for distance education in prelicensure nursing programs shows a lack of consistency across BON in program approval and licensure requirements for clinical and didactic faculty teaching in distance programs (Lowery & Spector, 2014). Thus, it is of utmost importance that nurse educators stay current in education and practice requirements specific to the BON in their state.

As regulatory bodies that maintain standards in nursing practice and nursing education, state boards of nursing often offer helpful, updated, evidence-based resources. The Oregon State Board of Nursing offers guidance for nurse educators on "Use of High Stakes Testing or Single Assessment Approaches in Nursing Education Programs" (available at: https://www.oregon.gov/osbn/Documents/IS_HighStakesTesting.pdf). These guidelines walk nurse educators through a systematic analysis of the

TABLE 2.4

Differences between Regulatory Bodies and Professional Organizations

Element of the Model	Regulatory Bodies	Professional Organizations
Primary purpose	Protect the public	To advance the profession
Organizational language	Board, Body, Commission, Division	Academy, association, guild, society
Membership	Mandatory for licensees	Voluntary
Coverage	Covers all those authorized to practice and use the protected title	Mostly for those associated with the professional organization and sometimes for broader professional practice
Cultural alignment	Impartial and evidentiary approach due to legal and public directive	Advocate for and promote the profession
Rights and responsibilities	Focused on public protection	Self-directed, usually broadly based
Typical activities	Identify minimum licensure, practice issues, education, discipline standards, maintain register, enforce discipline	Advocate for the profession, set standards, offer advanced credentials
Policy focus	Regulation policies	Professional and practice policy
Source of power	Legislation	Membership numbers, position statements, and visibility of work
Politically connected	No	Sometimes
Advocacy	Usually through formal consultative processes	Using various mobilization techniques advocacy may be broad-based
Leadership composition	Appointed board	Elected by membership
Accountability	To public via legislative and governmental structures	To members
Continuing professional development	Continuing competence of the practitioner	Career progression and advanced credentials

Adapted from Benton, D. C., Thomas, K., Damgaard, G., Masek, S. M., & Brekken, S. A. (2017). Exploring the differences between regulatory bodies, professional associations, and trade unions: An integrative review. *Journal of Nursing Regulation, 8*(3), 4–11.

appropriateness of assessment methodologies. The North Caroline State Board of Nursing recommends an evidence-based Student Practice Event Evaluation Tool (STEEP) that walks an educator through a logical process of reviewing an adverse event, using a Just Culture framework (available at: https://www.ncbon.com/education-resources-for-program-directors-just-culture-information). The Arizona State Board of Nursing offers a carefully curated list of resources to assist nurse educators in graduating "practice-ready" nurses. The bibliography of resources currently on the Arizona State Board of Nursing's website contains references from the last two years (available at: https://drive. google.com/file/d/1Tr88a5ztTzULS5dHcQiocsEIXp1vnmtC/view).

National Council of State Boards of Nursing (NCSBN)

The National Council of State Boards of Nursing (NCSBN) provides overarching leadership for the fifty US BON. NCSBN develops and administers licensing exams for Registered Nurses (RNs) and Licensed Practical Nurses (LPNs) or Licensed Vocational Nurses (LVN). And per NCSBN's home website, "NCSBN is an independent, not-for-profit organization through which nursing regulatory bodies act and counsel together on matters of common interest and concern affecting public health, safety, and welfare, including the development of nursing licensure examinations" (NCSBN, n.d.).

NCSBN offers syntheses and position statements on practice issues when it is determined that the focal area is a common interest or concern. For example, NCSBN conducted a study in 2019 to explore whether the metric of requiring first-time pass rates for the National Council Licensing Examination (NCLEX) at 80 percent is appropriate, and whether other metrics exist that might amend or replace this regulatory standard of 36 BON (NCSBN, 2019).

NCSBN offers an abundance of resources to provide updated information about licensure testing. With Next Generation NCLEX introduced in April 2023, NCSBN offered a variety of resources for nurse educators to become familiar with the changes to the licensing exam, so they were well equipped to best prepare their students. NCSBN regularly updates the NCLEX RN-Test Plan that provides in-depth detail about the specifics of a license test (available at: https://www.ncsbn.org/publications/2023-nclex-rn-test-plan). NCSBN's website includes resource videos for nurse educators and nursing students, for example, "The Next Generation NCLEX Uses Computer Adaptive Testing" (available at: https://www.ncsbn.org/video/the-next-generation-nclex-uses-computer-adaptive-testing-cat). NCSBN will often offer periodical educational resources when significant changes are anticipated in licensure testing. In preparation for the release of the Next Generation NCLEX in April 2023, NCSBN published a quarterly publication (Next Generation NCLEX News) that provided the latest data about the research to assess the changes to the NCLEX (available at: https://www.ncsbn.org/public-files/ngn_spring2023.pdf).

With increasing complexity around recommendations to improve quality and safety in health care, leaders across professional and regulatory organizations are beginning to collaborate in aligning models and priorities. The American Association of Colleges of Nursing (AACN) published Updated Essentials for Professional Nursing Education (2021) and is proactively identifying advantageous overlap with regulatory standards. Recommendations for regulatory bodies include revision of specific regulatory standards, updating of program assessment and measurement of student outcomes, and a renewed look at approval processes for nursing programs based on AACN's utilization of the competency-based education model in the updated Essentials (Giddens, 2022). This explicit call for overlap across accreditation and regulatory standards creates beneficial alignment for nurse educators.

The Joint Commission

The Joint Commission accredits health care organizations, with a primary focus on protecting patient safety. Per their mission statement, The Joint Commission "is a global driver of quality improvement... Through leading practices, unmatched knowledge and expertise, and rigorous standards, we help organizations across the continuum of care lead the way to zero harm" (The Joint Commission, 2023). The Joint Commission offers practice standards, often in response to their tracking of sentinel events. National Patient Safety Goals have long been based on patterns and trends identified in sentinel event reports. As an accrediting body for clinical agencies, The Joint Commission offers a wealth of practice standards that can be easily integrated into prelicensure and graduate nursing curricula.

As a regulatory body that enforces practice standards, The Joint Commission's website includes resources relevant to nurse educators. The Joint Commission has maintained a focus on patient safety for decades, and the wealth of resources available in the area of patient safety reflects this continued focus. Content areas with multiple resources include zero harm, emergency management, health care workforce safety and well-being, infection prevention and control, suicide prevention, and workplace violence prevention (available at: https://www.jointcommission.org/resources/patient-safety-topics/). The Joint Commission's more recent focus on addressing health equity is evident in robust, evidence-based resources specific to this focus. Nurse educators can find various resources on The Joint Commission's website including health equity standards, a Resource Center specific to health equity tools, and a continuing education to prepare one for Health Care Equity Certification (available at: https://www.jointcommission.org/our-priorities/health-care-equity/).

ACCREDITATION

Accreditation Standards

Accreditation is the process by which public standards are maintained in educational programs. A 2020 international consensus consortium examining the role of accreditation in health professions education defined accreditation as the process of formal evaluation of an educational program, institution, or system against defined standards by an auditing body to ensure quality assurance (Frank et al., 2020). Accreditation contributes to ensuring educational quality as it can enhance health care outcomes through its influence and the standardization of quality metrics in training programs. The accreditation process supports programs to continuously enhance the curriculum to align with population needs and improve learning environments (Frank et al., 2020). Across health professions education programs, there are core features that impact the purpose, structure, and processes of accreditation. Table 2.5 outlines ten common elements of accreditation across health professions education.

There are three primary accrediting bodies for nursing education programs: (1) the Commission on Collegiate Nursing Education (CCNE), overseen by AACN; (2) the Commission for Nursing Education Accreditation (CNEA), overseen by the National League for Nursing; and (3) the Accreditation Commission for Education in Nursing (ACEN). Despite the different emphases across these three accrediting organizations,

<table>
</table>

TABLE 2.5

Core Elements of Accrediting Agencies

Core Element	Explanation
Mandate	To review the quality of educational programs, institutions, or systems.
Criteria	Generally accepted measures or benchmarks used in making decisions about the quality of the program, institution, or system.
Application for initial accreditation	An initial request for accreditation by a program seeking to demonstrate adherence to the established standard and a decision on whether first-time accreditation is granted.
Self-study process	A program, institution, or system's internal process assessing alignment with externally established standards.
External assessment	External reviewers' process of determining the level of compliance of a program, institution, or system with established accreditation standards.
Accreditation reports	The final report by external evaluators regarding the level of compliance of a program, institution, or system with established standards.
Accreditation decision	The accrediting body's decision on accreditation status and its associated follow-up.
Accreditation cycle	Phases of an accreditation process identifying how often each program, institution, or system is reevaluated for compliance with the standard, including follow-up activities that must occur.
Site review model	The composition of an external site review team including processes for recruiting, assigning, and training the assessment team.
Accreditation administration	Supports for the administration and operationalization of the accreditation process.

Adapted from Frank, J. R., Taber, S., van Zanten, M., Scheele, F., & Blouin, D. (2020). The role of accreditation in 21st century health professions education: Report of an International Consensus Group. *BMC Medical Education, 20*(1), 1–9.

comparative analysis reveals multiple overlapping areas. All three sets of standards require educational programs to engage in continual assessment of program administration, program faculty, curricular elements, and program outcomes. For sustained accreditation, educational programs engage in regular self-study to produce a substantive self-study report used in site visits and program appraisal.

Accreditation for Advanced Practice Programs

Advance Practice RN (APRN) programs prepare advanced practice nurses who care for diverse populations across multitudes of clinical contexts. Due to this complex diversity, there are multiple models for ensuring educational quality in APRN programs. Where appropriate, overarching professional organizations, such as NCSBN or the National Organization of Nurse Practitioner Faculty (NONPF), offer guidelines for alignment across diverse APRN practices. For example, NCSBN developed common guidelines for APRN programs through its Consensus Model for Licensure, Accreditation,

Certification, Education (LACE) document (NCSBN, 2008). Although specific needs of populations or clinical settings may require adjustment, these inclusive guidelines facilitate collaboration across specialty practice organizations (Brown et al., 2022).

Some Advanced Practice RN (APRN) programs undergo their own accreditation process by accrediting agencies dedicated to that practice specialty. The Council on Accreditation (COA) solely accredits Certified Registered Nurse Anesthetist (CRNA) programs. COA's mission is to grant public recognition to nurse anesthesia programs and institutions that award post-master's certificates and master's and doctoral degrees that meet nationally established standards of academic quality and to assist programs and institutions in improving educational quality (COA, n.d.). CRNA programs go through cycles of accreditation, similar to prelicensure nursing programs. COA also directs educational requirements, recently deciding on standardizing the Doctor of Nursing Practice (DNP) degree for CRNAs (Madsen Gombkoto et al., 2014).

Nurse midwifery programs are accredited by the American College of Nurse Midwives (ACNM). ACNM's leadership as an accrediting body and professional organization is especially important for nurse midwives, as there are multiple pathways to becoming a midwife. ACNM was established to ensure standardization of nurse-midwifery education and promote excellence. The aim of ACME is to ensure that programs are performing at the highest level of quality and providing learning experiences that will lead to optimal outcomes for learners (ACME, n.d.). Along with establishing and maintaining accreditation standards for nurse-midwifery programs, ACNM offers leadership and recommendations in the areas of diversity of the nurse-midwifery workforce, policy, national advancement of midwifery, global engagement, and operational excellence.

CHAPTER SUMMARY

Teaching in a practice-based profession means that it is incumbent upon nurse educators to stay up to date with current practice standards. Employment of integrative teaching/learning strategies facilitates the growth and development of learners who are practice-ready. Effective integration is best facilitated through sustained collaborative efforts between education and practice, so as to maximally benefit learners. Reviews examining how to concurrently address priorities of theory and practice repeatedly emphasize the necessity of generative collaboration between academic lecturers and clinical educators (Berndtsson et al., 2020). As nurse educators work to continually update their teaching/learning strategies, a useful model is to remain mindful of how their course content, course design, learning activities, and evaluation methodologies attend to Benner's three apprenticeships. Additionally, ensuring one's course is in alignment with current recommendations from professional organizations, accrediting bodies and regulatory agencies ensures that one's learners are receiving a sound preparation for practice.

References

Accreditation commission for midwifery education (ACME). (n.d.). Retrieved January 6, 2023, from https://www.midwife.org/accreditation

Alter, J., & Coggshall, J. G. (2009). Teaching as a clinical practice profession: Implications for teacher preparation and state policy. Issue Brief. *National Comprehensive Center for Teacher Quality*. Retrieved from https://files.eric.ed.gov/fulltext/ED543819.pdf.

American Association of Colleges of Nursing. (2021). *The essentials: Core competencies for professional nursing education*. American Association of Colleges of Nursing.

American Association of Colleges of Nursing, Manatt Health. (2016). *Advancing healthcare transformation: A new era for academic nursing*. American Association of Colleges of Nursing. Retrieved from https://www.manatt.com/Insights/White-Papers/2016/Advancing-Healthcare-Transformation-A-New-Era-for-Academic-Nursing

Andiwatir, A., & Betan, Y. (2018). Letter to the Editor: Evidence-based practice for nursing profession: Barriers and teaching strategies solutions. *International Journal of Nursing Sciences*, 6(1), 123–124. https://doi.org/10.1016/j.ijnss.2018.11.009

Benner, P., Sutphen, M., Leonard, V., & Day, L. (2010). *Educating nurses: A call for radical transformation*. Jossey-Bass.

Benton, D. C., Thomas, K., Damgaard, G., Masek, S. M., & Brekken, S. A. (2017). Exploring the differences between regulatory bodies, professional associations, and trade unions: An integrative review. *Journal of Nursing Regulation*, 8(3), 4–11.

Berndtsson, I., Dahlborg, E., & Pennbrant, S. (2020). Work-integrated learning as a pedagogical tool to integrate theory and practice in nursing education—An integrative literature review. *Nurse Education in Practice*, 42, 102685. https://doi.org/10.1016/j.nepr.2019.102685

Bogard, K., Murry, V. M., & Alexander, C. M. (2017). *Perspectives on health equity and social determinants of health*. National Academy of Medicine (US). Retrieved March 12 from: https://nam.edu/wp-content/uploads/2017/12/Perspectives-on-Health-Equity-and-Social-Determinants-of-Health.pdf

Brown, A. M., Reyes, I., Zeno, R., & Whited, T. (2022). Alignment of pediatric nurse practitioner licensure, accreditation, certification, and education for employers. *The Journal for Nurse Practitioners*, 18(3), 316–319. https://doi.org/10.1016/j.nurpra.2021.11.020

Council on Accreditation (n.d.). About Us. Retrieved January 6, 2023 from: https://www.coacrna.org/about-coa/

Crider, M. C., & McNiesh, S. G. (2011). Integrating a professional apprenticeship model with psychiatric clinical simulation. *Journal of Psychosocial Nursing and Mental Health Services*, 49(5), 42–49. https://doi.org/10.3928/02793695-20110329-01

Diaz, K., Staffileno, B. A., & Hamilton, R. (2021). Nursing student experiences in turmoil: A year of the pandemic and social strife during final clinical rotations. *Journal of Professional Nursing*, 37(5), 978–984. https://doi.org/10.1016/j.profnurs.2021.07.019

Eldridge, N., Wang, Y., Metersky, M., Eckenrode, S., Mathew, J., Sonnenfeld, N., Perdue-Puli, J., Hunt, D., Brady, P. J., McGann, P., Grace, E., Rodrick, D., Drye, E., & Krumholz, H. M. (2022). Trends in adverse event rates in hospitalized patients, 2010–2019. *JAMA*, 328(2), 173–183. https://doi.org/10.1001/jama.2022.9600

Frank, J. R., Taber, S., van Zanten, M., Scheele, F., & Blouin, D. (2020). The role of accreditation in 21st century health professions education: report of an International Consensus Group. *BMC Medical Education*, 20(1), 1–9.

Giddens, J., Douglas, J. P., & Conroy, S. (2022). The revised AACN essentials: Implications for nursing regulation. *Journal of Nursing Regulation*, 12(4), 16–22. https://doi.org/10.1016/S2155-8256(22)00009-6

Hold, J. L., Ward, E. N., & Blake, B. J. (2014). Integrating professional apprentices into an end-of-life course. *The Journal of Nursing Education*, 53(2), 112–115. https://doi.org/10.3928/01484834-20140122-04

Kang, Y., & Hwang, H. (2023). The impact of changes in nursing practicum caused by COVID-19 pandemic on new graduate nurses. *Nurse Education Today*, 121, 105675. https://doi.org/10.1016/j.nedt.2022.105675

King, D., Tee, S., Falconer, L., Angell, C., Holley, D., & Mills, A. (2018). Virtual health education: Scaling practice to transform student learning: Using virtual reality learning environments in healthcare education to bridge the theory/practice gap and improve patient safety. *Nurse Education Today, 71*, 7–9. https://doi.org/10.1016/j.nedt.2018.08.002

L'Ecuyer, K. M., Lancken, S. V. D., Malloy, D., Meyer, G., & Hyde, M. J. (2018). Review of state boards of nursing rules and regulations for nurse preceptors. *Journal of Nursing Education, 57*(3), 134–141.

Lehane, E., Leahy-Warren, P., O'Riordan, C., Savage, E., Drennan, J., O'Tuathaigh, C., O'Connor, M., Corrigan, M., Burke, F., Hayes, M., Lynch, H., Sahm, L., Heffernan, E., O'Keeffe, E., Blake, C., Horgan, F., & Hegarty, J. (2019). Evidence-based practice education for healthcare professions: An expert view. *BMJ Evidence-Based Medicine, 24*(3), 103–108. https://doi.org/10.1136/bmjebm-2018-111019

Lowery, B., & Spector, N. (2014). Regulatory implications and recommendations for distance education in prelicensure nursing programs. *Journal of Nursing Regulation, 5*(3), 24–33.

Madsen Gombkoto, R. L., Walker, J. R., Horton, B. J., Martin-Sheridan, D., Yablonky, M. J., & Gerbasi, F. R. (2014). Council on accreditation of nurse anesthesia educational programs adopts standards for the practice doctorate and Post-graduate CRNA fellowships. *AANA Journal, 82*(3), 177–183.

National Academy of Medicine. (n.d.). About the National Academy of Medicine. Retrieved January 6, 2023 at https://nam.edu/about-the-nam/

National Council of State Boards of Nursing. (2021). *Report of findings from the 2021 RN nursing knowledge survey*. NCSBN. Last retrieved from: https://www.ncsbn.org/public-files/21_RN_KSA_FINAL.pdf

National Council of State Boards of Nursing. (2019). The NCSBN 2019 environmental scan: 40th anniversary edition. *Journal of Nursing Regulation, 9*(4, suppl), S1–S40. Last retrieved at: www.journalofnursingregulation.com/article/S2155-8256(18)30177-7/fulltext

National Council of State Boards of Nursing. (n.d.). Retrieved January 5, 2023, from https://www.ncsbn.org

National Councils of State Boards of Nursing APRN Advisory Committee & APRN Consensus Work Group. (2008). APRN consensus model-the consensus model for APRN regulation, licensure, accreditation, certification and education. Retrieved January 5, 2023, from https://www.ncsbn.org/aprn-consensus.htm

Noone, J. (2009). Teaching to the three apprenticeships: Designing learning activities for professional practice in an undergraduate curriculum. *The Journal of Nursing Education, 48*(8), 468–471. https://doi.org/10.3928/01484834-20090518-08

NQF: About us. (n.d.). Retrieved January 8, 2023, from https://www.qualityforum.org/About_NQF/

Packard, S. A., Polifroni, C., & Shah, H. S. (1994). Rules and regulations governing nursing education. *Journal of Professional Nursing, 10*(2), 97–104. https://doi.org/10.1016/8755-7223(94)90070-1

Salifu, D. A., Gross, J., Salifu, M. A., & Ninnoni, J. P. (2019). Experiences and perceptions of the theory-practice gap in nursing in a resource-constrained setting: A qualitative description study. *Nursing Open, 6*(1), 72–83. https://doi.org/10.1002/nop2.188

Scully, N. J. (2011). The theory-practice gap and skill acquisition: An issue for nursing education. *Collegian, 18*(2), 93–98. https://doi.org/10.1016/j.colegn.2010.04.002

Shekelle, P. G., Ortiz, E., Rhodes, S., Morton, S. C., Eccles, M. P., Grimshaw, J. M., & Woolf, S. H. (2001). Validity of the Agency for Healthcare Research and Quality clinical practice guidelines: How quickly do guidelines become outdated? *JAMA, 286*(12), 1461–1467. https://doi.org/10.1001/jama.286.12.1461

Shojania, K. G., Sampson, M., Ansari, M. T., Ji, J., Doucette, S., & Moher, D. (2007). How quickly do systematic reviews go out of date? A survival analysis. *Annals of Internal Medicine, 147*(4), 224–233. https://doi.org/10.7326/0003-4819-147-4-200708210-00179

Shulman, L. S. (1998). Theory, practice, and the education of professionals. *The Elementary School Journal, 98*(5), 511–526.

Tesseyman, S., Peterson, K., & Beaumont, E. (2022). The nurse apprentice and fundamental bedside care: An historical perspective. *Nursing Inquiry*, e12540. https://doi.org/:10.1111/nin.12540.

The Joint Commission. (2023). Who We Are. Retrieved January 5, 2023, from https://www.jointcommission.org/who-we-are/

Yang, S. Y. (2022). Impact of the COVID-19 pandemic on neonatal nursing practicum and extended reality simulation training needs: A descriptive and cross-sectional study. *International Journal of Environmental Research and Public Health*, *20*(1), 344. https://doi.org/10.3390/ijerph20010344

3

The Science of Learning

Joanne Noone, PhD, RN, CNE, FAAN, ANEF

CHAPTER OVERVIEW

This chapter summarizes current thought on how people learn, especially focusing on long-term retention and the importance of lifelong learning, and facilitating students to become self-directed learners in a professional practice discipline. Topics covered include scaffolding; social, emotional, and physical influences on learning; contextualized learning; and practices that facilitate integration and connection with prior learning and across concepts. These include reflection, information retrieval, interleaving, and explanation. The concept of testing as learning will be reviewed. Important resources for further exploration of the science of learning will be described.

WHAT IS LEARNING?

As educators, we are concerned about learning in the discipline of nursing. However, learning is essentially a biological process necessary for survival (Madrazo & Motz, 2005). We are learning all the time and throughout our lives. According to Ambrose and colleagues learning is "a *process* that leads to *change*, which occurs as a result of *experience* and increases the potential for improved performance and future learning...Learning involves change in knowledge, beliefs, behaviors, or attitudes" (Ambrose et al., 2010, p. 3). Physical changes occur in the brain because of learning. The aim of teaching is to facilitate learning by making and enhancing connections in the brain and to improve the transfer of knowledge to real-life situations. Learning requires memory and the ability to access that memory when needed (Brown et al., 2014). It is critical that nurse educators have a good working knowledge of learning science to facilitate learning that can endure and grow over a lifetime of practice. When we consider what nurses and others in a practice-based discipline need to know and remember, we think of a multitude of metacognitive skills needed to master the knowledge and skills of the discipline, readily retrieve information from memory when needed, make connections, and transfer knowledge to apply from one situation to another. Additionally, our learners must be self-directed to continue learning over a lifetime of practice.

Learning is thought to occur in three phases: encoding, storage, and retrieval. Learning and memory formation result from neuronal changes in the brain and the connections that occur among these neurons is called synaptic plasticity, which results in encoding of short-term memory (Owens & Tanner, 2017). Effortful learning facilitates encoding of memories and is discussed later in the section about the concepts of desirable versus undesirable difficulties in learning. Storage occurs during consolidation of memories. Consolidation of memories required for learning takes time and effort to strengthen neuronal networks that create long-term memory retention. Sleep is essential to consolidation and storage of memory (National Academies of Sciences, Engineering, and Medicine [NASEM], 2018). Retrieval is the process of moving long-term memories back into accessible short-term memory to use information. Retrieval is also an important process during learning since neuronal connections are strengthened during this process. Throughout this chapter, we will look at influences that facilitate or impair these different phases so we as educators can choose techniques and practices that best support effective long-term learning.

IMPORTANT CHARACTERISTICS FOR LIFELONG LEARNING

Nurse educators have long focused on lifelong learning as a key attribute of nursing education programs. There are teaching and learning principles that promote lifelong learning. In several of these strategies, learners can engage individually in their study habits and educators can also promote these strategies in their teaching practices to enhance lifelong learning.

Lifelong learners, especially in a practice discipline such as nursing, need to be able to retrieve information when needed. Students need to develop strategies that promote long-term learning and memory retention to enhance this characteristic. Peter Brown et al. (2014) identified certain study habits and teaching methods that primarily tend to facilitate short-term learning. Rereading and highlighting texts and cramming for tests are strategies that learners typically use because they are effective for short-term learning as strategies used to prepare for the next test. However, they are less useful for long-term memory retention. We will review methods and examples of information retrieval and spaced practice and other methods that tend to strengthen neural pathways to enhance further encoding and facilitate long-term learning. Frequent self-quizzing and testing built into courses, both no-stakes and low-stakes, can facilitate information retrieval (Agarwal & Bain, 2019). Lifelong learners also need to be able to transfer and apply knowledge to new settings and situations and make connections between like concepts and patterns. Teaching strategies, such as concept maps and concept-based clinical learning activities (see Chapter 11, *Concept-Based Learning in the Clinical Learning Environment*), which promote identifying patterns and making connections, can strengthen neural pathways.

To facilitate lifelong learning, learners also need to think about their own learning and how they learn, a process called metacognition. Becoming a self-directed learner includes establishing learning goals based on an awareness of what they know and don't know. Encouraging self-testing through the use of flashcards is a strategy that can help learners assess themselves and gain insight into what they know and identify their gaps in knowledge. Strategies that educators can use include in-class low-stakes testing and providing feedback indicating incorrect and correct responses on exams (Agarwal & Bain, 2019). We will look later at how methods that promote student processing of how they performed on an exam can assist learners to become aware of their own strengths and weaknesses, and help them identify gaps in learning to guide subsequent study

(Ambrose et al., 2010). These methods incorporate reflection, which is a method that learners can use, especially when structured to understand what they currently know, what they want to know, and what they want to remember about the topic under discussion.

SCAFFOLDING

Scaffolding is an instructional concept in which structure and support are intentionally provided to promote learning (Ambrose et al., 2010). Scaffolding can be especially useful to students entering a nursing program who may be unfamiliar with the ideas, information, and tacit knowledge of the discipline. Scaffolding can lower students' feeling overwhelmed or anxious, which may inhibit learning (Eyler, 2018). This is also recommended for students reentering an academic learning environment who may need refresher skills in areas such as literature searching and academic writing. Sakraida (2020) describes a scaffolded approach for reentering RN to BSN students focusing on developing library search and technical writing skills to facilitate research appraisal. In this example, modules on library searching and research appraisal prepare the learner for more complex research writing activities. Such support then diminishes as students progress, become more independent learners, and develop a knowledge base in the discipline. Coombs (2018) recommends purposefully designing scaffolding in the program of study using a backward design approach to facilitate student motivation and confidence. We discuss this process in Chapter 7, *Backward Design: Aligning Outcomes, Assessments, and Activities*.

Strategies recommended that illustrate scaffolding include breaking down assignments into smaller units that build upon one another and into a final summative assessment (Coombs, 2018) or that build from one course into another. This is especially useful when considering a large summative project, such as a capstone or clinical inquiry project. Peer and faculty feedback during these building block phases provides learner support as they revise and refine their learning. Peer feedback can also be helpful learning to the peer reviewer as they begin to see a range of examples of learning that may enhance their own learning. Modeling is another strategy that may be a helpful support early in learning by providing expert examples of an assessment or role modeling a behavior or skill by an expert, such as in a video exemplar or simulation. Faculty role modeling of professional behaviors or how to use a tool can provide helpful support (Sanders & Welk, 2005). Coram (2016) demonstrated improved clinical judgment scores in novice nursing students who watched a video of an expert nurse role modeling care. Scaffolding supports student success and socialization into the profession or specialty and aids in development of clinical judgment, skills, and clinical reasoning (Buterakos & Keiser, 2021; Herrington & Schneidereith, 2017; Holland, 2020).

SOCIAL AND EMOTIONAL INFLUENCES ON LEARNING

Lev Vygotsky's Sociocultural Learning Theory (Vygotsky, 1978) provides guidance in assisting educators to support effective education. This theory proposes that social interactions lead to learning and cognitive development through faculty guidance and collaboration with other learners. Vygotsky describes a "zone of proximal development" which is the gap or distance between the learner's current knowledge and ability to their potential capability to achieve the desired new learning. Setting our teaching goals for learners above their current ability is necessary to achieve new learning. If that gap is too wide or there are too many barriers for learners to navigate the distance success- fully, learning can be compromised. As educators, we can think about this zone of proxi- mal development and how we as faculty can assist learners to achieve their learning potential through an understanding of our learners' current knowledge, and considering social and emotional influences on learning.

Learning is a social process involving human interactions. Learners bring the influ- ence of their past and current social relationships into the current learning environment, through values, attitudes, and cultural influence. Learning can occur through modeling behaviors and adopting attitudes by observing others. Immordino-Yang and Damasio (2007) term emotional thought "the platform for learning" as it is a basic neurophysi- ological process necessary for survival in telling our brains what to pay attention to and remember. "Quite literally, it is neurobiologically impossible to think deeply about or remember information about which one has had no emotion because the healthy brain does not waste energy processing information that does not matter to the individual" (NASEM, 2018, p. 29). Positive emotions, such as motivation and a sense of belonging, can facilitate attention, memory, and learning. Negative emotions, such as higher levels of anxiety, or feeling isolated, impair memory and learning. Educators can consider the social and emotional influences of learning as they construct the nature of the learning environment, role model expected classroom and professional behaviors, support moti- vation and a sense of belonging in all learners, and attend to the expected challenges in learning goals for learners to achieve.

Stress

Stress can have positive and negative influences on learning. Low levels of stress, espe- cially if associated with emotions, can enhance the encoding of memories related to attending to the emotionally linked content but may impair encoding of material unre- lated to the emotion that may be ignored by the brain. For example, a learner is in a simulation caring for a client with a cardiovascular illness and is implementing motiva- tional interviewing (MI) techniques to assist the client with lifestyle changes. The client responds positively to the MI intervention and the learner is excited about how well the experience turned out. This learning about MI techniques, because of its association with emotion, may be more clearly encoded for this learner than other aspects of the simulation. Conversely, higher levels of stress and anxiety can impair learning since, as we recall from the fight or flight stress response, blood is shunted from the brain to our muscles to fight or flee. Thus, concentration can be decreased, impacting memory, in high stress situations. High stress around the time of memory retrieval, such as during examinations, can decrease retrieval or remembering of information (Vogel & Schwabe, 2016). It is wise to consider how to decrease negative emotions, such as fear, that may inhibit learning. Bjork coined the term "desirable difficulties," or creating challenges in the academic environment that enhance memory and information retrieval. Desirable difficulties are challenges that strengthen learning and can be overcome with learner effort. Examples of desirable difficulties we will look at later in this chapter include information retrieval, spaced practice, and interleaving. Bjork and Bjork (2014) also recommend reducing "undesirable difficulties," those that may interfere with learning unnecessarily. For example, an undesirable difficulty exists when learners do not have the necessary foundational skills for current learning goals, if the learning activity does not contribute to the knowledge needed to achieve the learning outcomes, or if the learning activity activates a high stress response.

Trauma-informed teaching practices, discussed in Chapter 5, *Creating Inclusive Learning Environments,* may facilitate creating a supportive learning environment. Another growing body of literature in nursing education to support nursing student well-being is focused on mindfulness interventions to decrease stress and anxiety and to promote resilience and healthy adaptive coping strategies. A recent meta-analysis of ten studies of mindfulness interventions in nursing education indicated they were effective in reducing stress, anxiety, and depression in nursing students (Chen et al., 2021). Such interventions may be of assistance in supporting student success during stressful periods of the curriculum such as during testing and simulation and may also assist in developing resilience and positive coping strategies early on in one's professional life (Hughes et al., 2021; Wheeler et al., 2021).

Mindset

An important concept to consider regarding social and emotional influences on learning is the learner's view of their own intelligence and how educators can enhance or support learner success and resilience. This concept has been initially developed and studied by Dweck et al. (2014), who identified the characteristics of a fixed mindset compared to a growth mindset. Those with a fixed mindset view their intelligence as static or a limited quantity while those with a growth mindset believe their intelligence to be malleable with hard work and effort. People with a fixed mindset tend to focus on proving their intelligence and avoid failure while a growth mindset is associated with resilience and viewing setbacks or failures as opportunities to learn. A growth mindset is associated with greater academic performance. Williams (2021), in a survey of 151 nursing students, identified that students with a growth mindset were more likely to use more effective learning strategies, such as peer teaching and quizzing, spaced studying rather than cramming, and use of flashcards, than those displaying a fixed mindset. Dweck et al. (2014, p. 6) describe the rationale behind this in that those "with a growth mindset earned higher grades because they valued learning more than looking smart…and tended to perceive academic setbacks as a call to increase their effort or to try new strategies. Students with a fixed mindset, on the other hand, were less likely to welcome challenges that could reveal shortcomings."

Faculty who view their students as having a fixed mindset negatively influence students' academic performance and experience. This is especially important to consider in students who have been historically underrepresented in nursing and may be experiencing stereotype threat, or what happens when people live out the negative stereotypes associated with their group. We will talk more about stereotype threat in Chapter 5, *Creating Inclusive Learning Environments.* Canning and co-authors (2019) conducted a recent longitudinal, seven-term study in one university setting of 150 science, technology, engineering, and mathematics faculty to determine the faculty's mindset and the influence of that mindset on 15,466 students' achievement and experience. The faculty's belief in a fixed mindset predicted poorer performance by students, especially for underrepresented minority students. Students in a faculty's class who endorsed a fixed mindset were less likely to report they did their best work in the course and were less likely to recommend the course to others, as compared to students who experienced a class in which the faculty facilitated beliefs in a growth mindset.

The good news is that simple interventions have been found to facilitate student adoption of a growth mindset and academic success, especially for those students who may be underperforming or at risk for stereotype threat. In a national study of 6,320 ninth-graders who were identified as low-achieving (Yeager et al., 2019), participants were randomized into an intervention or control group; the intervention group received a one-hour online module that shared information and stories about growth mindset and that intelligence increases with learning. Students who received the intervention outperformed the control group in core classes at the end of ninth grade. Lewis and colleagues (Lewis et al., 2020) in a study of 35 prelicensure nursing students, implemented a one-hour growth mindset intervention, exploring attributes of a fixed versus growth mindset, the neuroplasticity of the brain, and behaviors exhibited by growth mindset students. After the intervention, more students demonstrated growth mindset characteristics on assessment and were less likely to use less effective study strategies, such as re-reading the text and memorization.

Belonging

Faculty, in creating a sense of belonging and a caring environment, can impact student success. This is especially true for students historically underrepresented in nursing who may be more at risk for feeling isolated or that they do not belong either in college or in nursing. These negative stereotypes may impede student success by creating a cycle of isolation and self-beliefs that may impair performance and pose risks to student retention (Yeager & Walton, 2011). A scoping review of thirty studies addressing inclusivity within baccalaureate education (Metzger et al., 2020) summarized the results demonstrating that underrepresented students' experience of discrimination in all aspects of the learning community within nursing education can contribute to social isolation and a lack of belonging. In studies where a sense of belonging was facilitated, this "led to engagement, motivation, less stress in clinical setting, and confidence which increased chances of success and influenced future career decisions" (Metzger et al., 2020, p. 11).

It is important to address interventions at all levels of the learning experience, including at the campus and program level, and to align inclusivity initiatives with faculty actions so that students' experiences of belongingness are congruent with these initiatives. Additionally, brief interventions by faculty have also been helpful to impart a sense of belonging and may be especially powerful for underrepresented students. Walton and Cohen (2011) established the effectiveness of a brief intervention aimed at Black and white college freshmen that framed social adversity as common and transient as students enter college and not necessarily linked to one's social identity. The intervention consisted of reading more senior students' experiences that the lack of belonging diminished and confidence increased with time over the first year of college. This was then reinforced by participants in the intervention group writing about how their own experiences were similar to the readings. At three-year follow-up, Black students in the intervention group had higher GPAs and less uncertainty about their belonging than Black students in the control group, who received a one-hour intervention unrelated to belonging. The authors posit that similar findings were not seen in the white students because lack of belonging is not as high a threat for such students in a college setting. Yeager and Walton (2011) believe such interventions can complement and support more formal educational initiatives. Faculty warmth and simple techniques such as knowing students' names can contribute to a sense of belonging (Metzger et al., 2020, p. 11). Lang (2021) also recommends normalizing help-seeking behaviors. Gurung and Galardi (2022) evaluated syllabus tone (warm vs cold) and inclusion of a "Reach Out" statement regarding mental health in a syllabus and found that both a warm tone and inclusion of a statement facilitated students' intentions to seek help from the instructor. Interestingly, the warm-toned syllabus received greater endorsements from students to seek help than the statement promoting help-seeking from the instructor. According to the authors,

> The warm-toned syllabi differed from the cold-toned syllabi by providing a rationale for assignments, using positive or friendly language, sharing personal experiences, using humor, showing enthusiasm for the course, and conveying compassion (p. 3).

Motivation and Self-Efficacy

Nurse educators have the benefit of usually working with learners who are intrinsically motivated to achieve a career goal. There are several strategies that nurse educators can use to facilitate motivation, or persistence toward a goal, and related factors that influence motivation, such as interest, positive emotions, and self-efficacy. Learners' goals for learning, their beliefs in the value of learning, and their perceived self-efficacy in achieving outcomes all influence motivation as does their perception of a supportive learning environment (Ambrose et al., 2010). Attending to motivation is one of Ambrose and colleagues' seven key principles of smart teaching. "Students' motivation determines, directs, and sustains what they do to learn...When students find positive value in a learning goal or activity, expect to successfully achieve a desired learning outcome, and perceive support from their environment, they are likely to be strongly motivated to learn" (Ambrose et al., 2010, p. 5).

Attending to motivation can facilitate student engagement in learning. While learners may be motivated and value their end goal of completing their program of study and achieving their career goal, they may have difficulty seeing the value in course assignments and how these facilitate progress toward this overall goal. Nurse educators can assist in this process by making this link explicit in how the course activities assist in meeting these goals. They can select learning activities that connect with students' interests and also align with achieving course and program goals. For example, if a writing assignment is a specific assessment and activity within a course, allowing flexibility in the topic and student choice can facilitate students' interest and perceived value in the activity. "Flexibility lends a sense of control, which can contribute to a student's expectation of success" (Ambrose et al., 2010, p. 89). Providing authentic learning activities that represent what nurses need to be able to know and do can facilitate student engagement and motivation. Examples include developing academic-practice partnerships that could include service learning opportunities or evidenced-based practice partnerships (Noone, 2022). Lastly, incorporate a reflection activity that is structured toward facilitating motivation and expectations for future success. Brookfield (2017) recommends a learning audit in which students summarize their learning to aid them to see the value in their learning. Sample questions can be found in Table 3.1.

TABLE 3.1	
Questions and Prompts to Facilitate Motivation	
Questions and Prompt Focus	**Examples**
Learning Audit (Brookfield, 2017)	Regarding the topic, subject or course: What do you know about that you didn't know at the beginning of the term? What can you do that you couldn't do at the beginning of the term? What can you tell or demonstrate to someone that you couldn't at the beginning of the term?
Questions to facilitate students' identification of the value in their learning	Describe the most important clinical lesson you learned today that you want to remember for the future. Identify three actions you will do differently in future situation when you encounter a similar patient or completing a similar project.

To support learners' self-efficacy, educators can consider setting achievable desirable difficulties to facilitate learners' expectancies so that they can be successful in achieving course goals. Understanding learners' prerequisite knowledge, developing challenging yet achievable learning goals, providing practice opportunities to assist learners to develop mastery, and scaffolding learning to support success can all contribute to assisting learner self-efficacy so that goal achievement is possible. Lang (2021) and Ambrose et al. (2010) recommend sharing stories and one's passion for the profession which can engage students' curiosity and promote positive emotions towards learning. Sharing clinical stories can engage learners and connect them with authentic experiences. Communicating one's enthusiasm for the profession can ignite student curiosity and interest.

PHYSICAL INFLUENCES ON LEARNING

Just as social and emotional contexts influence learning, physical influences can impact learning as well. "A student whose basic needs—food, drink, sleep, shelter—are not met cannot learn as effectively as they might if these needs were fulfilled. Another way to think about this: A hungry brain cannot learn. A tired brain cannot think" (Eyler, 2018, p. 216). We will briefly consider factors that influence learning in nursing education; sleep, nutrition, and basic safety and security needs. Lack of sleep and proper nutrition can affect concentration and memory. Experiencing basic needs insecurity can trigger stress and anxiety that can impair learning (Silva et al., 2017).

The #RealCollege Survey (The Hope Center for College, Community, & Justice, 2021) is an annual survey of college student needs, surveying students from two-year and four-year colleges and universities. Their latest survey, from the Fall of 2020, collected information from over 195,000 college students in 42 states. Three in five students report experiencing basic needs insecurity, with 39 percent of students at two-year institutions reporting food insecurity compared to 29 percent of students at four-year institutions. Housing insecurity affected almost half of respondents (48 percent) with homelessness affecting

14 percent. Disparities exist for students of color with 75 percent of Indigenous students and 70 percent of Black and American Indian/Alaska Native students reporting basic security needs not being met compared to 54 percent of White students. Disparities also existed for first-generation students and those identifying as LGBTQ.

Students who report food or housing insecurity are at greater academic risk. Multiple studies have shown these risks to be associated with lower academic performance including lower GPAs and more failures (Maroto et al., 2015; Silva et al., 2017). Students with food and housing insecurity report more difficulty attending classes and having to choose between paying for food and housing over tuition and books.

Sleep deprivation has been reported in prelicensure and graduate nursing students especially as students balance work and personal life events, such as family caregiving, with the demands of school. Sleep deprivation can impair cognition that can affect learning and is also a patient safety issue that is compounded by novice or beginning learners (Thomas et al., 2017). Goldin (2017) in a study of 123 advanced practice nursing students, identified that GPA was negatively associated with employment and daytime sleepiness of students. Some strategies that may be used to support students' physical health can be found in Table 3.2.

TABLE 3.2

Strategies to Promote Physical Health

Strategy	Example and Rationale
Work with community agencies and student support services to provide links to resources for basic needs.	▸ Single Stop USA is an agency that connects students at participating community colleges to resources and benefits. A recent analysis of the effectiveness of this support demonstrated improved academic performance in student users of Single Stop (Daugherty et al., 2020).
Consider adoption of open access resources.	▸ While such resources can save students money and reduce overall debt, use of these resources have been associated with improved grades and academic success, especially for students of color (Colvard et al., 2018).
Consider safety issues in educational experiences for students.	▸ Maneval and Kurz (2016) recommend developing safety policies for students in community clinical setting. ▸ Thoughtfully consider night shift clinical experiences and their effect on student learning. Night shift rotations may be unavoidable to optimize clinical placements especially as students near program completion. However, such clinical experiences earlier in a program of study may interfere with critical learning due to sleep deprivation. Night-shift clinical experiences should be evaluated to examine if they align with meeting the desired student learning outcomes (Palese et al., 2017).
Integrate nurse well-being as a key part of student learning outcomes.	▸ This has been a recent recommendation of the 2020–2030 Future of Nursing Report (National Academies of Sciences, Engineering, & Medicine [NASEM], 2021) to combat physical and emotional health stressors that influence nurses' well-being. ▸ Developing a lifetime of healthy coping habits during these formative years can carry over to sustain graduates throughout their professional career.

CONTEXTUALIZED LEARNING

As noted earlier, learning is experiential and the more we can engage students in authentic learning experiences that resemble what nurses need to know and be able to do, the richer that learning becomes. This is more fully discussed in Chapter 8, *Strategies for Active and Authentic Learning*. Contextualized learning links knowledge within situations where learning can be applied to meaningful practice experiences. Nurse educators do a wonderful job of creating rich clinical learning experiences, including simulation, to promote authentic learning. Classroom learning can also be contextualized to replicate authentic practice and enhance learning through active learning strategies that promote engagement with clinical practice and lessen the practice-education, or theory-practice, gap that is discussed in Chapter 2, *Teaching in a Practice-Based Profession*. Active learning strategies are associated with improved student academic performance in multiple studies. Theobald et al. (2020) completed a systematic review of the impact active learning had on examination scores and failure rates. The systematic review explored 15 studies that studied exam scores including 9,238 students, and 26 studies that examined failure rates for 44,606 students in STEM majors. In comparing active learning to traditional lecturing, active learning reduced achievement gaps for minoritized students in examination scores by 33 percent and in passing rates by 45 percent.

Eyler (2018) posits these findings are related to the brain's increased focus and attention to what is perceived as relevant. The learner's brain perceives and attends to the relevance of active, experiential learning that is contextualized to actual practice (Eyler, 2018). It is also posited that active learning strategies use higher-order thinking skills in order to integrate new learning. Active learning strategies can influence other facilitators of learning previously discussed such as motivation and self-efficacy. Carstensen et al. (2020) implemented an active learning strategy that consisted of pre-class study questions, in-class polling, and collaborative learning with peer instruction for concepts students had difficulty with. Exam scores and student satisfaction improved with this implementation. Service learning and academic-practice partnerships are two suggested clinical learning strategies to more authentically replicate real-world learning experiences to narrow the theory-practice gap.

CONNECTION AND INTEGRATION

Nursing is a vast discipline with endless interconnections among patient experiences, physiological processes, and interventions. In this section, we will review the numerous strategies to enhance the connection between concepts and how to integrate new learning with prior learning. Methods to enhance coding into long-term retention through practice and retrieval can enhance the learning required for a practice discipline by requiring students to access memory to retrieve information.

Activating Prior Learning

Ambrose et al. (2010, p. 11) state, "Students learn more readily when they can connect new learning to what they already know." According to Brown et al. (2014, p. 73),

"Prior learning is a prerequisite for making sense of new learning, and forming those connections is an important task of consolidation," which is the strengthening process that helps to create long-term memory. It is important for the educator to understand that learners may not be able to effectively activate prior knowledge without assistance. Additionally, to build upon this knowledge, it is helpful for both the teacher and learner to identify if prior learning is sufficient preparation for the anticipated new learning and to identify misperceptions or gaps in knowledge. Ambrose et al. (2010) recommend that faculty explicitly describe the necessary prior knowledge either from the current course or previous courses and activate this learning through preassessments such as testing, reflection, or concept mapping. Pretests of prerequisite knowledge can occur through various means, such as completion of worksheets or web-based questions. Aggregate assessments can be evaluated prior to class. In that way, the faculty can evaluate results and focus on clarifying gaps in knowledge.

Concept maps, which are visual representations that learners draw either by hand or electronically to depict their understanding of the relationships of concepts of a topic, can be used for multiple purposes (Ambrose et al., 2010; Lang, 2021). Learners are usually asked to diagrammatically identify concepts in circles and then identify relationships by connecting the circles with lines. Similarly, reflective writing can activate prior learning through directed questions (Brown et al., 2014). Aids, such as concept maps or reflective writing, facilitate the retrieval of prior learning from memory, having it available for current learning.

Explanation

Providing intentional opportunities to facilitate student explanation can assist with connecting and integrating new learning. This can occur through self-explanation or explaining to others. Multiple methods can be used to encourage explanation including reflective writing, think-aloud strategies, and through teaching others, either teaching clients or peers. Such methods deepen learning by strengthening memory through recall and clarifying concepts as learners construct explanations into their own words or self-clarify concepts to explain to others (Lang, 2021).

Providing opportunities for oral or written self-explanation can occur in the classroom as well as in clinical situations. Written reflections to facilitate understanding can occur anytime throughout a class setting. Smith (2021) surveyed nursing students and faculty regarding the use of a guided reflection tool in the clinical setting that was based on facilitating clinical reasoning and judgment. Students perceived the benefit of reflection in assisting them to make sense and connections across patient care situations. Such written reflections were helpful for faculty to understand, clarify, and correct students' thinking processes.

"Think-aloud" (TA) strategies, particularly in simulated or laboratory learning environments, can promote student self-explanation and provide meaningful data to educators about student thinking processes. TA is a teaching strategy in which learners verbalize their thoughts. Students using TA strategies in a physical assessment class reported higher self-efficacy scores and had higher grades on physical assessment skills compared to learners not using TA (Verkuy et al., 2018). Learners reported benefits in being more prepared and aware of their knowledge gaps. Additionally, they reported more confidence in transferring these skills to actual patient care settings.

Peer teaching can deepen learning. In a study of peer instruction in undergraduate students, Fiorella and Mayer (2013) divided participants into three groups: a control group, a second group who were asked to prepare to teach about a topic but did not provide the actual instruction (called teaching expectancy), and a third group who both prepared and carried out the instruction. While both intervention groups had improved knowledge of the subject, the third group who actually carried out the teaching had the most persistent gains in knowledge. These findings of the benefits of teaching expectancy on knowledge with stronger benefits on learning with actual teaching were further supported by a meta-analysis of 28 studies on the topic (Kobayashi, 2019).

Practice

Facilitating practice opportunities to recall information and connect and integrate this information with new knowledge can promote learning. Memory is strengthened, in addition to the ability to recall information when needed and transfer this information to new situations, all vital skills for healthcare practitioners. Such practice opportunities can be beneficial for both developing knowledge and skills practice. We start off by defining some terms and looking at the science associated with recommended practice strategies. Examples from the literature and recommendations for implementation are provided below and in Table 3.3.

TABLE 3.3	
Strategies for Connections and Integration	
Strategy	**Description**
Activate Prior Learning	
Pretests of prerequisite knowledge can occur through various means, such as completion of worksheets or web-based or in-class pretest questions.	For a unit of instruction on cardiac disorders for undergraduate students, the prerequisite knowledge includes key understanding of cardiac anatomy, physiology, and cardiac assessment techniques. The faculty creates a preassessment worksheet to complete on these concepts prior to class and opens the session with a few polling questions. Aggregate assessment indicates good understanding of cardiac anatomy and assessment techniques, but the instructor determines there is a gap in understanding concepts of preload and afterload so the educator provides some clarification of these concepts prior to introducing new learning.
Activities to generate recall of prior learning with concept maps or reflective writing	➤ Learners can be asked to complete a concept map, either individually or in a group, of what they recall about a topic. ➤ Use reflective writing, such as asking students to recall what they remember about a topic or what they learned from a previous class

TABLE 3.3

Strategies for Connections and Integration *(Continued)*

Strategy	Description
Explanation	
Self-explanation through oral and written reflection and think-aloud (TA) strategies	➤ Pose a question that requires students to write an explanation of a concept, how concepts interrelate, or how they are similar or different from each other.
	➤ Encourage learners to first answer from recall without using resources as that helps to encourage memory retrieval and to uncover faulty thinking.
	➤ Use TA strategies; ask learners to verbalize their thoughts as they complete an assigned task, assessment, or intervention
	➤ TA can also happen retrospectively during debriefing sessions to encourage learners to explain their thinking processes during certain parts of the simulation or task completion.
Teaching others—peer teaching	A peer instruction technique developed by Eric Mazur (Schell & Butler, 2018) uses a combination of classroom polling of discussion or test questions, first completed individually, and then describes using peer teaching to facilitate learning. This technique encourages grouping of students who have different answers to discuss and come to a new, shared understanding.
Practice	
Retrieval practice	➤ Multiple strategies can be used to facilitate retrieval: polling questions, reflection, verbalization, and simulation-based mastery practice.
	➤ Frequent testing is therefore recommended, with these assessments being formative and either low stakes or no stakes.
	➤ Provide feedback with rationale on correct and incorrect answers for all assessment enhances learning.
	➤ Cumulative exams, versus discrete unit exams, are recommended as they facilitate retrieval practice of information over a longer period and encourage learners to make connections between concepts.
Spaced practice	➤ More frequent testing in a course spaces out learning through assessment rather than cramming for a midterm or final.
	➤ Avoid mass practice "front-loading" of skills.
Interleaving	➤ Mixing up learning works particularly well with math problems and skills development (Shellenbarger & Robb, 2021).
	➤ It is also very appropriate to provide some focused blocked practice opportunities especially when students are learning a new skill (Lang, 2021). Learners may not be ready to focus on understanding more complex nuances of concepts or skills when they are new to a subject or concept.
	➤ As students progress in a course or program, however, mixing of interleaving and block practice will facilitate long-term learning.

> Retrieval practice: "Retrieval practice is the act of calling information to mind that has previously been encoded or learned rather than rereading or rehearing it" (Martinelli et al., 2019, p. 914). This is also referred to as the "testing effect" or "test-enhanced learning." Multiple studies demonstrate the effectiveness of this strategy in long-term memory retention as compared to more passive strategies, such as rereading and highlighting texts (Green et al., 2018). According to Brown et al. (2014, pp. 28–29), "Repeated recall appears to help memory consolidate into a cohesive representation in the brain and to strengthen and multiply the neural routes by which the knowledge can later be retrieved." These neural pathways are strengthened by the movement of information back and forth from long-term to short-term memory. Testing, whether by written or practical examinations, is considered a learning opportunity rather than solely an assessment of learning. Brown et al. (2014) recommend that the type of retrieval practice designed match how that knowledge will be used later. Consequently, providing opportunities for retrieval practice for performing psychomotor skills will be most effective prior to a practice assessment. Since this strategy of retrieval is more effective than more passive study habits, such as reading and highlighting the text, sharing this information with learners and encouraging more active study habits (such as recall from flash cards) is recommended.

> Spaced practice versus massed practice. Spacing, or distributed, learning and retrieval of information over time facilitates learning and academic performance compared to mass practice and this has implications for how learners study and how educators schedule learning and assessment activities. Spaced learning and practice allow some forgetting, which is actually beneficial as it helps memory formation. Allowing time between learning helps to consolidate learning that occurs during sleep. More frequent quizzing has also been reported to reduce student anxiety (Brown et al., 2014). This also has implications for supporting students' study habits to avoid cramming as a primary study method and encouraging spaced retrieval practice. Cramming and massed practice may help with short-term memory and performing well on an examination given in the near future but long-term retention with this practice declines over time in comparison to spaced practice (Agarwal & Bain, 2019). Learners may tend to see the benefit of cramming based on their narrowed focus on their performance on a particular examination. Therefore, they may need assistance in evaluating the evidence related to successful study habits in order to adopt them. Educators can model this through spaced vs. massed skills practice and testing.

> Interleaving. Interleaving is the instructional strategy of mixing up retrieval practice and learning at least two or more concepts, skills, etc., as compared to blocked practice or focusing on one area or task for learning (Brown et al., 2014; Lang, 2021). While this may appear to the learner as more effortful, performance in learning improves, it is thought, because the learner encodes and retrieves a more complex understanding of the similarities and differences of concepts being discussed. In addition, each time the learner returns to retrieve previously learned material, memory is strengthened. Interleaving also more realistically represents authentic clinical practices as nurses commonly are dealing with multiple tasks, assessments, client presentations, etc., at the same time. This facilitates integration

of learning and transfer to new settings and contacts. Focusing on blocked practice, or one area for learning, cues the learner and narrows the possibilities of options to consider. Intentional planning of blocked and interleaved learning activity is recommended to best support initial learning and retrieval of information to transfer to new settings (Lang, 2021). Similar to other retrieval strategies, blocked practice may be more effortless and preferred by the learner. Supporting learners to understand that more effortful learning is linked to more available and more long-term retention is recommended.

TESTING AS LEARNING

We have reviewed throughout this chapter that testing has multiple benefits in addition to summative assessment used to evaluate competency. Low-stakes or no-stakes quizzing can promote information retrieval, connect prior learning to new topics, and identify gaps in understanding. In this section, we look at the benefits to learners in reviewing tests and explore methods that structure self-understanding of one's own thinking processes, known as metacognition. Facilitating students' understanding of how they learn and study involves their assessment of their strengths and weakness, as well as reflecting on what strategies are most effective. Faculty can provide feedback about students' future study and test-taking plans and connect them with available resources to help them improve. Exam wrappers are an example of a strategy to review how students prepared for and completed a test and are structured short activities that learners can complete after each exam. This tool has demonstrated improvement in student metacognitive abilities, test performance, and study habits, such as a reduction in cramming (Sethares & Asselin, 2022). Ambrose et al. (2010) recommend having students complete this activity immediately after the test. Faculty can then review individual and aggregate results and provide feedback prior to the next exam. A structured class discussion can focus on sharing strategies and highlighting best practice study habits as well as less helpful ones. Box 3.1 provides a sample exam wrapper.

CHAPTER SUMMARY

Understanding how learning occurs as well as key positive and negative influences of learning are critical in the intentional design of a course structure and learning activities. Long-term memory retention and the ability to retrieve that knowledge over a career when needed are crucial in a practice discipline that depends on lifelong learning. Learning is the brain changing through the construction of neural connections that result in memory formation during the processes of encoding, storage, and retrieval. For nursing education, the aim of teaching is to create the best environment for those brain changes to occur to facilitate the transfer of this learning to authentic nursing practice situations. Integration of new learning and connection with prior learning occurs during consolidation of memories during the storage phase and occurs over time since consolidation is facilitated by sleep. Long-term memory retention is strengthened by facilitating the retrieval of knowledge. These have implications for structuring study

BOX 3.1

Sample Exam Wrapper

Name: _____

This activity is designed to give you a chance to reflect on your exam performance and, more importantly, on the effectiveness of your exam preparation. Please answer the questions sincerely. Your responses will be collected by your teacher to plan and discuss various pre-exam strategies to best support your learning. We will hand back the sheet in advance of your next exam to inform and guide your preparation for that exam.

Part One:

1. Approximately how much effort did you spend preparing for this exam?

    1   2   3   4   5   6

  Low effort   Moderate   High Effort

2. Approximately how much time did you spend preparing for this exam? _____
3. When did you start studying for this exam (in days)? _____
4. Did you study individually or in a group? _____
5. Approximately how many hours/days before the exam did you stop studying? _____

Part Two:

1. What percentage of your test preparation time was spent in each of these activities (make sure the percentages add up to 100 percent)?
   a. Reading the textbook the first time _____
   b. Rereading the textbook _____
   c. Reading the lecture slides the first time _____
   d. Rereading the lecture slides the first time _____
   e. Reading your notes from the class _____
   f. Other practice (flashcards, etc.) _____
      i. Please list: _____
   g. Other? _____
      i. Please list: _____
2. Now that you have looked over your graded exam, estimate the percentage of points you lost due to each of the following:
   a. I did not know content or concepts _____
   b. I changed my answer _____
   c. I misread the question _____
   d. I did not understand words in the question or answer _____
   e. I had difficulty choosing between two answers _____
   f. I ran out of time _____
   g. I marked the answer incorrectly _____
   h. I read too much into the question
      i. Other? _____
         i. Please list: _____

Part Three:

1. Based on your findings above, what three things can **you** do differently in preparing for the next exam?
   a. _____ b. _____ c. _____
2. What three things can **we** do to support your learning and improve your test performance?
   a. _____ b. _____ c. _____

practices and learning. The specific practices of retrieval practice, spaced practice, and interleaving are all recommended strategies to facilitate learning.

All aspects of the learning environment contribute to learning, including campus climate that facilitates belonging and faculty beliefs about their students and learning, such as beliefs in a growth mindset. There are social, emotional, and physical influences on learning, and connecting students to additional resources to support them can enhance student success. Additionally, faculty should consider all elements of a course to contribute to learning, such as testing, and structure opportunities to capture learning at every opportunity. Some recommended resources for further learning about learning science can be found in Box 3.2.

BOX 3.2

Recommended Resources about Learning Science

Some references that have guided the development of this chapter are:

➤ *How Learning Works* (2010): Ambrose et al. (2010) from Carnegie Mellon University describe the research and associated teaching strategies for seven principles of teaching. Their associated website at the Carnegie Mellon University Eberly Center Teaching Excellence & Educational Innovation at https://www.cmu.edu/teaching/ provides a wealth of resources on teaching principles and assessment. Their seven principles focus on the assessment of prior knowledge to provide a foundation for further learning or to identify gaps in understanding; integration of knowledge, making connections across concepts, fostering student motivation, and providing practice opportunities with goal-directed feedback to improve the quality of learning; understanding that there are social and emotional influences on learning that exist within the individual learner but also within the course climate that faculty can influence; and, becoming a self-directed learner is key to improving performance.

➤ *Make it Stick: The Science of Successful Learning* (2014): Dr. Peter Brown et al. (2014) provide an in-depth review of the research behind current knowledge in learning science, especially on long-term memory retention and accessing that memory, both critical for the discipline of nursing. They emphasize the importance of information retrieval and spaced practice as key to learning (topics revisited later in this chapter more fully). Brown and colleagues outline learning practices that should be avoided as they contribute mostly to short-term memory retention, such as rereading or outlining the text and mass practices. Examples of massed practice include cramming for tests and scheduling day-long skills days.

➤ The Small Teaching series: This series consists of two books: *Small Teaching: Everyday Lessons from the Science of Learning* by James Lang (Lang, 2021) and the companion book, *Small Teaching Online: Applying Learning Science in Online Classes* by Flower Darby and James Lang (Darby & Lang, 2019). Each of these books focuses on current knowledge of learning science with practical applications that can be easily implemented in traditional face-to-face, hybrid, and online learning environments.

➤ *Powerful Teaching: Unleash the Science of Learning* (Agarwal & Bain, 2019): Written by Pooja Agarwal and Patrice Bain (a college and a K-12 educator, respectively), who participated in the research studies described in *Make it Stick*, these researchers have continued their collaboration in this book on practical strategies to implement in the classroom focused on Retrieval Practice, Spacing, Interleaving, and Feedback-Driven Metacognition. Their accompanying website, https://www.retrievalpractice.org/, provides additional teaching tips and guides and educators can subscribe free to updated information.

References

Agarwal, P. K., & Bain, P. M. (2019). *Powerful teaching: Unleash the science of learning.* Jossey-Bass.

Ambrose, S. A., Bridges, M. W., DiPietro, M., Lovett, M. C., & Norman, M. K. (2010). *How learning works.* John Wiley & Sons.

Bjork, E. L., & Bjork, R. A. (2014). Making things hard on yourself, but in a good way: Creating desirable difficulties to enhance learning. In M. A. Gernsbacher & J. Pomerantz (Eds.), *Psychology and the real world: Essays illustrating fundamental contributions to society* (2nd ed., pp. 59–68). Worth.

Brookfield, S. (2017). *Becoming a critically reflective teacher.* (2nd ed.). Jossey-Bass.

Brown, P. C., Roediger, H. L. III, & McDaniel, M. A. (2014). *Make it stick: The science of successful learning.* Harvard University Press.

Buterakos, R. M., & Keiser, M. (2021). Scaffolding role development and clinical reasoning for online AG-ACNP students. *Journal for Nurse Practitioners, 17*(5), 615–618. https://doi.org/10.1016/j.nurpra.2020.12.031

Canning, E. A., Muenks, K., Green, D. J., & Murphy, M. C. (2019). STEM faculty who believe ability is fixed have larger racial achievement gaps and inspire less student motivation in their classes. *Science Advances, 5*(2), eaau4734. https://doi.org/10.1126/sciadv.aau4734

Carstensen, S. S., Kjaer, C., Möller, S., & Bloksgaard, M. (2020). Implementing collaborative, active learning using peer instructions in pharmacology teaching increases students' learning and thereby exam performance. *European Journal of Pharmacology, 867*, 172792. https://doi.org/10.1016/j.ejphar.2019.172792

Chen, X., Zhang, B., Jin, S. X., Quan, Y. X., Zhang, X. W., & Cui, X. S. (2021). The effects of mindfulness-based interventions on nursing students: A meta-analysis. *Nurse Education Today, 98*, 104718. https://doi.org/10.1016/j.nedt.2020.104718

Colvard, N. B., Watson, C. E., & Park, H. (2018). The Impact of open educational resources on various student success metrics. *International Journal of Teaching and Learning in Higher Education, 30*(2), 262–276.

Coombs, N. M. (2018). Educational scaffolding: Back to basics for nursing education in the 21st century. *Nurse Education Today, 68*, 198–200. https://doi.org/10.1016/j.nedt.2018.06.007

Coram, C. (2016). Expert role modeling effect on novice nursing students' clinical judgment. *Clinical Simulation in Nursing, 12*(9), 385–391. https://doi.org/10.1016/j.ecns.2016.04.009

Darby, F., & Lang, J. M. (2019). *Small teaching online: Applying learning science in online classes.* John Wiley & Sons.

Daugherty, L., Johnston, W. R., & Tiffany Berglund, T. (2020). *Connecting college students to alternative sources of support: The single stop community college initiative and postsecondary outcomes.* RAND Corporation. Retrieved from https://www.rand.org/pubs/research_reports/RR1740-1.html

Dweck, C. S., Walton, G. M., & Cohen, G. L. (2014). Academic tenacity: Mindsets and skills that promote long-term learning. Retrieved from https://k12education.gatesfoundation.org/resource/academic-tenacity-mindsets-and-skills-that-promote-long-termlearning/.

Eyler, J. (2018). *How humans learn: The science and stories behind effective college teaching.* West Virginia University Press.

Fiorella, L., & Mayer, R. E. (2013). The relative benefits of learning by teaching and teaching expectancy. *Contemporary Educational Psychology, 38*, 281–288. https://doi.org/10.1016/j.cedpsych.2013.06.001

Goldin, D. S. (2017). *Factors that predict levels of sleepiness of advanced practice nursing students.* Doctoral dissertation. Nova Southeastern University. Retrieved from https://nsuworks.nova.edu/hpd_con_stuetd/43

Green, M. L., Moeller, J. J., & Spak, J. M. (2018). Test-enhanced learning in health professions education: A systematic review: BEME Guide No. 48. *Medical Teacher, 40*(4), 337–350. https://doi.org/10.1080/01421 59X.2018.1430354

Gurung, R. A. R., & Galardi, N. R. (2022). Syllabus tone, more than mental health statements, influence intentions to seek help. *Teaching of Psychology, 49*(3), 218–223. https://doi.org/10.1177/0098628321994632

Herrington, A., & Schneidereith, T. (2017). Scaffolding and sequencing core concepts to develop a simulation-integrated nursing curriculum. *Nurse Educator, 42*(4), 204–207. https://doi.org/10.1097/NNE.0000000000000358

Holland, T. (2020). Educational strategies to foster empathy utilizing simulation pedagogy. *International Journal of Caring Sciences, 13*(3), 1589–1595.

The Hope Center for College, Community, and Justice. (2021). *#RealCollege 2021: Basic needs insecurity during the ongoing pandemic*. Retrieved from https://www.natcom.org/sites/default/files/publications/NCA_CBrief_Vol11_8.pdf

Hughes, V., Cologer, S., Swoboda, S., & Rushton, C. (2021). Strengthening internal resources to promote resilience among prelicensure nursing students. *Journal of Professional Nursing, 37*(4), 777–783. https://doi.org.liboff.ohsu.edu/10.1016/j.profnurs.2021.05.008

Immordino-Yang, M. H., & Damasio, A. R. (2007). We feel, therefore we learn: The relevance of affective and social neuroscience to education. *Mind, Brain and Education, 1*(1), 3–10.

Kobayashi, K. (2019). Learning by preparing-to-teach and teaching: A meta-analysis. *Japanese Psychological Research, 61*(3), 192–203. https://doi.org/10.1111/jpr.122212019

Lang, J. M. (2021). *Small teaching: Everyday lessons from the science of learning* (2nd ed.). John Wiley & Sons.

Lewis, L. S., Williams, C. A., & Dawson, S. D. (2020). Growth mindset training and effective learning strategies in community college registered nursing students. *Teaching & Learning in Nursing, 15*(2), 123–127. https://doi.org/10.1016/j.teln.2020.01.006

Madrazo, G. M., & Motz, L. L. (2005). Brain research: Implications to diverse learners. *Science Educator, 14*(1), 56–60.

Maneval, R. E., & Kurz, J. (2016). "Nursing Students Assaulted": Considering student safety in community-focused experiences. *Journal of Professional Nursing, 32*(3), 246–251. https://doi.org/10.1016/j.profnurs.2015.11.001

Maroto, M. E., Snelling, A., & Linck, H. (2015). Food insecurity among community college students: Prevalence and association with grade point average. *Community College Journal of Research and Practice, 39*, 515–526. https://doi.org/10.1080/10668926.2013.850758

Martinelli, S. M., Isaak, R. S., Schell, R. M., Mitchell, J. D., McEvoy, M. D., & Chen, F. (2019). Learners and luddites in the twenty-first century: Bringing evidence-based education to anesthesiology. *Anesthesiology, 131*(4), 908–928. https://doi.org/10.1097/ALN.0000000000002827

Metzger, M., Dowling, T., Guinn, J., & Wilson, D. T. (2020). Inclusivity in baccalaureate nursing education: A scoping study. *Journal of Professional Nursing, 36*(1), 5–14. https://doi.org/10.1016/j.profnurs.2019.06.002

National Academies of Sciences, Engineering, and Medicine. (2021). *The future of nursing 2020–2030: Charting a path to achieve health equity*. The National Academies Press. https://doi.org/10.17226/25982

National Academies of Sciences, Engineering, and Medicine. (2018). *How people learn II: Learners, contexts, and cultures*. The National Academies Press. https://doi.org/10.17226/24783

Noone, J. (2022). Engaged students: Essential to achieve distinction in nursing education. In M. Adams, & T. Valiga (Eds.), *Achieving distinction in nursing education*. National League for Nursing.

Owens, M. T., & Tanner, K. D. (2017). Teaching as brain changing: Exploring connections between neuroscience and innovative teaching. *CBE Life Sciences Education*, *16*(2), fe2. https://doi.org/10.1187/cbe.17-01-0005

Palese, A., Basso, F., Del Negro, E., Achil, I., Ferraresi, A., Morandini, M., Moreale R., & Mansutti, I. (2017). When are night shifts effective for nursing student clinical learning? Findings from a mixed-method study design. *Nurse Education Today*, *52*, 15–21.

Sakraida, T. J. (2020). Writing-in-the-discipline with instructional scaffolding in an RN-to-BSN Nursing Research Course. *Journal of Nursing Education*, *59*(3), 179–180. https://doi.org/10.3928/01484834-20200220-15

Sanders, D., & Welk, D. S. (2005). Strategies to scaffold student learning: applying Vygotsky's Zone of Proximal Development. *Nurse Educator*, *30*(5), 203–207. https://doi.org/10.1097/00006223-200509000-00007

Schell, J. A., & Butler A. C. (2018). Insights from the science of learning can inform evidence-based implementation of peer instruction. *Frontiers in Education*, (3), 1–13. https://doi.org/10.3389/feduc.2018.00033

Sethares, K. A., & Asselin, M. E. (2022). Use of exam wrapper metacognitive strategy to promote student self-assessment of learning: an integrative review. *Nurse Educator*, *47*(1), 37–41. https://doi.org/10.1097/NNE.0000000000001026

Shellenbarger, T., & Robb, M. (2021). *Make it stick: "Small Teaching" for big learning*. National League for Nursing Education Summit.

Silva, M. R., Kleinert, W. L., Sheppard, A. V., Cantrell, K. A., Freeman-Coppadge, D. J., Tsoy, E., Roberts, T., & Pearrow, M. (2017). The relationship between food security, housing stability, and school performance among college students in an Urban University. *Journal of College Student Retention: Research, Theory & Practice*, *19*(3), 284–299. https://doi.org/10.1177/1521025115621918

Smith, T. (2021). Guided reflective writing as a teaching strategy to develop nursing student clinical judgment. *Nursing Forum*, *56*(2), 241–248. https://doi.org/10.1111/nuf.12528

Theobald, E. J., Hill, M. J., Tran, E., Agrawal, S., Arroyo, E. N., Behling, S., Chambwe, N., Cintrón, D. L., Cooper, J. D., Dunster, G., Grummer, J. A., Hennessey, K., Hsiao, J., Iranon, N., Jones, L., 2nd, Jordt, H., Keller, M., Lacey, M. E., Littlefield, C. E., Freeman, S. (2020). Active learning narrows achievement gaps for underrepresented students in undergraduate science, technology, engineering, and math. *Proceedings of the National Academy of Sciences of the United States of America*, *117*(12), 6476–6483. https://doi.org/10.1073/pnas.1916903117

Thomas, C. M., McIntosh, C. E., Lamar, R. A., & Allen, R. L. (2017). Sleep deprivation in nursing students: The negative impact for quality and safety. *Journal of Nursing Education and Practice*, *7*(5), 87–93. https://doi.org/10.5430/jnep.v7n5p87

Verkuyl, M., Hughes, M., & Fyfe, M. C. (2018). Using think aloud in health assessment: A mixed-methods study. *The Journal of Nursing Education*, *57*(11), 684–686. https://doi.org/10.3928/01484834-20181022-10

Vogel, S., & Schwabe, L. (2016). Learning and memory under stress: implications for the classroom. *NPJ Science Learn*, *1*, 16011. https://doi.org/10.1038/npjscilearn.2016.11

Vygotsky, L. (1978). *Mind and society: The development of higher mental processes*. Cambridge University Press.

Walton, G. M., & Cohen, G. L. (2011). A brief social-belonging intervention improves academic and health outcomes among minority students. *Science, 331*, 1447–1451.

Wheeler, J., Dudas, K., & Brooks, G. (2021). Anxiety and a Mindfulness Exercise in Healthcare Simulation Prebriefing. *Clinical Simulation in Nursing*, *59*, 61–66. https://doi.org/10.1016/j.ecns.2021.05.008

Williams, C. (2021). Nursing students' mindsets and choice of learning strategies. *Nurse Educator*, *46*(2), 92–95. https://doi.org/10.1097/NNE.0000000000000870

Yeager, D. S., & Walton, G. M. (2011). Social-psychological interventions in education: They're not magic. *Review of Educational Research*, *81*(2), 267–301.

Yeager, D. S., Hanselman, P., Walton, G. M., Murray, J. S., Crosnoe, R., Muller, C., Tipton, E., Schneider, B., Hulleman, C. S., Hinojosa, C. P., Paunesku, D., Romero, C., Flint, K., Roberts, A., Trott, J., Iachan, R., Buontempo, J., Yang, S. M., Carvalho, C. M., . . . Dweck, C. S. (2019). A national experiment reveals where a growth mindset improves achievement. *Nature*, *573*(7774), 364–369. https://doi.org/10.1038/s41586-019-1466-y

4

Faculty Development: Preparing to Teach

Susan Gross Forneris, PhD, RN, CNE, CHSE-A, FAAN
Barbara J. Patterson, PhD, RN, FAAN, ANEF

CHAPTER OVERVIEW

This chapter focuses on the requisite preparation, development, and support needed for faculty to flourish in their teaching role in order to implement the best practices outlined in this book. Topics are grounded in the pedagogy of teaching and include faculty development in learning science, the art of dialogue in teaching, and faculty as learners to prepare a nursing workforce that can critically think to deliver safe and effective care in the current complex health care environments to achieve health equity. An illustration of the application of a novel approach to faculty development with an exemplar of teaching social determinants of health is shared.

FACULTY PREPARATION AND DEVELOPMENT TO TEACH

In nursing practice, the term "professional development" (PD) is most often associated with clinical staff development to describe the role of competence of clinicians regarding the goal of improving professional practice and population health through patient care (Brunt & Russell, 2022). The specialty practice of academic nursing education, PD for educators is generally termed faculty development and refers to ongoing professional learning for educators. Professional learning for educators often includes nursing practice content. However, this chapter focuses on the professional development of the pedagogy of teaching and learning. The emphasis is on preparing educators to teach. The terms professional development and faculty development may be used interchangeably.

Role development as a nurse educator has been guided by eight evidence-based nurse educator core competencies first articulated in 2007 and further supported with empirical literature in 2019 (Halstead, 2007, 2019; NLN, n.d.). These competencies formed a framework for certification as a nurse educator (CNE®) and the academic preparation and development of educators. Halstead (2019) stated "faculty who demonstrate the competencies in their educator role will facilitate achievement of student learning outcomes and ultimately influence the quality of care delivered to patients" (p. 169). Recognizing the specialized role competencies of the academic clinical nurse educator, Shellenbarger (2019) provided a detailed analysis and synthesis of relevant literature to guide this educator group. Shellenbarger (2019) highlights the complex role and unique practice area of the clinical nurse educator. She notes that evidence-based competencies and tasks help educators prepare students for the rigors of clinical practice. In 2020, Christensen and Simmons included the academic clinical nurse educator in their scope of practice book acknowledging these educators' experience in clinical and academic nursing education practice.

Academic nurse educators are considered practicing in the full scope of the educator role when engaged in all of the core competencies (Christensen & Simmons, 2020). However, to achieve these competencies, the preparation and development of faculty is crucial. Miller et al. (2022) identify PD for faculty or faculty development as including "any modality that increases the pedagogical knowledge of a faculty member" (p. 151) through exploration of specific pedagogical topics. At the organizational level, PD is a cost-effective investment in faculty, promotes job satisfaction (Smith et al., 2023), and has the potential to create a collegial atmosphere leading to improved recruitment and retention of faculty (DeFelippo & Dee, 2022; Jeffers & Mariani, 2017; Young-Brice et al., 2022).

Similar to Halstead (2019), Miller et al. (2022) also argue that PD can dramatically improve one's teaching and is an effective way to facilitate positive outcomes for students. In higher education, Wright et al. (2018) argued that there is growing evidence for a strong connection between faculty development and student learning. Faculty development requires continuous quality improvement (Valiga, 2019). However, there is an identified gap in the nursing education literature focused on the effectiveness of faculty development programs designed "to help faculty increase their effectiveness in facilitating learning" (Caputi & Frank, 2019, p. 35). This gap supports the need for robust research studies specifically examining the link between faculty development and student academic success.

Professional development in nursing academia is not well addressed in the literature despite what is reported as a great desire for development by nurse educators (Oprescu et al., 2017). In an integrative review, Smith et al. (2023) reported the number of articles on professional development for nurse educators was small ($n = 13$) and that the PD needs of nurse educators are heterogeneous. Their findings indicated that nurse educators have multiple roles and varied personal and institutional needs; therefore, continuing PD is necessary during different phases of one's career.

Nursing as a profession has discussed the shortage and lack of qualified nurse educators for over two decades necessitating the hiring of educators who have limited preparation to teach. Multiple solutions have been offered to address this lack of preparation and development for nurse educators (see Table 4.1). Although a variety of mechanisms and topics have been suggested to partially remedy the lack of preparation and development for the nurse educator, there remains limited empirical evidence on their effectiveness, sustainability, and one's knowledge acquisition. As noted in their findings, Jeffers and Mariani (2017) concluded that mentoring relationships were not always successful.

TABLE 4.1

Faculty Development Initiatives

Authors (Year)	Strategy	Description
Young-Brice et al. (2022)	Onboarding and orientation program: Teaching Excellence Program (TEP)	Based on Meleis' transition theory, newly hired faculty met individually and in as a cohort 11 times. They received electronic teaching resources. University speakers spoke on various topics.
Mackessy-Lloyd et al. (2019)	Online mentorship	Based on Meleis' transition theory, using a learning management system, strategies included group texting (Groupme), online discussion, and access to resources.
NLN (2022)	Mentoring toolkit	Provides a review of literature with recommended practices for mentors and mentees.
Fitzwater et al. (2021)	Simulation learning	Based on Meleis' transition theory, a literature review on simulation use for faculty as learners and transition to the teaching role support was reported.
Walker et al. (2022)	Fitness initiative	Promoting a contemporary view of faculty development, a fitness initiative included a variety of monthly fitness activities to highlight the inclusion of self-care in faculty development.
Reese and Ketner (2017)	Nurse educator institute	A statewide online program with a workbook to practice skills was developed to build a foundation for learning theories, curriculum, evaluation, and performance improvement. A certificate and continuing education credits were offered upon completion.
Cooley and De Gagne (2016)	Internship program	Guided by Kolb's experiential learning theory, a qualitative study was designed to gain insight into novice educators' experiences. Data-supported mentorship & internship programs.
O'Connor et al. (2019)	Diversity, equity, and inclusion institute	A 3-day program was conducted to create an inclusive environment to facilitate crucial conversations on -isms, practice skills, and transform a class activity.
Smallheer et al. (2021)	Day-long workshop	Quality improvement project using Kirkpatrick's model of evaluation—day-long interactive workshop using trigger films, group discussion, and interactive theater.

Preparation of Academic Nurse Educators

There is a plethora of literature reporting that new faculty lack the preparation and knowledge necessary to teach (Bullin, 2018; Han et al., 2022; Kalensky & Hande, 2017; Oermann, 2017; Randall & Randall, 2021; Ross & Dunkler, 2019). Advocates of pedagogical preparation of nurse educators abound (Booth et al., 2016); however, there remains a lack of consensus and divergent views regarding the educational preparation of the academic nurse educator (Booth et al., 2016). While the Doctor of Philosophy degree (PhD) or equivalent is the required degree in the majority of institutions of higher education, few academic nurse educators are formally prepared to teach (Bullin, 2018). The findings of Bullin's (2018) integrative review concluded that while there is an expectation of the delivery of quality nursing education, the associated preparation for this role remains wanting. Bullin noted that the goal of delivering effective nursing education is more than nursing content knowledge. It is the "pedagogical knowledge that engages and informs that knowledge" (Bullin, 2018, p. 10).

Being unprepared to teach can have numerous professional outcomes (Young-Brice et al., 2022). These include the impact on the recruitment and retention of educators which ultimately impacts the nursing workforce at large. Garner and Bedford (2021) conducted a phenomenological study exploring the experiences of early-career faculty and the feeling of being unprepared to teach. One of their themes was "ownership for ongoing learning." They stated that self-regulation theories place responsibility for learning on both the individual and the institution. As novice educators:

> . . . [they] learn and transition to early-career nursing faculty, they become active, deliberate learners, taking a significant role in self-regulated decision making . . . [and] taking a self-guided approach to professional development. (Garner & Bedford, 2021, p. 2)

The implications of their findings supported ongoing mentorship and the need to standardize adequate nurse faculty preparation for the educator role prior to assuming that role. These findings also highlighted a move from traditional learning to the individual's role in their professional development.

Ongoing learning reinforces the sixth NLN nurse educator core competency of "pursu[ing] continuous quality improvement in the nurse educator role" (Halstead, 2019). This consists of participating in PD opportunities to increase one's effectiveness in the educator role and development of the educator competencies. Identified research gaps included how to prepare novice nurse educators and how to help them effectively develop into professional nurse educators. Role development needs of nurse faculty, at every level of employment, require attention. For this competency, "formal academic preparation for the nurse educator role was not addressed" (Halstead, 2007, p. 136) in the review of the literature.

Development of Academic Nurse Educators

With career longevity and advancement, educators' development needs subsequently shift and change (Seldin, 2006). Simultaneously, their learning needs evolve, and nursing education, the student population, and nursing practice changes. Thus, there remains a need for continued faculty development, enhancement of expertise, and tailoring of learning experiences to promote faculty growth and career satisfaction. Oermann (2017) eloquently stated ". . . for effective teaching in nursing, and our need to build our scholarship of teaching and learning, we cannot expect nurse educators to be prepared 'on the job'—it is not fair to the faculty, students, or school" (p. 1). While there is general agreement that academic nurse educators need pedagogical development in teaching strategies, curriculum, and evaluation methods, many faculty lack systematic approaches to guide their professional development (Kalensky & Hande, 2017).

Some faculty development programs in the nursing literature have focused on specific content and areas of practice that need to be developed. Reported programs include gender-associated incivility (Smallheer et al., 2021), social determinants of health (Noone, 2022), culturally sensitive teaching (Leibold et al., 2022), online teaching (Lee et al., 2010; Quinco et al., 2022), gerontology content (McCleary et al., 2009), informatics (Forman et al., 2019), simulation (Fitzwater et al., 2021), and learning communities (Drummond-Young et al., 2010). Despite the significance of these programs, they remain content driven. Faculty need to learn *how* to teach the content.

Recommendations for pedagogical content knowledge for the nurse educator have been relatively consistent (Crider, 2022) with a common practice of learning pedagogical content/material through traditional workshops and didactic lectures with discussion. Unfortunately, didactic lecture decontextualizes the pedagogical knowledge that educators want and need to apply in their practice. In 2015, Benner articulately argued that "in a practice discipline, 'how' to use knowledge is equally important as the knowledge presented in formal decontextualized forms" (p. 2).

Faculty development needs to both prepare and develop nursing faculty as educators, which is more than specific knowledge and different types of delivery strategies. Oermann (2017) noted "although faculty development and continuing education programs combined with mentors will meet some of the needs of novice faculty, these programs do not provide the depth of understanding needed" (p. 1). Thus, while the essential elements and content of faculty development programs may be driven by the mission of the school/university, excellence in teaching and learning is more than content delivery for the educator as a learner. Teaching is a social process and faculty must have opportunities to apply what they learn in safe environments to achieve excellence in their teaching practice.

Two articles were located that proposed strategies to create cognitive learning opportunities for faculty development. In a participatory action research project, Randall and Randall (2021) had participants share teaching challenges, and the stories were used to create a script for critical incident videos. One theme that surfaced from the focus groups was "teaching learning to learn." The theme reflected "the participants' desire to understand and teach students ways to learn more effectively . . . . instructors need to make ways in which students learn to 'think like a nurse' more visible" (Randall & Randall, 2021, p. 85).

Another alternative strategy for faculty preparation and development included an Experimental Teaching Course (Johnson-Crowley, 2004). The author argued that using the same approaches and models for teacher preparation has shown limited success in promoting educator competence and confidence and the promotion of educational understanding of the teaching and learning process is crucial. Using a constructivist model for the design of program courses, students were able to identify and examine their beliefs about teaching and learning contributing to a growth in confidence and competence in teaching and a sense of empowerment.

Nurse educators must develop confidence and competence in all aspects of their academic role. Miller et al. (2022) recommend that all PD workshops be active learning centers "where participants learn through doing" and the best workshops are those where participants can "envision how to apply the strategies" to their own practice (p. 155). They note that participants must learn the information to be most effective. To develop competence in the educator role, alternative methods of preparation and development are needed that promote educator understanding of the teaching and learning process and move beyond content and skill development. The next section includes the application of neuroscience principles and the educator as learner that offer a novel approach to preparing and developing nurse educators beyond content and delivery approaches to achieve understanding.

SHIFTING THE FOCUS: A PRIMER FOR FACULTY PREPARATION AND DEVELOPMENT IN CONTEMPORARY NEUROSCIENCE

Given the growing interest in neuroscience and learning, or educational neuroscience, strong arguments have been rendered for the inclusion of education in this area for all educators (Doukakis & Alexopoulos, 2021), both in their preparation and professional development. The connections between the brain and learning seem obvious; "the brain is the main organ of learning, so a deeper understanding of the brain would appear highly relevant to education" (Goswami, 2008, p. 381). Likewise, Agarwal and Bain (2019) have argued that by incorporating the science of learning into educator preparation programs, colleges and universities can add scientific rigor, encourage tougher standards for certification, enhance decision-making based on student data (rather than simply "the more data, the better"), and ultimately move us toward a higher-quality education system (p. 282).

Nevertheless, there is limited empirical literature assessing the outcomes of the preparation of educators in neuroscience (Privitera, 2021). Doukakis and Alexopoulos (2021) stated that the benefit of the preparation of educators "in educational neuroscience is the transformation of their knowledge which will eventually result in improving student knowledge and learning" (p. 52). Knowledge of how the brain works has been linked to teacher effectiveness and perception of their ability to influence student learning.

Over the past ten years, the National League for Nursing published vision statements with a call to action focused on faculty preparation to support learner development of high-level reasoning skills throughout a program of study (NLN, 2015a, 2015b). In response to this call, the NLN published a series of nurse educator resources grounded in contemporary neuroscience (Forneris & Fey, 2016, 2018, 2021). These resources focus less on teaching content, but instead, on the use of brain science strategies that guide students in using the content (Forneris & Fey, 2021).

Brain-based learning is changing the face of education today (Agarwal, 2019; Doyle & Zakrajsek, 2019; Pan & Rickard, 2018; Pelletier et al., 2021; Weidman & Baker, 2015). This newer evidence originating in the discipline of education counters the prevailing thinking in nursing education that teaching as one was taught is not effective with today's learn-ers. Reporting on emerging technologies for teaching and learning, the *Horizon Report* serves as a reference planning guide for higher education and has been a driver of inno-vation and change in the education discipline (Pelletier et al., 2021). These reports support the increased use of learning technologies that include artificial intelligence, blended and hybrid learning, and learning analytics (Pelletier et al., 2021). The science of learning is at the heart of educational best practices with cognitive principles that continue to stand firm: (a) the ability for learners to think about and pay attention to meaning, and (b) the importance of the nature of deliberate practice in the learning of new information (Deans for Impact, 2021).

In the next section of this chapter, the foundational brain science principles will be explored through an experiential lens with you, the reader, as both the educator and the faculty learner.

Dialogue in Teaching: Setting the Context for Learning

Grounded in contemporary neuroscience, the use of dialogue is rooted in critical theory as a foundation to engage learner perspectives, thinking, and reasoning. Setting the stage for this learning dialogue requires a thoughtful approach. Educators must con-sider factors that will successfully set the context for learning.

The optimal context for learning is creating a space where you and the student learn-ers feel safe; a safe space to share how you and the student learners understand con-tent, share thinking, and can admit to not knowing something. Setting this space for learning as a safe container, requires attending to both emotion and cognition. Evidence in neuropsychology and neuroscience suggests that emotion can significantly impact cognitive abilities (Dweck, 2016; Edmondson, 2019; Lerner et al., 2015; Okon-Singer et al., 2015; Pessoa, 2015). Both student learners and educators alike come to a learning encounter using a filter of past experiences. These past experiences hold biases and assumptions that have accumulated over time. This filter of "accumulated past experience" influ-ences how we select the data to which we are paying attention; interpret this data; and finally influence how we prioritize actions when making a judgment and then acting on that judgment. Past experiences trigger emotions and shape how we construct knowl-edge (Forneris & Fey, 2018, 2021). The challenge in any learning encounter is the level of engagement. Engagement is influenced by emotional activation; too little emotion and engagement will be limited, while too much emotion may overwhelm engagement and impair thinking and decision-making.

A teaching strategy that blends feedback and reflection is a powerful way to learn, a critical dialogue. Critical dialogue is a purposeful conversation that explores perceptions and thought processes, provides feedback, and generates a "back and forth" sharing of perspectives on the part of both the student learner and the educator (Forneris & Fey, 2021). It is a dialogue grounded in curiosity. As a faculty learner reading this section on engag-ing a critical dialogue, consider the role of a detective, or in the context of learning, a cognitive detective. As a cognitive detective, curiosity guides the questions you ask with the goal of understanding how a student learner is making sense of the content being used during the learning encounter. You need time and practice uncovering, rehears-ing, and connecting knowledge and thinking, and when action is taken, articulating the rationale for action. If you only transmit content, your student learners will never rehearse, use the content, and encode it for later retrieval out of long-term memory.

When you experience dialogue that involves curiosity and respect and transparency in thinking you are likely motivated and engaged. Your level of curiosity will help you to diagnose learning needs more accurately. In the discipline of nursing, the overall goal is to develop into a skilled practitioner with the ability to self-monitor one's own thinking, knowledge, and practice. Dialogue has been shown to be a most powerful strategy for learning and achievement (Forneris & Fey, 2021). This small shift to curiosity moves the passive action of transmitting content to an active dialogue of examining and sharing perspectives.

Beginning with the End in Mind

Over the last decade, teaching and learning strategies have become quite sophisticated. With the shift from "teaching content" to "teaching learners how to use the content," educators are required to be more thoughtful in their approach to choosing teaching strategies that will help learners build their own learning foundations. Every learning encounter is driven by an anticipated outcome; a learning objective that guides the educator in (a) the selection and use of specific teaching strategies; and (b) discerning how a learner is managing the content. Every course, class, and lesson plan is guided by outcomes. Outcomes drive the what and how of teaching and assist educators to determine the best approach to engage the learner and guide their achievement. Nurse educator preparation that begins with the end in mind, guided by outcomes, assures a thoughtful approach to creating a curious and engaging learning space for students. This strategy is more thoroughly discussed in Chapter 7, *Backward Design: Aligning Outcomes, Assessments, and Activities*.

Addressing Content through Neuroscience Strategies

"When it comes to educator preparation, every future teacher must have a deep understanding of desirable difficulties, metacognition, and the critical importance of retrieval" (Agarwal & Bain, 2019, p. 282). The following section explores each of these brain science concepts and their importance in the teaching and learning process for nurse faculty preparation and development.

Desirable Difficulty

Operationalizing neuroscience strategies in teaching catapults the educator beyond the transmitter of content and the learner beyond memorization. Neuroscience teaching strategies create durable, flexible learning with desirable difficulty (Bjork, 1994, 2013) on one end of the trajectory, and on the other end, with the achievement of the desired outcome. Creating a learning environment that embraces desirable difficulty, without pushing the learner over the edge, opens the door to natural learner errors made in the spirit of learning and can be powerful triggers to reflective learning and solid encoding of information into long-term memory.

As discussed in Chapter 3, learning in its simplest form requires an understanding of the learning sequence whereby a learner first attends to outside information in sensory memory. Once attended, it transfers from short-term memory (where it is consciously processed) to long-term memory (where it is stored and then retrieved when needed later). The key is to focus on the teaching and learning strategies that help learners to consciously process information in short-term memory, so the information is properly encoded for later use.

As a faculty learner, you can be seduced into believing you have learned, for example, when you have a sense of understanding content, like the content on desirable difficulty. You may read, highlight, and re-read and then easily retrieve from memory and recite the definition of desirable difficulty. Or that feeling of familiarity with a topic, like desirable difficulty, that is triggered by something you hear, or experience, only to be limited in just how much you can explain or interpret. The dilemma is that you can be lured into a false sense of having learned when you use strategies that generate quick improvement of performance only to fail when attempts at retrieving that same knowledge later are not successful: performance versus learning. Bjork (1994, 2013) would suggest that while performance is observable in the moment, it may not be a true indicator of learning that has been encoded and permanently stored for accurate retrieval and use over time.

Your ability to both store and retrieve knowledge and its appropriate utility is what defines learning. Bjork (1994, 2013) makes an important point; strategies that rapidly increase your ability to retrieve knowledge differ from strategies that maximize the gain of storage strength. As in the example above, when you read, highlight, and re-read content and then immediately demonstrate that you can quickly retrieve and articulate the information, you may be misinterpreting storage strength with retrieval strength. You may likely prefer this easy learning over a perceived more difficult learning that would maximize storage strength and accurate retrieval for later use.

Desirable difficulty, also known as the productive struggle (Bjork, 1994, 2013), is the generation of a challenging learning condition such that your productive struggle with the content results in more durable and flexible learning. With desirable difficulty, emphasis is placed on the word desirable. Simply put, strategies that help you trigger the necessary encoding and retrieval processes that support learning, comprehension, and remembering are desirable. If you do not have the background knowledge or skills to respond to a learning strategy, the learning is difficult and therefore not desirable. In this case, the chance of encoding and later retrieving the knowledge is diminished (Bjork, 1994, 2013).

Strategies that generate this productive struggle are strategically generated by the educator and include varying the condition of learning, so the struggle is meaningful. For example, as a faculty learner, at this moment you are reading about desirable difficulty in this chapter. A change in the condition of learning might include taking out a blank piece of paper and without resources, writing down everything you understand about desirable difficulty. With another learning condition change; a few days later, you challenge yourself to discuss, with a colleague, how desirable difficulty is being used in a course you teach. A few weeks later, you intentionally work with your educator teaching team to create a learning activity that embraces the concept of desirable difficulty. Varying the learning condition over time by challenging both retrieval of your knowledge on how you understand the concept of desirable difficulty with additional examples of how you might use it in one of your classes will generate a more productive struggle.

You will discover and better cement your memory pathway. The struggle of not quite remembering and then using an activity that actively engages you to continue to use and make sense of new learning creates both the desire and the struggle.

Metacognition

Simply put, metacognition is the process of thinking about your thinking. Reflecting on content, questioning how the content is understood, and being aware of how you see and think about the content, you are thinking about your thinking to make sense of the content. Nurse educators focus their efforts on teaching learners to think like a nurse; yet the challenge is to create learning encounters that provide opportunities for (a) educator role modeling; and (b) learner rehearsal. Gaining a deeper appreciation for strategies that unlock exploration of thinking and the sharing of that thinking will generate critical thinkers.

Reconsider the previous section on desirable difficulty and the examples provided of the varying learning conditions with which you, as a faculty learner, might have engaged to learn about this concept. Now consider the following: you were able to successfully define desirable difficulty when you wrote it down on the blank sheet of paper. You went over it and re-read your notes and resources the night before you were planning to meet with a colleague to discuss how desirable difficulty is being used in the courses you teach. However, on the day of the conversation, you do not easily remember some of the main points you thought you had mastered.

What happened here? Engaging in metacognitive thinking is self-directed. As a faculty learner in this moment, you choose what to accomplish, and how you monitor your progress to achieve and then evaluate achievement. Your ability to be accurate about this learning trajectory is paramount to effective learning. The important feature of metacognition is the ability as a learner to truly recognize and accurately determine when you have learned. Weidman and Baker (2015) used the term metacomprehension or the awareness one has about their own level of comprehension of a topic. They suggest that when you have a high level of metacomprehension, you demonstrate strategies that include spending more self-directed learning time on topics or concepts not well understood as opposed to topics you feel you have mastered.

Metacognition will be enhanced when you (a) accurately assess whether you are achieving the learning outcomes; and (b) intentionally engage in opportunities to rehearse your thinking on outcomes not being achieved. Opportunities to rehearse and more accurately assess your own learning will improve both your metacomprehension and metacognition. As emphasized earlier, in the discipline of nursing, the overall goal is to develop a skilled practitioner with the ability to self-monitor one's own thinking, knowledge, and practice.

Retrieval Practices

The goals of nurse educators are to prepare future practitioners who can quickly access and use nursing knowledge to inform decision-making in a future real-life situation. Understanding and using brain science helps one to engage cognition. How you retrieve information to improve your cognition is paramount. The key to embracing the brain science concept of retrieval is understanding that good retrieval practice is the struggle of not quite remembering and then returning and actively engaging in making sense again of the material. Spacing the time frame before your return to the content will assist in the transfer of this content into long-term memory (Agarwal, 2019; Weidman & Baker, 2015).

Consider the activity used around desirable difficulty. Reading and re-reading the section and your notes on desirable difficulty is a common method to study and learn this concept. A week later you are asked to explain desirable difficulty and provide an example that illustrates its use in a nursing course you teach. You are employing a retrieval strategy. Weidman and Baker (2015) have argued that retrieval practice is not simply restudying content. Deeper learning will occur if content is revisited in a spaced-out manner stretching the time interval for rehearsing and metacognition (Agarwal, 2019). Spacing content provides opportunities to practice recalling relevant information and is a form of retrieval practice. When you are required to extract and use your content knowledge in the moment, the struggle of not quite remembering makes learning durable (Forneris & Fey, 2021).

Weidman and Baker (2015) suggested that using intentional strategies that assist you to recall content in the moment is what enhances the encoding and transfer into long-term memory. This would also suggest that teaching something once may not be effective. Unfortunately, this is a common teaching practice governed by a long-held belief that content that you can recall once indicates learning has occurred. Strategic use of retrieval practices that help you to manage cognitive load and space out the time frame when content is again revisited, creates a more meaningful approach for the transfer of learning to long-term memory.

Blocked Spacing vs. Interleaving

Blocked spacing and interleaving are both forms of retrieval practice and when used effectively create opportunities to recall and use existing content knowledge. Blocked spacing is the presentation of a chunk of content that is spaced out *over* a period. Interleaving is the presentation of chunks of content switching back and forth *within* a set period. Time is the important differentiator, *over time* versus *within a period of time* (Agarwal, 2019; Weidman & Baker, 2015).

Using Table 4.2, let's explore how you as a faculty learner might better understand *over time* versus *within a period of time* using the previous examples of desirable difficulty and metacognition. When learning using a blocked approach, you can see that the concepts of desirable difficulty and metacognition are split up between weeks 1 and 2. Using an interleaved approach, you would experience a varied approach discussion on desirable difficulty and metacognition within the same week or within even the same class.

Both strategies use similar forms of retrieval practices, yet the effects differ. They both use a form of spacing to provide some time for forgetting so you can enhance your memory with opportunities to recall the information. With the example of interleaving, you would experience a switching back and forth between the topics of desirable difficulty and metacognition within the same period of time. The forgetting time is less and is interrupted by the addition of new content. Inductive reasoning is enhanced as you

TABLE 4.2

Retrieval Practices of Metacognition and Desirable Difficulty

Retrieval Practice	Week 1	Week 2
Blocked	Desirable difficulty	Metacognition
	Desirable difficulty	Metacognition
	Desirable difficulty	Metacognition
	Desirable difficulty	Metacognition
Interleaved	Metacognition	Desirable difficulty
	Metacognition	Desirable difficulty
	Desirable difficulty	Metacognition
	Desirable difficulty	Metacognition

move from desirable difficulty to metacognition without completely understanding one before moving to the next. This strategy is effective when the topics are similar and are mixed; learning to differentiate in the moment. When topics are different, (e.g., metacognition and test item analysis), interleaving would not be an effective strategy. Learning is enhanced when the content can be themed and mixed to enhance differentiation when switching between topics. The key is that you are using bits of content from each topic as you move to the whole of understanding (Argawal, 2019; Firth et al., 2019).

As suggested by Agarwal (2019), every educator must have a deep understanding of desirable difficulty, metacognition, and retrieval. With intentional consideration, the three practices work together to create a dynamic learning encounter that fosters deep learning. Beginning with the end in mind, guided by learning outcomes, one employs all practices to structure and create an opportunity for learners to make meaning.

SETTING THE COURSE FOR FACULTY DEVELOPMENT

In the previous chapter sections both context and content were presented; setting a context for learning, and how the content of learning can be strategically presented to enhance learning. As the faculty learner, you had the opportunity to read and reflect on both. In this final section, we explore how to move forward and use this content to change your teaching and learning practice, setting the course.

Faculty as Learner

In a descriptive study by Patterson and Forneris (2023), nurse educators involved in a 10-week/30-hour faculty intensive, were studied to determine how the learning of neuroscience strategies impacted nurse educator teaching practice. The intensive was specifically designed for faculty to experience, as learners, neuroscience strategies in action. The neuroscience concepts, retrieval practices, metacognition, and desirable difficulty, were experienced by the faculty while they were engaged in learning about them (i.e., the topic of retrieval practices included the facilitator role-modeling a retrieval strategy while they engaged the faculty learners in a retrieval activity). The faculty, as learners, explored the content of neuroscience principles while they were experiencing them. As a faculty educator participant in the intensive course program, they were the learner.

Cognitive Shift

Faculty as learner was an important role in the exploration and experience of neuroscience teaching and learning (Patterson & Forneris, 2023). Teaching and learning concepts were at the center of the intensive experience and included setting a safe learning space (the context) to explore neuroscience principles (the content). The neuroscience principles were the framework that engaged the faculty learner and provided the occasion to experience the context and content of learning. As learners, a student-centered approach using neuroscience principles, which they were simultaneously learning, created an opportunity to deepen their understanding. The blending of context and content informed the learning lens; as learners, they valued intentional experiential learning encounters. Patterson and Forneris (2023) concluded that faculty learners made a cognitive shift in the way they thought about teaching. The safe, intentional, immersive learning environment as the context to explore the content of neuroscience teaching created an informed new understanding of teaching; a cognitive shift from teaching with *teaching in mind* to teaching with *learning in mind*.

Learning in Mind

The study findings (Patterson & Forneris, 2023) supported that the cognitive shift occurred because the educators had experienced learning. As learners, they understood and embraced the shift needed to redirect their teaching practice in a new and informed manner. Patterson and Forneris (2023) found that the faculty learners emphasized the importance of adopting a critical perspective, examining the whys in their own thinking as well exploring the whys in their students' thinking. This was articulated as a shift from teaching to learning; the educator must focus on how the content is being perceived and used. In other words, *coming to the learning space with learning in mind.*

The faculty-as-learner experience emphasized the importance of being responsible for one's learning; responsibility was understood and embraced when, as faculty learners, they experienced active engagement. The experience clarified for them why neuroscience strategies work and motivate learners. They could articulate how educators ensure learning and were empowered to begin teaching using those same neuroscience strategies.

Teaching and learning blend along a continuum. Building faculty expertise in teaching with neuroscience strategies to secure higher-level reasoning in student learners is imperative in today's nursing education environments. These strategies are successful because the teaching is focused on how educators guide student learners to use the content. It is not about teaching the content; it is imperative educators teach the student how to use the content for learning.

BRAIN SCIENCE CONSIDERATIONS: PREPARING EDUCATORS TO TEACH SOCIAL DETERMINANTS OF HEALTH

The exemplar set out in Table 4.3 outlines considerations for faculty preparation to teach the social determinants of health guided by the foundational brain science principles previously discussed.

TABLE 4.3	
Exemplar: Faculty Development to Teach Social Determinants of Health Using Brain Science Principles	
Brain Science Principle	**Teaching Approach**
Desirable difficulty	**CLASS SESSION 1:** As educator learners enter the classroom, they are provided a sheet listing the social determinants of health. Working in small groups, they assess the influence of the determinant (i.e., strongly deters health; moderately deters health, neutral; strongly supports health, moderately supports health) based on the World Health Organization (n.d.) definition of health. Small groups discuss rationale for choices as they work together. Large group conversations compare and contrast social determinants of health influencers across small groups and their impact on nursing practice.
Retrieval practices	**CLASS SESSION 2:** As educator learners enter the classroom, they are randomly assigned a patient persona and a description of the town where the persona lives. The personas they are given are designed to provide an opportunity for the learners to explore the different dimensions of the social determinants of health as they relate to their assigned identity. Educator learners are asked to recall the social determinants of health activity in which they were previously involved, specifically their recollections of the social determinants of health. Educator learners then independently assess the social determinants of their personas. Educator learners then move into small groups on the basis of the towns/cities where their personas reside. Discussions ensue in these small groups comparing their persona assessments. Guided questions are used to facilitate small group conversations.
Metacognition	**CLASS SESSION 2:** (End of class classroom assessment technique) The last 20 minutes of class time: Write a reflection as follows: ➤ Consider the persona and assigned town/city. Select two social determinants that you assessed. ➤ Describe why you believe these determinants influence health for your persona. ➤ As a professional nurse, how does this influence your overall practice considerations?

Adapted from Richardson, J. W. (2020). An active learning approach to teaching social determinants of health. *Pedagogy in Health Promotion: The Scholarship of Teaching and Learning, 1–8*. https://doi.org/10.1177/2373379920933311j

CHAPTER SUMMARY

In this chapter, we focused on faculty development and the importance of preparing and developing faculty to teach, recognizing with faculty development the faculty member is the faculty learner. This chapter included the requisite preparation, development, and support. The education literature supports the need for intentional opportunities for faculty as a learner to experience "how to teach" throughout their preparation as educators. These learning experiences inform our knowing and in turn, with an experiential new lens, positively impact how we implement teaching our students moving forward.

References

Agarwal, P. K. (2019). Retrieval practice & Bloom's taxonomy: Do students need fact knowledge before higher order learning? *Journal of Educational Psychology*, *111*(2), 189–209. https://doi.org/10.1037/edu0000282

Agarwal, P. K., & Bain, P. (2019). *Powerful teaching: Unleash the science of learning*. John Wiley & Sons, Incorporated.

Benner, P. (2015). Curricular and pedagogical implications for the Carnegie study, educating nurses: A call for radical transformation. *Asian Nursing Research*, *9*(1), 1–6. https://doi.org/10.1016/j.anr.2015.02.001

Bjork, R. A. (1994). Memory and metamemory considerations in the training of human beings. In J. Metcalfe & A. Shimamura (Eds.), *Metacognition: Knowing about knowing* (pp. 185–205). MIT Press.

Bjork, R. A. (2013). Desirable difficulties perspective on learning. In H. Pashler (Ed.), *Encyclopedia of the mind*. Sage.

Booth, T. L., Emerson, C. J., Hackney, M. G., & Souter, S. (2016). Preparation of nurse educators. *Nurse Education in Practice*, *19*, 54–57. https://doi.org/10.1016/j.nepr.2016.04.006

Brunt, B., & Russell, J. (2022). Nursing professional development standards. In *StatPearls Publishing*. https://www.ncbi.nlm.nih.gov/books/NBK534784

Bullin, C. (2018). To what extent has the doctoral (PhD) education supported academic nurse educators in their teaching roles: An integrative review. *BMC Nursing*, *17*(6), 1–18. https://doi.org/10.1186/s12912-018-0273-3

Caputi, L., & Frank, B. (2019). Competency I: Facilitate learning. In J. A. Halstead (Ed.), *NLN Core competencies for nurse educators: A decade of influence* (pp. 17–44). National League for Nursing.

Christensen, L. S., & Simmons, L. E. (2020). *The scope of practice for academic nurse educators & academic clinical nurse educators* (3rd ed.). National League for Nursing.

Cooley, S., & De Gagne, J. (2016). Transformative experience: Developing competence in novice nurse faculty. *Journal of Nursing Education*, *55*(2), 96–100. https://doi.org/10.3928.01484834-20160114-07

Crider, C. (2022). Pedagogical content knowledge for nurse educators: An intersection of disciplines. *Teaching and Learning in Nursing*, *17*(4), 449–454. https://doi.org/10.1016/j.teln.2022.01.001

Deans for Impact. (2021). *Learning by scientific design*. https://deansforimpact.org/resources/learning-by-scientific-design/

DeFelippo, A. M., & Dee, J. R. (2022). Vitality in the academic workplace: Sustaining professional growth for mid-career faculty. *Innovative Higher Education*, *47*, 565–585. https://doi.org/10.1007/s10755-021-09589-z

Doukakis, S., & Alexopoulos, E. (2021). Online learning, neuroscience and knowledge transformation opportunities for secondary students. *Journal of Higher Education Theory and Practice*, *21*(3), 49–57. https://doi.org/10.33423/jhetp.v21i3.4141

Doyle, T., & Zakrajsek, T. (2019). *The new science of learning: How to learn in harmony with your brain* (2nd ed.). Stylus Publishing.

Drummond-Young, M., Brown, B., Noesgaard, C., Lunyk-Child, O., Maich, N. M., Mines, C., & Linton, J. (2010). A comprehensive faculty development model for nursing education. *Journal of Professional Nursing, 26*(3), 152–161. https://doi.org/10.1016/j.profnurs.2009.04.004

Dweck, C. (2016). *Mindset: Changing the way you think to fulfill your potential* (Updated ed.). Random House.

Edmondson, A. C. (2019). *The fearless organization: Creating psychological safety in the workplace for learning, innovation, and growth.* Wiley.

Firth, J., Rivers, I., & Boyle, J. (2019). A Systematic review of interleaving as a concept learning strategy: A study protocol. *Social Science Protocols,* (2), 1–7.

Fitzwater, J., McNeill, J., Monsivais, D., & Nunez, F. (2021). Using simulation to facilitate transition to the nurse educator role: An integrative review. *Nurse Educator, 46*(5), 322–326. https://doi.org/10.1097/NNE.0000000000000961

Forman, T., Armor, D., & Miller, A. (2019). A review of clinical informatics competencies in nursing to inform best practices in education and nurse faculty development. *Nursing Education Perspectives, 41*(1), e3–e7. https://doi.org/10.1097/01.NEP.0000000000000588

Forneris, S. G., & Fey, M. (Eds.). (2018). *Critical conversations: The NLN guide for teaching thinking.* National League for Nursing.

Forneris, S. G., & Fey, M. (Eds.). (2021). *Critical conversations (Volume 2): From monologue to dialogue.* National League for Nursing.

Forneris, S. G., & Fey, M. K. (2016). *The NLN Guide for Teaching Thinking.* National League for Nursing. http://www.nln.org/docs/default-source/professional-development-programs/nln-guide-to-teaching-thinking.pdf?sfvrsn=2

Garner, A., & Bedford, L. (2021). Reflecting on educational preparedness and professional development for early-career nurse faculty: A phenomenological study. *Nurse Education in Practice, 53*(2021), 103052. https://doi.org/10.1016/j.nepr.2021.103052

Goswami, U. (2008). Principles of learning, implications for teaching: A cognitive neuroscience perspective. *Journal of the Philosophy of Education, 42*(3–4), 2008. https://doi.org/10.1111/j.1467-9752.2008.00639.x

Halstead, J. A. (2007). *Nurse educator competencies: Creating an evidence-based practice for nurse educators.* National League for Nursing.

Halstead, J. A. (2019). *NLN Core competencies for nurse educators: A decade of influence.* National League for Nursing.

Han, H. R., D'Aoust, R., Gross, D., Szanton, S., Nolan, M., Campbell, J., & Davidson, P. (2022). Preparing future nursing faculty: Integrating enhanced teaching and leadership development curricula into PhD education [Editorial]. *Journal of Advanced Nursing, 78,* e3–e5. https://doi.org/10.1111/jan.14982

Jeffers, S., & Mariani, B. (2017). The effect of a formal mentoring program on career satisfaction and intent to stay in the faculty role for novice nurse faculty. *Nursing Education Perspectives, 38*(1), 18–22. https://doi.org/10.1097/01.NEP.0000000000000104

Johnson-Crowley, N. (2004). An alternative framework for teacher preparation in nursing. *The Journal of Continuing Education in Nursing, 35*(1), 34–43. https://doi.org/10.3928/0022-0124-20040101-11

Kalensky, M., & Hande, K. (2017). Transition from expert clinician to novice faculty: A blueprint for success. *The Journal for Nurse Practitioners, 13*(9), e433–e439. https://doi.org/10.1016/j.nurpra.2017.06.005

Lee, D., Paulus, T., Loboda, I., Phipps, G., Wyatt, T., Myers, C., & Mixer, S. (2010). A faculty development program for nurse educators learning to teach online. *TechTrends: Linking Research and Practice to Improve Learning, 54*(6), 20–28. https://www.learntechlib.org/p/65615/

Leibold, N., Schwartz, L., & Gordon, D. (2022). Culturally responsive teaching in nursing education: A faculty development project. *Creative Nursing, 28*(3), 154–160. https://doi.org/10.1891/CN-2021-0044

Lerner, J. S., Li, Y., Valdesolo, P., & Kassam, K. S. (2015). Emotion and decision making. *Annual Review of Psychology, 66,* 799–823. https://doi.org/10.1146/annurev-psych-010213-115043

Mackessy-Lloyd, E. L., Frith, K., & Dickson, M. (2019). Enhancing the teaching experiences of adjunct nursing faculty in an associate degree nursing program through a focused online mentoring intervention. *International Journal of Nursing and Health Care Research, 2*(2), 1–10. https://doi.org/ 10.29011/IJNHR-071.1000071

McCleary, L., McGilton, K., Boscart, V., & Oudshoorn, A. (2009). Improving geron- tology content in baccalaureate nursing education through knowledge transfer to nurse educators. *Nursing Leadership, 22*(3), 33–46. https://doi.org/10.12927/ cjnl.2009.21153

Miller, S. H., DeMolle, D., Menge, K., & Voorhees, D. H. (2022). Faculty-led profes- sional development: Designing effective workshops to facilitate change. In E. M. D. Baer, K. M. Layou, & R. H. Macdonald (Eds.), *Catalyzing change: STEM faculty as change agents. New Directions for Com- munity Colleges* (Vol. 199, pp. 149–161). John Wiley & Sons. https://doi.org/10.1002/ cc.20530

National League for Nursing (n.d.). Core competencies for academic nurse educa- tors. Retrieved from https://www.nln.org/ education/nursing-education-competencies/ core-competencies-for-academic-nurse- educators

National League for Nursing. (2015a). *A vision for teaching with simulation*. NLN Vision Series. https://www.nln.org/docs/ default-source/uploadedfiles/about/ nln-vision-series-position-statements/ vision-statement-a-vision-for-teaching-with- simulation.pdf?sfvrsn=e847da0d_0

National League for Nursing. (2015b). *Debriefing across the curriculum*. NLN Vision Series. https://www.nln.org/docs/ default-source/uploadedfiles/about/ nln-vision-series-position-statements/nln- vision-debriefing-across-the-curriculum. pdf?sfvrsn=e8bbdb0d_0

National League for Nursing. (2022). *NLN mentoring toolkit*. https://www.nln.org/docs/ default-source/default-document-library/ nln-mentoring-toolkit-2022.pdf

Noone, J. (2022). Preparing nurse educators to teach social determinants of health using

backward design. *Journal of Nursing Education, 61*(9), 511–515. https://doi. org/10.3928/01484834-20220705-05

O'Connor, M. R., Barrington, W. E., Buchanan, D. T., Bustillos, D., Eagen-Torkko, M., Kalkbrenner, A., Laing, S. S., Reding, K. W., & de Castro, A. B. (2019). Short-term outcomes of a diversity, equity, and inclusion institute for nursing faculty. *The Journal of Nursing Education, 58*(11), 633–640. https://doi.org/ 10.3928/01484834-20191021-04

Oermann, M. H. (2017). Preparing nurse faculty. It's for everyone [Editorial]. *Nurse Educator, 42*(1), 1. https://doi.org/10.1097/ NNE.0000000000000345

Okon-Singer, H., Hendler, T., Pessoa, L., & Shackman, A. J. (2015). The neurobiology of emotion-cognition interactions: Fundamental questions and strategies for future research. *Frontiers in Human Neuroscience, 9*, 58. https://doi.org/10.3389/fnhum.2015.00058

Oprescu, F., McAllister, M., Duncan, D., & Jones, C. (2017). Professional development needs of nurse educators. An Australian case study. *Nurse Education in Practice, 27*, 165–168. https://doi.org/10.1016/j.nepr.2017.07.004

Pan, S. C., & Rickard, T. C. (2018). Transfer of test-enhanced learning: Meta-analytic review and synthesis. *Psychological Bulletin, 144*(7), 710–756. https://doi.org/10.1037/bul0000151

Patterson, B., & Forneris, S. (2023). Faculty as learner: Neuroscience in action. *Journal of Nursing Education, 62*(5), 291–297.

Pelletier, K., Brown, M., Brooks, D. C., McCormack, M., Reeves, J., Arbino, N., Bozkurt, A., Crawford, S., Czerniewicz, L., Gibson, R., Linder, K., Mason, J., & Mondelli, V. (2021). *EDUCAUSE hori- zon report, teaching and learning edi- tion*. https://library.educause.edu/ resources/2021/4/2021-educause-horizon- report-teaching-and-learning-edition

Pessoa, L. (2015). Précis on the cognitive- emotional brain. *Behavioral and Brain Sciences, 38*, 1–66. https://doi.org/10.1017/ S0140525X14000120

Privitera, A. J. (2021). A scoping review of research on neuroscience training for teachers. *Trends in Neuroscience and Education, 24*, 100157. https://doi. org/10.1016/j.tine.2021.100157

Quinco, D., Cabanilla, A., & Cadosales, M. N. Q. (2022). Meta-synthesis on faculty development during the Covid-19 pandemic. *Journal of Positive School Psychology*, *6*(8), 981–991.

Randall, C. S., & Randall, C. E. (2021). Critical incident videos: Developing a cognitive strategy in simulation for faculty development. *Journal of Nursing Education*, *60*(2), 81–89. https://doi.org/10.3928/01484834-20210120-05

Reese, C., & Ketner, M. B. (2017). The nurse educator institute: An innovative strategy to develop nursing faculty. *Nurse Educator*, *42*(5), 224–225. https://doi.org/10.1097/NNE.0000000000000380

Richardson, J. W. (2020). An active learning approach to teaching social determinants of health. *Pedagogy in Health Promotion: The Scholarship of Teaching and Learning*, 1–8. https://doi.org/10.1177/2373379920933311j

Ross, J. G., & Dunkler, K. S. (2019). New clinical nurse faculty orientation: A review of the literature. *Nursing Education Perspectives*, *40*(4), 210–215. https://doi.org/10.1097/01.NEP.0000000000000470

Seldin, P. (2006). Tailoring faculty development programs to faculty career stages. *To Improve the Academy*, *24*, 137–146. https://doi.org/10.1002/j.2334-4822.2006.tb00455.x

Shellenbarger, T. (2019). *Clinical nurse educator competencies: Creating an evidence-based practice for academic clinical nurse educators*. National League for Nursing.

Smallheer, B., Gedzyk-Nieman, S., Molloy, M., Clark, C., Gordon, H., & Morgan, B. (2021). Faculty development workshop on gender-associated incivility in nursing education. *Nursing Forum*, *56*(4), 1044–1051. https://doi.org/10.1111/nuf/12615

Smith, J., Kean, S., Vauhkonen, A., Eloneen, I., Silva, S. C., Pajari, J., Cassar, M., Martín-Delgado, L., Zrubcova, D., & Salminen, L. (2023). An integrative review of continuing professional development needs for nurse educators. *Nurse Education Today*, *121*(2023), 1–11. https://doi.org/10.1016/j.nedt.2022.105695

Valiga, T. M. (2019). Competency VI: Pursue continuous quality improvement in the nurse educator role. In J. A. Halstead (Ed.), *NLN Core competencies for nurse educators: A decade of influence* (pp. 123–134). National League for Nursing.

Walker, C., Humphrey, S., & Chandler, V. (2022). Expanding nursing faculty development through a fitness initiative. *Building Healthy Academic Communities Journal*, *6*(2), 16–26. https://doi.org/10.18061/bhac.v6i2.8940

Weidman, J., & Baker, K. (2015). The cognitive science of learning: Concepts and strategies for the educator and learner. *Neuroscience in Anesthesiology and Perioperative Medicine*, *121*(6), 1586–1599. https://doi.org/10.1213/ANE.0000000000000890

Wright, M., Horii, C. V., Felton, P., Sorcinelli, D., & Kaplan, M. (2018). Faculty development improves teaching and learning. *POD Speaks Issue #2*. https://podnetwork.org/content/uploads/POD-Speaks-Issue-2_Jan2018-1.pdf

Young-Brice, A., Farrar-Stern, K., & Malin, M. (2022). Comprehensive onboarding and orientation to support newly hired faculty in a nursing program. *Nurse Educator*, *47*(6), 347–351. https://doi.org/10.1097/NNE.0000000000001242

2

Best Teaching Practices

5

Creating Inclusive Learning Environments

Teri A. Murray, PhD, PHNA-BC, RN, FAAN, ANEF

CHAPTER OVERVIEW

This chapter will review strategies for creating a culturally inclusive and responsive learning environment. The focus of this chapter will be on course design and interactions with learners that promote inclusion, equity, and belonging. Principles for identifying and responding to microaggressions in the classroom and clinical learning environments will be presented. Strategies for discussion of difficult topics will be reviewed.

INTRODUCTION
Diversity, Equity, Inclusion, and Justice

Creating an inclusive learning environment mandates an understanding of diversity, equity, inclusion, and justice (DEIJ). While the individual terms that comprise DEIJ have been used extensively in the literature, a brief definition is warranted since understanding the terms may vary from individual to individual. *Diversity* focuses on representation of perceived differences, often concerning aspects of one's social identity and the intersection of multiple and complex features of those identities. When discussing diversity as it relates to the learning environment, the aim of having a diverse learning environment is to expose students to varying perspectives and worldviews. This exposure can provide students with the knowledge, skills, and ability to function in a multicultural and pluralistic society. Thus, having diverse students within the classroom provides the students with the opportunity to partake in teaching and learning situations through various cultural lenses and engage more effectively in intercultural and multicultural environments (Aoun, 2017).

It is important that all students feel seen and heard in the classroom setting to realize the benefits of diverse perspectives and views. *Inclusion*, then, is when faculty intentionally incorporate educational strategies that foster a sense of connectedness and belonging by promoting meaningful interactions among students in the learning environment representing different characteristics, perceptions, and experiences (Metzger et al., 2020). Inclusion is where the students see themselves as active members of the learning environment. Their backgrounds, insights, and contributions are valued as part of the learning environment's creativity and productivity (Ackerman-Barger et al., 2016). Inclusion and belonging are closely tied to increased academic success, improved grade point averages, and retention (Kivlighan et al., 2018; Pentaraki & Burkholder, 2017).

Equity recognizes the different positions and spaces one occupies in life and acknowledges that some students are more advantaged than others. Equality is about fairness, wherein every student is treated the same. Equity involves providing individuals with the resources needed to be successful with the understanding that some student populations have historically been disenfranchised and entrenched in inequitable systems. Faculty with an equity mindset recognize the historical and contemporary patterns of educational disenfranchisement that have negatively impacted students and their learning experiences.

Justice involves dismantling practices and policies with disparate impacts on historically excluded groups (Stewart, 2017). Family income, wealth, and social position play a role in the educational opportunities available to students. These factors can support the additional enrichment opportunities and supplemental supports that help some students get ahead more than others. Justice examines the inequities that stem from the differential distribution of power and resources that privilege some students and disadvantage others. Justice demands envisioning policies and practices that produce equitable outcomes (Stewart, 2017).

The Pedagogy of Social Justice

The degree to which social justice influences the teaching-learning process remains understudied and often misunderstood since social justice is conceptually ambiguous and means different things to different people (Reagan & Hambacher, 2021). However, it is theorized that the pedagogy of social justice recognizes the significant disparities in the distribution of educational opportunities, resources, achievement, and positive outcomes between students from historically excluded groups compared to their non-Hispanic White counterparts (Cochran-Smith et al., 2009). For example, more affluent school districts, which are often located in predominantly White neighborhoods, have more qualified and experienced teachers, greater technological adjuncts for teaching, lower teacher-to-student classroom ratios, and more curricular and extracurricular enrichment opportunities to support learning as compared to students in less affluent and under-resourced schools. In educating for social justice, Whiteness is decentered; that is, the teaching counteracts the normative culture of Whiteness and affirms the multiple perspectives and lived experiences of students from marginalized cultures (Carter Andrews et al., 2021). When teaching for social justice, the teacher addresses societal inequities within their classrooms with the overall goal of improving student learning and enhancing every student's chance to succeed academically.

Traditional pedagogical approaches in nursing education often rely on didactic and teacher-centric methods that expect students to adapt to this learning approach, invariably giving little consideration to students whose learning styles might be cognitively or culturally different. Classroom dynamics shape the learning atmosphere and include the decisions regarding classroom practices, interactions with students, and the ability to connect with students. These dynamics also include how the faculty manages and organizes the classroom, their approach to their work, and how the faculty interprets what's happening in the classroom. The pedagogy of social justice recognizes how social identities and system inequities impact students in the academic setting. Accordingly, creating inclusive learning environments can transform the historical pedagogical practices in nursing education that have harmed or disadvantaged students from historically excluded or marginalized groups (Charania & Patel, 2022). Inclusive, just learning environments ensure that all students are treated equitably and feel welcomed, valued, and respected in the classroom, clinical, or laboratory settings.

Psychological Safety

Psychological safety is achieved when students feel their identity, perspectives, and contributions to the learning environment are valued (Lain, 2018). In psychologically safe environments, students feel comfortable taking the initiative, interacting with others, and speaking out without fear of humiliation, embarrassment, or being punished (Clark, 2020). Psychological safety is based on a mutual belief that it is okay to express ideas and concerns, speak up with questions, and admit that you lack understanding about some course materials—all without the fear of consequences (Gallo, 2023). A psychologically safe environment is necessary for students to establish feelings of trust and belonging and is vital for student learning.

Factors that can threaten the psychological safety of students include feelings of invisibility, lack of acknowledgment, humiliation, microaggressions, discrimination, and the lack of diversity in the classroom environment. Consequently, when psychological safety is lacking, the student expends more energy coping than learning. This, ultimately, contributes to poor academic performance and often leads to stereotype threat and imposter syndrome (Lain, 2018).

Stereotype Threat

In stereotype threat, stereotypic reputations of intellectual inferiority, often based on a group's social identity, can undermine performance on intellectual testing despite not having any actual difference in their cognitive ability (Croizet et al., 2004). When faculty are evaluating students, and the student believes the faculty perceive them as cognitively inferior, their performance suffers. When the student fears confirming an allegation of inferiority conveyed by the negative stereotype, the fear triggers psychological and physiological processes that expend extra cognitive and emotional load creating a disruptive mental workload (Spencer et al., 2016; Smith, 2020; Stewart & Valian, 2018; Croizet et al., 2004). These mechanisms drain cognitive energy or create cognitive interference and result in lowered performance. Strategies that faculty can employ to reduce stereotype threat include conveying to students that diversity is valued; supporting the student's sense of belonging; having diverse representations in course materials; facilitating multicultural interactions among students; and exposing students to successful role models with similar social identities that refute negative stereotypes (Carr et al., n.d.).

Imposter Syndrome

Imposter syndrome is described as feelings of inadequacy, self-doubt, and intellectual fraudulence that persist despite previous achievements and successes (Murray & Noone,

2022; Corkindale, 2008). With imposter syndrome, the student will feel a sense of inadequacy coupled with fear of being exposed as a fraud or imposter, not really belonging in the setting (Murray & Noone, 2022; Chrousos & Mentis, 2020; Mullangi & Jagsi, 2019). The consequences of imposter syndrome in students can lead to psychological stress and anxiety. Since imposter syndrome is an internalized problem, faculty members can assist by encouraging students, if aware of the syndrome, to get counseling and also offer the student positive affirmations. Imposter syndrome disproportionately affects students of color in predominantly White institutions (Murray & Noone, 2022; Chrousos & Mentis, 2020; Mullangi & Jagsi, 2019; Cokley et al., 2017).

UNIVERSAL DESIGN FOR LEARNING

Definition and Historical Roots

Universal Design (UD) was introduced by Ronald Mace, an architectural designer who believed that all products and environments should be designed with the most usability and the least adaptability for use by everyone (Kearney, 2022). Universal Design is a proactive approach based on principles to achieve the following aim: Build structures that can be accessed by anyone regardless of ability, age, size, or other attributes (Yerkey, 2022). Universally designed structures work for everyone, not just those with challenges of accessibility. Universal Design, initially conceived to allow students with physical disabilities to access mainstream classroom settings, has now been applied to the educational environment as the Universal Design for Learning (UDL). UDL recognizes that all students have varied and diverse learning needs. UDL maximizes learning for students and demonstrates how curricula can provide genuine learning opportunities for all students through a proactive design.

UDL guides faculty in the design of curricular goals, materials, instructional strategies, and assessments of student achievement (CAST, 2022). The proactive design of UDL makes the teaching-learning process more effective for a broad range of learners (Jung, 2021). The UDL guidelines are based on scientific insights into how people learn and offer concrete strategies and principles that ensure that learning is accessible, meaningful, and challenging for all students (CAST, 2022). UDL offers guidelines on making classroom environments welcoming, responsive, supportive, and flexible through multiple means of engagement, representation, and action and expression (Jung, 2021). Difficulties in student learning often originate from the design of the educational activity rather than the student's inability to learn to grasp the concepts. UDL recognizes that variability and diversity within students are normal and can be planned for within the educational design (Yerkey, 2022). The UDL approach creates equity in the learning environment.

UDL Neural Networks and Principles

The UDL is based on neuroscience research that identified three primary neural networks in the brain that influences learning: Affective, Recognition, and Strategic. The Affective network attends to the student's interest, motivation, effort, and willingness to engage in the teaching-learning process (CAST, 2022). It is the reason or the "why" behind learning. It is what motivates and answers the question, "why is learning this

TABLE 5.1

Universal Design for Learning Neural Networks

Affective (Why)	Recognition (What)	Strategic (How)
Engagement	Representation	Action and Expression

The "Why" of Learning	The "What" of Learning	The "How" of Learning
➤ Interest	➤ Perception	➤ Physical action
➤ Motivation	➤ Comprehension	➤ Expression and communication
➤ Effort		➤ Executive function
➤ Self-regulation		

Reprinted with permission from CAST (2022). *About universal design for learning*. Retrieved from https://www.cast.org/impact/universal-design-for-learning-udl.

necessary?" The Affective network, the "why" of learning, commits the learner to the educational process, including the goals and outcomes (Gilmore et al., 2022). The Recognition network involves the student's perception and comprehension of incoming materials (CAST, 2022). It is the "what" of learning. What knowledge, skills, or abilities should I be learning? It deals with cognition. The Recognition network considers how the learner comprehends the information they have been exposed to during the teaching-learning process. The Strategic network, the "how" of learning, involves action, expression and communication, and the use of an executive function (CAST, 2022). The Strategic network deals with the information-processing component of learning. The "how" I can demonstrate what I have learned focuses on how the learners process and apply the information. Table 5.1 illustrates how the three neural networks (Affective, Recognition, and Strategic), in conjunction with the three principles of UDL (Engagement, Representation, Action & Expression), work together to promote student learning. For the application of Universal Design for Learning Principles, see Chapter 6, *Frameworks to Engage Diverse Learners*.

Definition and the Empirical Basis for Equity-Focused Teaching

More than two decades of empirical evidence support the assertion that feelings of exclusion, whether conscious, unconscious, or subconscious, have a tremendous impact on students' ability to learn, their working memory, and their ability to perform in academic situations (Tanner, 2013). Equity-focused teaching is based on research that shows how the relationships between classroom climate and the student's sense of belonging, including stereotype threat and imposter syndrome, impact the teaching-learning process (Center for Research on Teaching & Learning [CRLT], 2021). In an equity-focused teaching environment, all students have equitable access to learning, feel valued, respected, and supported by the faculty and the learning community, and are mutually engaged in the teaching-learning process (CRLT, 2021). Thus, equity-focused teaching is designed to create an inclusive learning environment based on five principles: critical engagement of difference, structured interactions, academic belonging, transparency, and flexibility (CRLT, 2021).

The Five Principles of Equity-Focused Teaching

The first principle, *critical engagement of difference*, is when the faculty member is aware of the different identities and experiences of the students in their classroom and leverages those differences as an asset for learning to spark rich and varied dialogues among students (CRLT, 2021). Embedded in this principle is that faculty members have a critical consciousness and interrogation of their beliefs, values, social identity, privilege, and power that invites an understanding of their social location and position relative to their students (Reed et al., 2022). This consciousness should enable the faculty member to recognize that students' learning needs and abilities are shaped by their differences in identity and lived experiences and therefore adjust their pedagogical approaches accordingly.

Structured interactions, the second principle, enable students to get to know each other and have exposure to cognitive diversity. To engage all students in the teaching-learning process, the faculty member creates group norms for communication and provides opportunities for peer-to-peer exchanges and small-group learning (CRLT, 2021). Understanding how other students think, learn, and process information can enhance student learning. Structured interactions can lay the groundwork for future collaborations among students on team projects or clinical assignments.

Faculty members should listen to the concerns of students who convey feelings of unwelcomeness or lack of belonging. To *foster belonging* (the third principle), the faculty member should recognize the student's need to legitimately feel a part of the learning environment. Faculty members can help students authenticate themselves as potential members of the nursing profession by ensuring their teaching materials show diverse images, representations, and perspectives (CRLT, 2021).

The fourth principle of *transparency* involves ensuring that students are clear about course expectations, methods of evaluation, and what's required to be successful in the course. The learning materials should be diverse, inclusive, and representative of multiple social identities, including race, ethnicity, gender, gender identity, sexual orientation, ability, socioeconomic status, and others. The faculty member can also normalize help-seeking behaviors so that students feel comfortable approaching the faculty for help.

Lastly, *flexibility* is being student-centered and appropriately responding and adapting to circumstances that might occur within the teaching-learning situation (CRLT, 2021). It involves faculty understanding the unique challenges that students from historically excluded backgrounds face in the classroom and as future nurses (Charania & Patel, 2022). Faculty can be flexible while still holding the student accountable (Table 5.2). Flexibility

TABLE 5.2

Equity-Focused Teaching Application Strategies

Acknowledge Differences	Structure Interactions	Create a Sense of Belonging	Be Transparent	Provide Flexibility
➤ Acknowledge the varying identities of the students in the classroom and how that diversity contributes to the richness of the learning environment.	➤ Call students by their preferred names (correctly pronounced) and pronouns.	➤ Cultivate a learning environment that reflects and respects students' values.	➤ Communicate the course/clinical objectives, the assignments and how they will be graded, testing, and minimum grade requirements.	➤ Assess learning needs.
➤ Ask students to be mindful of their and other identities in the classroom.	➤ Encourage the active involvement and participation of all students.	➤ Integrate diverse examples, names, and sociocultural contexts when teaching and in all course materials.		➤ Build flexibility in student assignments and assessments.
➤ Normalize that students will have a range of backgrounds and identities.	➤ Assign group work to facilitate student interaction, such as think, pair, and share activities.	➤ Structure classroom and clinical discussions to include a range of voices.	➤ Allow time in class for students to clarify the expectations and ask questions about tests or assignments.	➤ Use various teaching-learning strategies (lecture, problem-based, case-based, and active learning exercises).
➤ Establish a norm for respectful interactions within the classroom.	➤ Be explicit about the need for and value of diverse perspectives.	➤ Use language in the syllabus that builds community, such as "we."	➤ Be intentional in promoting access and equity for all students.	➤ Solicit feedback from students regarding teaching-learning approaches.
➤ Reflect upon ways your identity has shaped your relationship to your work and to nursing.	➤ Provide students the opportunity to reflect with peers on what they've learned in class.	➤ Incorporate a welcoming statement in the syllabus that highlights the value of diverse perspectives.		➤ Invite students to share their expectations about the learning environment.
➤ Select course materials and readings (authors, images, etc.) that reflect the diversity of contributors to nursing.	➤ Promote civil discourse among students.			

is one way of being sensitive to the student's situation and working with the student so that it does not impair their ability to learn.

Application of Equity-Focused Teaching Principles to Nursing Education

Specific strategies by the faculty member can effectively promote learning by working toward a more inclusive, fair, and equitable classroom community for all students (Tanner, 2013). According to the *Boyer 2030 Commission Report*, students are most successful when evidence-based inclusive pedagogical practices are used, such as active learning strategies, which include low-stakes and ungraded assignments enriched by the faculty member's formative and summative assessment (The Association for Undergraduate Education at Research Universities [UERU], 2022). The use of the flipped classroom is a strategy that maximizes classroom effectiveness. The flipped classroom enables the student to engage in higher-order activities, such as small group discussion and group problem-solving—which are more engaging, expand their learning, and help to address inequities that hinder student success (UERU, 2022). Furthermore, the flipped classroom has the potential to create a supportive learning environment that may benefit the student's sense of belonging, leading to greater academic success. This technique is reviewed in depth in Chapter 8, *Strategies for Active and Authentic Learning*. The *Boyer 2030 Commission Report* emphasized that evidence-based inclusive practices should be an institutional norm, where their presence in the classroom is expected. The absence of inclusive practices is understood to be substandard, unprofessional, and unacceptable (UERU, 2022). In other words, inclusive teaching practices are a hallmark of excellence in teaching and support equity (UERU, 2022).

Intentionality is a must. Faculty must be proactive and intentional in creating an equity-focused learning environment. Ideally, maximum impact results when the entire program of study is equity-focused and active learning strategies are threaded throughout the curriculum. Creating equity-minded learning environments also begins with faculty educating themselves about the historical context of exclusionary practices in higher education and simply not blaming inequities and failures on an individual student's social, cultural, and educational background (Acosta, 2020). Creating equity-minded learning environments further requires shifting from screening individual student performance to investment in student performance via deconstructing habits, structures, policies, and practices that sustain inequities (Acosta, 2020).

TRAUMA-INFORMED TEACHING PRACTICES
Definition of Trauma

The U.S. Department of Health and Human Services, Substance Abuse and Mental Health Service Administration (SAMHSA) defined trauma as "an event, series of events, or set of circumstances experienced by an individual that is physically or emotionally harmful or threatening, and that has lasting adverse effects on the individual's functioning and wellbeing (2014, p. 7)." Trauma may be caused by a particular event, recurring events, or instances that occur over long periods of time. For example, being overlooked or devalued by a faculty member can traumatize a student. It's also important to note that a particular event may be experienced as traumatic by one person but not by someone else. Hence the effects of traumatic events vary by individual, and the adverse effects of trauma can be short-term, have a delayed onset, or be long-lasting. Considering the impact of trauma on individuals is important for both clinical and academic environments. It is important to recognize that trauma shapes a person's experience, and organizations that provide health care and education should be attuned to the fact that individuals may have had traumatic experiences. Therefore, they should interact with persons within those institutions in ways that are culturally sensitive and transparent and establish a rapport (McClinton & Laurencin, 2020).

The Effects of Trauma on Learning

The long-lasting effects of trauma are often played out in educational environments and manifested as difficulty in managing cognitive processes such as memory, holding attention, thinking, behavioral irregularities, or mood control (SAMSHA, 2014). Since trauma also affects the student's executive functioning and self-regulation skills, students may have difficulty planning, remembering, and focusing on what they need to learn (McMurtrie, 2020). Trauma can cause a shift in the neural networks mentioned in the UDL section of this chapter. Once this occurs, a trauma-informed approach is needed to help students feel safe, connected, empowered, inspired, and ready to engage, learn, and strive (Imad, 2021). Some populations, particularly those that have been historically excluded or marginalized, have higher rates of traumatic experiences and adversity (Brown et al., 2021). Faculty with a trauma-informed mindset accept that students have varied life experiences, and some of those experiences include trauma; therefore, it is essential for them to adopt trauma-informed educational principles (Najjar, 2023). Trauma-informed principles should be implemented as universal precautions because it is difficult to determine who has been exposed to trauma (McClinton & Laurencin, 2020).

Principles of Trauma-Informed Teaching

It is imperative that faculty understand, become more trauma aware, and be responsive to the impact of the trauma experienced by students to engage in trauma-informed educational practices. Being trauma-informed is understanding the ways in which traumatic experiences impact the lives of students and applying that understanding when designing pedagogical approaches (Carello & Butler, 2015). In a clinical setting, trauma-informed care (TIC) is a framework used to mitigate the effects of trauma and avoid retraumatization (Brown et al., 2021). Both trauma-informed care and trauma-informed teaching adhere to the following six principles: (1) Fostering a sense of safety, (2) building open and trusting relationships, (3) cultivating community and belonging, (4) recognizing power imbalances to enhance collaboration and mutuality, (5) empowering through voice and choice, and (6) being attuned to cultural, historical, and gendered contexts (Imad, 2021; SAMHSA, 2014).

Application of Trauma-Informed Teaching to Nursing Education

Fostering a Sense of Safety

The first step in fostering safety so that students feel psychologically safe, respected, and valued is to create a supportive learning environment. Oftentimes, first-generation college students (FGS) have limited knowledge of the collegiate experience and often feel insecure. FGSs frequently lack familiarity with course expectations and terminology, such as the syllabus and plagiarism, and may feel they do not belong in the setting (imposter syndrome). The students may be reluctant to contact the faculty members to express their uneasiness or uncertainty regarding class expectations. Uncertainty regarding expectations is minimized when faculty ensure students have a clear understanding of course requirements. Faculty should emphasize what students need to succeed in the course, including the syllabus. Faculty should treat students in a positive manner and show grace, humility, and positive intent when helping the student to understand course expectations. Faculty members must be aware of their biases and understand that issues surrounding bias and discrimination are real in today's academic environments (McClinton & Laurencin, 2020). Students from historically excluded groups face unique obstacles, and faculty can be extremely supportive by meeting with students individually to help them learn how to navigate both the course and educational terrains. This can be done by informing students of resources, including study skills, time management counseling, and health care resources within the campus environment (Schuyler et al., 2021).

Building Open and Trusting Relationships

Open, transparent, and trusting communications go a long way and help to build solid relationships with students. Faculty can explain to students the "whats" and "whys" behind course assignments and how the assignments are connected to course objectives. All syllabi should indicate the office hours of the faculty member. This allows all students, specifically FGS who may not be adept at navigating the college environment, to be aware of when the faculty is available to meet with them. In addition, using office hours, virtual or in-person, faculty can set up informal check-in sessions with students and let them know that they are there to support them and offer guidance. This action can enhance a student's sense of safety and support and helps build a trusting relationship with the faculty.

Cultivating Community and Belonging

Faculty members play a major role in helping students feel connected to the campus community and the learning environment. With a focus on inclusion, the faculty member must recognize the value that all students bring to the setting. Equally important is that faculty foster a community of belonging so that students also feel a sense of connection to each other. One way faculty members can do this is by facilitating student introductions in class so students can meet one another to begin building a sense of community. Faculty can begin the first day of class or clinical with ice-breaking exercises so that students get to know each other beyond their names. For example, you can ask students to tell one thing about themselves they feel comfortable sharing that others may not know. Another exercise asks students to state three things about themselves, one true statement and two false statements. The other students must guess which statement is true. Faculty can also design assignments that enhance interactions and support from peers, such as group assignments; think, pair, and share opportunities; or group-based clinical case presentations. Faculty can assign peer mentors or a buddy system within the course to help students build relationships. Creating a sense of community where students feel welcomed and valued is essential. Strengthening the sense of classroom community begins with building connections and relationships with students, fostering student-to-student interactions, and having an awareness and respect for the student's intercultural differences and discovering their similarities (Frazer et al., 2021).

Recognizing Power Imbalances to Enhance Collaboration and Mutuality

The power dynamic typically seen in faculty-student roles can be overcome when faculty engage students in the teaching-learning process by co-creating course materials. Co-creating deconstructs the traditional education models wherein the teacher transmits the knowledge, and the students absorb it. Co-creation recognizes that as adult learners, students have knowledge and experience they bring to the learning environment. bell hooks (1994) describes this as teaching that enables transgressions, a movement beyond the traditional boundaries. Classrooms as communal places enhance the likelihood of collective effort in creating and sustaining a learning community (hooks, 1994). Co-creating can provide meaningful learning experiences that disrupt power imbalances through collaborating with students instead of strictly adhering to faculty-directed classroom activities. This learning environment creates a sense of community, promotes high levels of student engagement, incorporates the students' voices, and creates a meaningful learning experience (Lubicz-Nawrocka & Bovill, 2021).

The syllabi and instructional strategies can be co-created with students to establish mutuality. Faculty can start by using a warm tone in the syllabus. For example, when discussing course pedagogy, faculty could use terms such as "we" rather than "I." Other ways faculty can co-create the course with students are to (1) engage students in creating classroom discussion norms, (2) have students find articles and evidence-based practice studies to present findings in the classroom, (3) ask students to present content, and (4) obtain students' input on how the course could be improved or redesigned. Lastly, the faculty should always seek formative feedback from students regarding course design and materials so that mid-course revisions can be made if needed. The faculty should let students know their input on summative evaluations will be used for future course improvements.

Empowering through Voice and Choice

The careful selection of assignments and course activities can foster empowerment. Providing students with choices in assignments or how they demonstrate their ways of knowing the content is consistent with the UDL Neural Network of Strategy; that is, selecting from various assignment options. The faculty can also assist students with goal setting and teach students self-advocacy skills. For example, if a student is unable to complete an assignment, the student should know in advance how the assignment will be made up (McMurtrie, 2020). Being flexible when working with students is part of empowering students with voice and choice. Faculty can collaborate with students on how missed assignments should be made up and on low-stakes assessments to catch up on what was missed. Since traumatic events affect memory, faculty can remind students of assignment due dates, re-emphasize concepts, and scaffold learning so students will know what they are learning and how it serves as the foundation for what they will learn next (McMurtrie, 2020).

Being Attuned to the Cultural, Historical, and Gendered Contexts

Inclusive teaching requires intentionality along with the acknowledgment that inequities exist within student populations. Therefore, faculty should engage in self-reflection activities that help them to recognize their implicit and explicit biases related to the social identities and lived experiences of students. Then, assume a culturally humble stance. When considering cultural, historical, and gendered contexts, faculty should be willing to adopt policies that are responsive to the needs of students who have been historically and systematically excluded from higher education. When these factors are considered, students may become less concerned about imposter syndrome or less likely to experience stereotype threat because course policies and practices are centered on the margins. Stringent, harsh, and inflexible course policies serve to retraumatize students. Trauma-informed pedagogy informs us that trauma and stress negatively impact students. Faculty should remember that "students are not information-receiving machines; they are living, feeling, human beings (Baker, 2022, para 13)."

A trauma-informed approach is when faculty members are attuned to whether their pedagogical practices breach safety or trust, enhance peer support, create a collaborative environment, offer the student a degree of autonomy, and consider the historical and social contexts of the student (Najjar, 2023). When faculty show students their humanity and acknowledge theirs, it lets students know the faculty sees them and that they matter (Imad, 2021).

Additionally, equity impact assessments are used to determine how different groups, specifically racial, ethnic, or gendered, will be affected by proposed policies, actions, and decisions (Keleher, 2009). They're designed to eliminate, prevent, or minimize inequitable or discriminatory treatment of persons who fall within certain groups. Some organizations have created Equity Impact Analysis toolkits. One example of a Toolkit can be found in Table 5.3, which consists of a series of six questions. These statements are especially important because when the impact is not assessed, the possibility of harm or inequity could be replicated.

MICROAGGRESSIONS

Microaggressions are the brief and commonplace daily, verbal, behavioral, and environmental indignities or insensitivities that communicate hostile, derogatory, or negative

TABLE 5.3

Example of an Equity Impact Assessment Toolkit

Focus	Questions
Impact	➤ What are the policies under consideration, and what would be the expected outcome of implementing the policy? ➤ Who benefits or is harmed by this policy? Are there unintentional consequences? If so, what strategies are in place to mitigate harm?
Assessment	➤ What data are available to support or refute the need for the policy, and how readily available are the data? ➤ Have the stakeholders who have a vested interest in this policy been engaged?
Implementation and evaluation	➤ What is the strategy for implementation? ➤ Who is accountable for the evaluation and outcomes of the project?

Source: Illinois State Board of Education, n.d.

racial, gender, sexual orientation, and religious slights and insults to members of marginalized groups, whether intentional or unintentional (Sue & Spanierman, 2020; Murray, 2020; Sue et al., 2019). Microaggressions can also be delivered through media images, mascots, monuments, and symbolism. Acts of microaggression differ from everyday rudeness or acts of incivility because the microaggressions tend to be constant and continuous, cumulative, and serve to remind the person that they are a member of a historically marginalized and excluded group (Sue et al., 2019). Microaggressions can be further divided into categories (Table 5.4). Although the nuanced distinctions can be confusing, the

TABLE 5.4

Types of Microaggressions

Type	Definition
Microassaults	The deliberate conscious form of racial attacks manifested as discriminatory verbal abuse against an individual.
Racial microaggressions	The everyday slights, insults, and invalidations that occur against people of color by well-intentioned White people who may be unaware that they have engaged in racially demeaning behavior.
Racial macroaggressions	Institutional-level or cultural racism.
Microinsults	Comments that are insensitive and disparaging such as "Are you the nursing assistant or the patient care technician? You couldn't really be the nurse."
Microinvalidations	Dismissive and exclusionary practices, such as scheduling a student assignment with the due date on a non-dominant cultural holiday.

Adapted from Ehie et al., 2021; Sue et al., 2019.

major point is to understand that microaggressions are harmful and can cause traumatic stress, which impacts the biological, emotional, cognitive, and behavioral functioning of individuals.

The Experience of Microaggressions (Perpetrator, Target, Bystander)

The person initiating the microaggression, the perpetrator, may unknowingly cause harm, leaving the target of the microaggression feeling uncomfortable, diminished, and hurt. Typically, the perpetrator will make a derogatory comment, intended or unintended. When called out by the target regarding the comment, the perpetrator's response is often that it was not intended the way it was interpreted. The perpetrator might believe the target is overreacting and overly sensitive, causing a feeling of being gaslit. *Gaslighting* is when the perpetrator manipulates the situation to the extent that it makes the target feel as if they imagined the offense or took the situation out of context. Gaslighting leaves the victim with feelings of self-doubt, confusion, and anxiety. Oftentimes, gaslighting enables microaggressions to go unaddressed because the behavior or comments are disguised in ways that cover the offense. See Table 5.5 for specific strategies to address microaggressions.

Bystanders are individuals who witness the microaggression and can intervene, condone, or do nothing. Upstanders are bystanders who stand up against the perpetrator's action. Bystanders can diffuse the situation by interrupting the perpetrator, asking someone in authority to intervene, writing notes or taking a video of the situation, or assisting the target in speaking up against the act (American Psychological Association, 2022).

Microaggressions in Campus, Classroom, and Clinical Settings

Microaggressions can play out in a variety of ways in academic settings (Sue, 2010) as seen in Table 5.6. When students find the academic environment invalidating, characterized by persistent patterns of being overlooked, under-respected, and devalued, they tend to underperform despite having the ability to succeed (Murray, 2020; Sue & Spanierman, 2020). Table 5.7 highlights the microaggressions that can occur in the classroom.

One of the first things faculty can do is to ensure they are pronouncing the student's name correctly (Najjar et al., 2023). The correct pronunciation of the student's name fosters a sense of respect. Learning a student's name can also foster the student's sense of belonging. There are resources to assist faculty in the correct pronunciation of student names (Najjar et al., 2023).

Faculty members should endeavor to understand the reality of microaggressions and be aware of their choice of words, behaviors, and actions when interacting with students in the classroom. It is important to understand that student perspectives matter and develop habits of cultural humility. Cultural humility is the process of self-awareness, being open, and incorporating self-reflection and critique when interacting with others (Tervalon & Murray-Garcia, 1998). Faculty members must be intentional in the development of

TABLE 5.5

Microaggressions—Calling In and Calling Out

Calling in is an invitation to meet with an individual on a person-to-person basis or with a small group to bring the microaggression to the person's attention.	**Calling out** is bringing public attention to a person, group, or organization's acts of microaggression.
What should I consider before calling in behavior?	**What should I consider before calling out behavior?**
‣ The degree of influence you have on the person. ‣ The degree of safety and freedom from psychological harm you will have with the person in a private meeting. ‣ The degree of openness and the level of commitment the person has to foster a respectful, diverse, and inclusive environment.	‣ The degree of urgency. Is there an immediate need to hit the "pause" button to prevent causing further harm? ‣ The degree of the power dynamic between you and the person committing the microaggression. ‣ The degree to which previous private attempts to call in the person have been unsuccessful.
Examples	**Examples**
Clarify: ‣ Can you help me understand what you meant by your comment? ‣ Did I hear you say_____? Communicate the impact: ‣ Are you aware of the effect of a comment of that nature? ‣ Statements like _____ make me feel uncomfortable or really hurt. ‣ Do you understand your comment and how it makes others feel? How could the meaning of your words be interpreted differently by others? Teach: ‣ Do you understand the difference between "intent" and "impact?" ‣ The more appropriate term to use is _____. Direct confrontation: ‣ Comments of that nature are not tolerated within this environment.	Clarify: ‣ It sounded like you said_____. Is that what you meant? Communicate the impact: ‣ Was your comment meant to be funny? I don't find it very funny. ‣ I want to tell you how your comment landed with me. Direct confrontation: ‣ Your comments are inconsistent with the values of this organization.

What to Do When Someone Calls Me In or Out?

‣ Take a deep breath. You may have emotions that range from apprehension to embarrassment to panic.

‣ Decrease your discomfort by not making it about you. Recognize that your actions or words have harmed a person. Focus on the target of the microaggression and not your feelings.

(continued)

TABLE 5.5

Microaggressions—Calling In and Calling Out *(Continued)*

> Listen attentively to the person's concerns to gain insight into their perspective. Make sure the person feels like you heard them.
> Take responsibility for your words and actions.
> Thank the person for bringing the situation to your attention.
> Apologize and vow to be more aware of your words and actions.
> Give yourself time to reflect on the situation and to process your thoughts and emotions.
> Follow up with the person to express your concern for their well-being.
> Work toward understanding the harmful aspects of bias and creating an environment of inclusion and psychological safety.
> Stop beating yourself up about the misstep.
> Continue to evolve in understanding diverse perspectives and social and historical injustices.
> Strive to be better and more culturally humble.

Adapted from Knight, R. (2020). You've been called out for a microaggression. What do you do? *Harvard Business Review*. Retrieved from https://hbr.org/2020/07/youve-been-called-out-for-a-microaggression-what-do-you-do and Office for Equity, Diversity, Inclusion, and Belonging (OEDIB), Harvard University. (2023). *Calling in and calling out guide*. Retrieved from https://edib.harvard.edu/calling-and-calling-out-guide.

TABLE 5.6

Microaggressions on Campus

Type	Examples
Microaggressions	> Faculty, staff, and students may unknowingly invalidate students from historically excluded groups on campus and in the classroom.
	> Microaggressions can be seen in the curriculum (culturally biased textbooks, lectures, teaching, and teaching materials) that may have misinformation or portray students from underrepresented groups in an unfavorable light.
Lack of belonging	> Students from underrepresented groups may not feel that classroom environments are conducive to learning despite classroom resources and faculty expertise available within the classroom setting.
Dominant culture perspective	> The campus climate may be situated in the normative White culture with little attention to the needs/likes of various other groups, including the cafeteria food choices, music selected for campus functions, and the types of activities celebrated.
	> Student support services may be offered from a primarily White European perspective, and not necessarily attend to the needs of historically excluded groups. That is, tutoring services may be offered in the evenings when some students may have to work or when there is no public transportation.
	> Programs, policies, and practices may be grounded in a privileged perspective and put students who are from marginalized backgrounds at a disadvantage.
	> Students from diverse backgrounds and identities are deemed as "othered," which implies that certain backgrounds are considered normal or normative.

TABLE 5.7

Microaggressions in the Classroom

Description	Examples
Prejudging academic ability	➤ Setting low expectations for students from certain groups or backgrounds ➤ Ascription of intelligence ➤ Believing that a student's dialect or language skills are problematic ➤ Stating how a non-White student is articulate or well-spoken
Devaluing culture, heritage, and religious traditions	➤ Scheduling assignments, projects, and exams on cultural or religious holidays ➤ Disregarding religious traditions ➤ Expressing Eurocentric and ethnocentric views ➤ Failing to learn to pronounce or continuing to mispronounce student names ➤ Pointing students out based on their background ➤ Expecting students to be the spokesperson for their racial/ethnic/cultural group
Criminalizing behavior	➤ Referring to undocumented students as "illegals" ➤ Making assumptions about students and their backgrounds ➤ Banning certain ethnic clothing or head coverings such as hats or hoodies and certain hairstyles
Disregarding income inequality	➤ Assigning class projects that disregard socioeconomic status and penalize students with fewer financial resources ➤ Assuming all students have access to and are proficient with the use of computers, technology, and applications for communications related to academic assignments ➤ Excluding students from accessing certain activities due to the expense of the activity
Making politically charged statements	➤ Expressing racially charged political opinions in class ➤ Using inappropriate political and partisan humor in class that degrades members from other groups ➤ Hosting debates in class that place students holding opposing views in bad predicaments
Dismissing difference	➤ Conveying only heteronormative examples in class ➤ Calling on, engaging, and validating one gender, class, or race of students while ignoring other students during class ➤ Requiring students with non-visible disabilities to identify themselves in class ➤ Use of heteronormative or binary gender metaphors ➤ Assuming the gender identity of students ➤ Misusing pronouns after the student indicates their pronoun

Source: Murray, 2020; Lynch, 2019; Sue, 2010.

the following skills: self-awareness, capacity for empathy and perspective-taking, which is a structural change in the way the self is viewed in relation to others, active listening, and inquiry while being undergirded in the ethical code as outlined in the American Nurses Association (Hughes et al., 2020).

When students are the victims of microaggressions in the classroom, they should be encouraged to seek campus support services, such as meeting with a faculty member, counselor, or academic advisor. Often students seek out classmates with similar backgrounds, social, cultural, or ethnic backgrounds to share their concerns. This helps students muster up a collective sense of identity and to support shared experiences in addition to coping strategies to face the insults and slights experienced in the classroom (Murray, 2020; Sue & Spanierman, 2020). See Table 5.8 for what faculty can do when microaggressions occur in the clinical setting.

TABLE 5.8

When Microaggressions Happen in the Clinical Setting

When	Actions
Preparation	▸ Faculty members should foster a culture of mutual respect among staff and patients in the clinical environment. While orienting students to the clinical environment, it should be stressed that everyone should be treated respectfully. This includes the health care staff, fellow students, and patients.
	▸ Before entering the clinical setting, the faculty and students should participate in diversity, equity, and bias training that includes basic knowledge and skills-based strategies. The skill-based strategies can be accomplished by role-playing scenarios that address possible situations students may encounter in the clinical setting. This could entail describing a situation where a patient or another healthcare provider uses a racial epithet. Helping the students to work through how to handle such situations is imperative. Does the student call out the behavior? What factors should the student consider when the perpetrator is a patient, visitor, or staff member?
	▸ Faculty should establish a safe, trusting relationship with students so that students will be comfortable approaching the faculty if they have been the target of microaggressions or other forms of discrimination by staff or patients.
During	▸ Because of power differentials within clinical environments coupled with the students' unfamiliarity with the health care setting, faculty should be mindful and attuned to the occurrence of microaggressions.
	▸ While there is no "right way" to handle these types of situations; use strategies identified in Table 5.5.
After	▸ Debriefing situations outside the clinical environment is necessary. Students must be able to reflect on the situation and express their concerns in a non-threatening environment.
	▸ Provide students with additional resources and referrals if needed for additional training and counseling related to bias and microaggressions. There are many internet resources and toolkits to help students consider the pros and cons of calling in and calling out acts of microaggressions.

Source: Wheeler, D. J., Zapata, J., Davis, D., & Chou, C. (2019). Twelve tips for responding to microaggressions and overt discrimination: When the patient offends the learner. *Medical Teacher, 41*(10), 1112–1117.

COURAGEOUS AND INCLUSIVE CONVERSATIONS

Faculty and students enter classroom discussions with their own ideas, beliefs, and values. Those beliefs are often shaped by circumstances beyond their control, such as age, gender, ethnicity, ability, culture, socioeconomic status, religion, and other social identities based on lived experience. Inclusive classroom environments acknowledge and value differences and are respectful of others who may have dramatically different life experiences. Courageous and inclusive conversations, embedded with a healthy dose of cultural humility, can provide faculty and students with the skills to develop cultural fluidity, which makes for an inclusive learning environment. Cultural fluidity, also known as cultural agility, is the ability to interact with others in the space between categories and ideologies (Hughes et al., 2020). Cultural agility, cultural agility goes beyond valuing diversity and diverse perspectives; it is the ability to perceive situations through various cultural lenses (Aoun, 2017).

Establishing Ground Rules

Prior to engaging in potentially controversial topics, faculty members should consider how the topic or subject is connected to the learning objectives of the class and explain the connection to students. Then, the faculty should ensure there are group discussion guidelines in place before introducing controversial topics, "hot topics," or content known to evoke tensions. Guidelines can serve as group norms to help students engage in respectful dialogues. Ideally, guidelines should be co-created with students on the first day of class or clinical. Once guidelines are developed and discussed, students should be asked to commit to them. When students and faculty have a culturally humble approach in classroom environments, then a psychologically safe and respectful learning environment is easier to attain. These environments have the potential to improve learning outcomes and promote academic success (Smith & Foronda, 2019). Examples of ground rules are:

> Assume the other person has positive intent.
> Act in humility but hold self and others accountable.
> Actively listen and respect the opinion of others; allow the person to finish their comments uninterrupted.
> Attempt to understand other perspectives and be nonjudgmental.
> Seek clarification as necessary.

CHAPTER SUMMARY

This chapter focused on strategies to create inclusive learning environments that foster a sense of connectedness, engage students in the teaching-learning process, and promote meaningful interactions between students and faculty—all of which are necessary to create an environment whereby students can be successful. First, the principles of Universal Design for Learning, Equity-Focused Teaching, and Trauma Informed Care were discussed, along with specific application strategies. Next, this chapter provided information on microaggressions and what to do when microaggressions occur in the classroom or clinical setting. Finally, since inclusive learning environments require open and honest communication, the chapter ends with how to have those courageous and inclusive conversations by establishing ground rules which ideally should be developed during the first classroom on clinical encounter in partnership with students.

References

Ackerman-Barger, K., Valderama-Wallace, C., Latimore, D., & Drake, C. (2016). Understanding health professions students' self-perceptions of stereotype threat susceptibility. *Journal of Best Practices in Health Professions Diversity, 9*(2), 1232–1246.

American Psychological Association. (2022). Bystander intervention tip sheet. Retrieved from https://www.apa.org/pi/health-equity/bystander-intervention.pdf.

Aoun, J. E. (2017). *Robot-proof: Higher education in the age of artificial intelligence.* MIT Press.

Baker, K. J. (2022). Mays Imad on trauma-informed pedagogy. *The National Teaching and Learning Forum, 31*(2), 5–6. https://doi.org/10.1002/ntlf.30313.

Brown, T., Berman, S., McDaniel, K., Radford, C., Mehta, P., Potter, J., & Hirsh, D. A. (2021). Trauma-Informed Medical Education (TIME): Advancing Curricular Content and Educational Context. *Journal of the Association of American Medical Colleges, 96*(5), 661–667. https://doi.org/10.1097/ACM.0000000000003587.

Carello, J., & Butler, L. D. (2015). Practicing what we teach: Trauma-informed educational practice. *Journal of Teaching in Social Work, 35*, 262–278.

Carr, P., David, P. M., Grossman, P., Nak-kyung Kim, S., Lizcano, R., Logel, C., & Materman, H. (n.d.). Empirically validated strategies to reduce stereotype threat. Retrieved from https://ed.stanford.edu/sites/default/files/interventionshandout.pdf.

Carter Andrews, D. J., He, Y., Marciano, J. E., Richmond, G., & Salazar, M. (2021). Decentering Whiteness in teacher education: Addressing the questions of who, with whom, and how. *Journal of Teacher Education, 72* (2), 134–137.

CAST. (2022). About universal design for learning. Retrieved from https://www.cast.org/impact/universal-design-for-learning-udl.

Center for Research on Teaching & Learning (CRLT), University of Michigan. (2021). Equity-focused teaching. Retrieved from https://crlt.umich.edu/equity-focused-teaching.

Charania, N. A. M. A., & Patel, R. (2022). Diversity, equity, and inclusion in nursing education: Strategies and processes to support inclusive teaching. *Journal of Professional Nursing, 42*, 67–72. https://doi.org/10.1016/j.profnurs.2022.05.013.

Chrousos, G. P., & Mentis, A. A. (2020). Imposter syndrome threatens diversity. *Science, 367*(6479), 749–750.

Clark, T. R. (2020). *The 4 Stages of Psychological Safety: Defining the Path to Inclusion and Innovation.* Berrett-Koehler Publishers.

Cochran-Smith, M., Shakman, K., Jong, C., Terrell, D. G., Barnatt, J., & McQuillan, P. (2009). Good and just teaching: The case for social justice in teacher education. *American Journal of Education, 115*(3), 347–377. https://doi.org/10.1086/597493.

Cokley, K., Smith, L., Bernard, D., Hurst, A., Jackson, S., Stone, S., Awosogba, O., Saucer, C., Bailey, M., & Roberts, D. (2017). Impostor feelings as a moderator and mediator of the relationship between perceived discrimination and mental health among racial/ethnic minority college students. *Journal of Counseling Psychology, 64*(2), 141–154. https://doi.org/10.1037/cou0000198.

Corkindale, G. (2008). Managing yourself: Overcoming imposter syndrome. *Harvard Business Review.* Retrieved from https://hbr.org/2008/05/overcoming-imposter-syndrome.

Croizet, J.-C., Despres, G., Gauzins, M.-E., Huguet, P., Leyens, J.-P., & Meot, A. (2004). Stereotype threat undermines intellectual performance by triggering a disruptive mental load. *Personality and Social Psychology Bulletin, 30*(6), 721–731.

Ehie, O., Muse, I., Hill, L., & Bastien, A. (2021). Professionalism: Microaggression in the healthcare setting. *Current Opinion in Anaesthesiology, 34*(2), 131–136. https://doi.org/10.1097/ACO.0000000000000966

Frazer, C., Reilly, C. A., & Squellati, R. E. (2021). Instructional strategies: Teaching nursing in today's diverse and inclusive landscape. *Teaching and Learning in Nursing, 16*(3), 276–280.

Gallo, A. (2023). What is psychological safety? *Harvard Business Review*. Retrieved from https://hbr.org/2023/02/what-is-psychological-safety

Gilmore, J. P., Halligan, P., & Browne, F. (2022). Pedagogy as social justice-Universal Design of Learning in nurse education. *Nurse Education Today*, *118*, 105498. https://doi.org/10.1016/j.nedt.2022.105498.

Harvard Diversity Inclusion & Belonging. (n.d.). *Calling in and calling out guide*. Retrieved from https://edib.harvard.edu/calling-and-calling-out-guide.

hooks, b. (1994). *Teaching to transgress: Education as the practice of freedom*. Routledge Taylor and Francis Group.

Hughes, V., Delva, S., Nkimbeng, M., Spaulding, E., Turkson-Ocran, R. A., Cudjoe, J., Ford, A., Rushton, C., D'Aoust, R., & Han, H. R. (2020). Not missing the opportunity: Strategies to promote cultural humility among future nursing faculty. *Journal of Professional Nursing*, *36*(1), 28–33. https://doi.org/10.1016/j.profnurs.2019.06.005.

Illinois State Board of Education. (n.d). *Equity impact analysis toolkit*. Retrieved from https://www.isbe.net/Documents/EIAT-flyer.pdf.

Imad, M. (2021). Transcending adversity: Trauma-informed educational development. *To Improve the Academy*, *39*(3), 1–23. https://doi.org/10.3998/tia.17063888.0039.301.

Jung, L. A. (2021). Lesson planning with universal design for learning. *Educational Leadership*, *21*, 38–43.

Kearney, D. B. (2022). Universal design for learning (UDL) for inclusion, diversity, equity, and accessibility (IDEA). eCampus. Retrieved from https://ecampusontario.pressbooks.pub/universaldesign/

Keleher, T. (2009). Racial equity impact assessment. Race Forward. Retrieved from https://www.raceforward.org/sites/default/files/RacialJusticeImpactAssessment_v5.pdf.

Kivlighan, D. M., III, Abbas, M., Gloria, A. M., Aguinaga, A., Frank, C., & Frost, N. D. (2018). Are belongingness and hope essential features of academic enhancement groups? A psychosociocultural perspective. *Journal of Counseling Psychology*, *65*(2), 204.

Knight, R. (2020). You've been called out for a microaggression. What do you do? *Harvard Business Review*. Retrieved from https://hbr.org/2020/07/youve-been-called-out-for-a-microaggression-what-do-you-do

Lain, E. C. (2018). Racialized interactions in the law school classroom: Pedagogical approaches to creating a safe learning environment. *Journal of Legal Education*, *67*(3), 780–801. https://www.jstor.org/stable/26890967.

Lubicz-Nawrocka, T., & Bovill, C. (2021). Do students experience transformation through co-creating curriculum in higher education? *Teaching in Higher Education*, 1–17. https://doi.org/10.1080/13562517.2021.1928060

McClinton, A., & Laurencin, C. T. (2020). Just in TIME: Trauma-Informed Medical Education. *Journal of Racial and Ethnic Health Disparities*, *7*(6), 1046–1052. https://doi.org/10.1007/s40615-020-00881-w.

McMurtrie, B. (2020). *What does trauma-informed teaching look like?* The Chronicle of Higher Education. Retrieved from https://www.chronicle.com/newsletter/teaching/2020-06-04.

Metzger, M., Dowling, T., Guinn, J., & Wilson, D. T. (2020). Inclusivity in baccalaureate nursing education: A scoping study. *Journal of Professional Nursing*, *36*(1), 5–14. https://doi.org/10.1016/j.profnurs.2019.06.002.

Mullangi, S., & Jagsi, R. (2019). Imposter syndrome: Treat the cause, not the symptom. *JAMA*, *322*(5), 403–404. https://doi.org/10.1001/jama.2019.9788.

Murray, T. A. (2020). Microaggressions in the classroom. *Journal of Nursing Education*, *59*(4), 184–185. https://doi.org/10.3928/01484834-20200323-02.

Murray, T. A., & Noone, J. (2022). Advancing diversity in nursing education: A groundwater approach. *Journal of Professional Nursing*, *41*, 140–148. https://doi.org/10.1016/j.profnurs.2022.05.002.

Najjar, R. H. (2023). A trauma-informed approach provides framework for achieving health equity. Campaign for Action. Retrieved from https://campaignforaction.org/trauma-informed-approach-provides-framework/

Najjar, R., Noone, J., & Reifenstein, K. (2023). Supporting an inclusive environment through correct name pronunciation. *Nurse Educator*, *48*(1), 19–23. https://doi.org/10.1097/NNE.0000000000001285.

Pentaraki, A., & Burkholder, G. J. (2017). Emerging evidence regarding the roles of emotional, behavioural, and cognitive aspects of student engagement in the online classroom. *European Journal of Open, Distance and E-Learning*, *20*(1), 1–21.

Reagan, E. M., & Hambacher, E. (2021). Teacher preparation for social justice: A synthesis of the literature, 1999–2019. *Teaching and Teacher Education*, *108*. https://doi.org/10.1016/j.tate.2021.103520.

Reed, L., Bellflower, B., Anderson, J. N., Bowdre, T. L., Fouquier, K., Nellis, K., & Rhoads, S. (2022). Rethinking nursing education and curriculum using a racial equity lens. *The Journal of Nursing Education*, *61*(8), 493–496. https://doi.org/10.3928/01484834-20220602-02.

Schuyler, S. W., Childs, J. R., & Poynton, T. A. (2021). Promoting success for first-generation students of color: The importance of academic, transitional adjustment, and mental health supports. *Journal of College Access*, *6*(1), Article 4. Available at: https://scholarworks.wmich.edu/jca/vol6/iss1/4

Smith, A., & Foronda, C. (2019). Promoting cultural humility in nursing education through the use of ground rules. *Nursing Education Perspectives*, *42*(2), 117–119. https://doi.org/10.1097/01.NEP.0000000000000594.

Smith, D. (2020). *Diversity's promise for higher education: Making it work* (3rd ed.). Johns Hopkins University Press.

Spencer, S. J., Logel, C., Davies, P. G. (2016). Stereotype threat. *Annual Review of Psychology*, *67*, 415–437.

Stewart, A. J., & Valian, V. (2018). *An inclusive academy: Achieving diversity and excellence*. Massachusetts Institute of Technology, MIT Press.

Stewart, D. (2017). Colleges need a language shift, but not the one you think (essay). Language of appeasement. *Inside Higher Ed*. Retrieved from https://www.insidehighered.com/views/2017/03/30/colleges-need-language-shift-not-one-you-think-essay.

Sue, D. W. (2010). *Microaggressions in everyday life: Race, gender, and sexual orientation*. John Wiley & Sons.

Sue, D. W., & Spanierman, L. (2020). *Microaggressions in Everyday Life*. John Wiley & Sons.

Sue, S., Alsaidi, S., Awad, M. N., Glaeser, E., Calle, C., & Mendez, M. (2019). Disarming racial microaggressions: Microintervention strategies for targets, white allies, and bystanders. *American Psychologist*, *74*(1), 128–142.

Tanner, K. D. (2013). Structure matters: Twenty-one teaching strategies to promote student engagement and cultivate classroom equity. *CBE-Life Sciences Education*, *12*, 322–331.

Tervalon, M., & Murray-García, J. (1998). Cultural humility versus cultural competence: A critical distinction in defining physician training outcomes in multicultural education. *Journal of Health Care for the Poor and Underserved*, *9*(2), 117–125. https://doi.org/10.1353/hpu.2010.0233.

The Association for Undergraduate Education at Research Universities (UERU). (2022). *The equity-excellence imperative: A 2030 Blueprint for undergraduate education at U.S. Research Universities*. The Boyer 2030 Commission. Retrieved from https://ueru.org/boyer2030.

The U.S. Department of Health and Human Services, Substance Abuse and Mental Health Service Administration (SAMHSA). (2014). *SAMHSA's concept of trauma and guidance for a trauma-informed approach*. Office of Policy, Planning and Innovation, Substance Abuse and Mental Health Services Administration.

Wheeler, D. J., Zapata, J., Davis, D., & Chou, C. (2019). Twelve tips for responding to microaggressions and overt discrimination: When the patient offends the learner. *Medical Teacher*, *41*(10), 1112–1117.

Yerkey, E. (2022). Universal design for learning: Removing barriers through options. *Journal of Neuroeducation*, *3*(1).

6

Frameworks to Engage Diverse Learners

Holly Fiock, MSEd

Glenise McKenzie, PhD, MN, RN

CHAPTER OVERVIEW

This chapter discusses the intentional use of frameworks to engage diverse learners in meaningful learning activities. Topics include dimensions of learner engagement, structural and individual factors influencing engagement, learner outcomes, and best practices to stimulate learner engagement. Frameworks reviewed will include the Community of Inquiry Model, Universal Design for Learning, and Quality Matters, among others.

LEARNER ENGAGEMENT IN THE CONTEXT OF NURSING EDUCATION

Preparing prelicense and new nurses to practice and lead within diverse, fast-paced, high-acuity, and technology-enhanced settings is critically important to the health of our nation. Nurse educators are therefore tasked with developing engaging and meaningful teaching practices that help learners situate content and concepts within the context of "real world" practice (Benner et al., 2010; Crookes et al., 2013). Nurse educators are instrumental to student success; based on their decisions about teaching methods and practices students are more engaged in meaningful learning (Bernard, 2015; Crookes et al., 2013).

Nurse educators and administrators have recognized the importance of nurse-learner engagement for many decades. In their Hallmarks of Excellence (2019), the National League for Nursing (NLN) (2023) specifically equates engaged learners ("students are excited about learning and exhibit a spirit of inquiry as well as a commitment to lifelong learning") with excellence in nursing education (p. 1). Many colleges and universities with schools of nursing also demonstrate commitment to improving student engagement by participating in and learning from the National Survey of Student Engagement (NSSE), a cross-disciplinary survey of undergraduate students in their first and again in their final year of baccalaureate education (2018). The NSSE measures student engagement in four core areas with a total of ten engagement indicators: (1) academic challenge (higher-order learning, reflective and integrative learning, learning strategies, quantitative reasoning); (2) learning with peers (collaborative learning, discussions with diverse others); (3) experiences with faculty (student-faculty interaction, effective teaching practices); and (4) campus environment (quality of interactions, supportive environment; National Survey of Student Engagement [NSSE], 2018). While the NSSE is administered to all baccalaureate students from participating colleges and universities, nursing-specific data is available. Nurse education researchers, utilizing secondary analyses of NSSE survey data, have described student perceptions of engagement indicators and provided related insights on strengths and potential opportunities for nurse educators related to student engagement. While nursing students consistently endorsed higher levels of "Academic Challenge," they did not perceive themselves as being engaged in active and collaborative learning as compared to students from other majors (Johnson, 2015; Popkess & McDaniel, 2011). In another cross-sectional study using the NSSE survey, Clynes et al. (2020) explored nursing students' perceptions of institutional support of engagement and found nursing students reported low levels of student-faculty interaction and collaborative learning. The authors also asked two open-ended questions to explore students' thoughts on their experience with engagement at their institution. The authors identified three themes related to what students found most supportive to their engagement: "Student-Lecturer Interactions" (lecturers who are approachable and interested in students as individuals); "Collaborative Learning" (active group work); and "Teacher and Institutional Support" (small classes, skills and practical sessions, and lecturers with clinical experience). Student engagement components hold relevance and opportunity for professional nursing organizations, nurse educators, and learners. The purpose of this chapter is to introduce components of student engagement in the context of nursing and recommend evidence-based teaching practices for engaging nurse learners in meaningful learning.

DEFINITION AND DIMENSIONS OF LEARNER ENGAGEMENT

Learner engagement, as defined in a concept analysis of nurse education literature, is "a dynamic process marked by a positive behavioral, cognitive, and affective state exhibited in the pursuit of deep learning" (Bernard, 2015). Student engagement is multidimensional (behavioral, affective, and cognitive) occurring within sociocultural contexts (interactions with diverse peers, faculty, staff, and health care communities) (Groccia, 2018; Kassab, 2022). Positive learner engagement in the behavioral dimension relates to what a learner is "doing" (participation, effort, and "showing up" for learning). Emotional engagement is what the learner is "feeling" (positive and negative affective reactions including interest, enjoyment, and a sense of belonging) (Pentaraki & Burkholder, 2017). In the cognitive dimension (what the student is "thinking"), engagement is reflected by investment in learning and integrating learning into real-world situations (Bernard, 2015; Hudson, 2015; Pentaraki & Burkholder, 2017). The dimensions of learner engagement are conceptualized as interdependent and to some extent malleable, with instructors in a key position to positively influence the antecedents and moderators of student engagement (Kassab et al., 2022; Pedler et al., 2020). A few examples of how instructors can influence positive student engagement include promoting a community where learners are able to collaborate with peers in a safe, no-risk environment, providing and incorporating real-world activities, and ensuring students feel emotionally and physically safe (Kassab et al., 2022; Pedler et al., 2020). Additional dimensions of student engagement are discussed

TABLE 6.1

Antecedents, Mediators, and Dimensions of Engagement

Social-Cultural Context
Includes: Student agency; peer, staff, faculty, mentor relationships; learning environment

Antecedents	Mediators	Dimensions	Indicators/Outcomes
Institutional	➤ Motivation	**Behavioral engagement**	➤ Positive academic outcomes
A. Structural	➤ Self-efficacy	Includes academic and social participation	
➤ Culture	➤ Reflectivity		➤ Persistence
➤ Policies	➤ Sense of belonging	**Affective engagement**	➤ Creating ties to an institution
➤ Curriculum		Both positive and negative interactions with teachers, peers, academics, and school	
➤ Assessment			➤ Willingness to do the work
B. Psychosocial		**Cognitive engagement**	➤ Critical thinking
➤ Workload		Incorporates thoughtfulness and willingness to exert the effort necessary	➤ Master difficult skills
➤ Support systems			➤ Teamwork
Student			➤ Collaboration
➤ Language			
➤ Cultural identities			
➤ Prior knowledge			
➤ Lived experience			
➤ Professional aspirations			

in the literature, especially by educational researchers in the health and psychology disciplines. For example, Kassab et al. (2022) proposed a health professional framework for enhancing engagement through partnership with students as both "customers and partners" in education. They argue for two additional dimensions; agentic engagement (student agency and choice) and sociocultural engagement (fostering of peer, staff, and faculty relationships). For the purpose of this overview, the important concepts of student agency and peer, staff, and faculty relationships are integrated as part of the sociocultural context of student engagement in nursing education. Refer to Table 6.1 for a summary of these concepts.

WHAT INFLUENCES STUDENT ENGAGEMENT?

Antecedents or drivers of engagement on multiple dimensions are described at the institutional (system) level and at the student (individual) level (Trowler et al., 2022). Learners in today's nursing classrooms and clinical settings are beginning to reflect the increasing diversity of the U.S. population where over 40 percent of Americans self-report as racially or ethnically diverse (U.S. Census Bureau, 2021). As such, nursing students bring diversity in language, cultural identities, prior knowledge, skills, lived experience, and professional aspirations, which may impact their academic and clinical engagement

(Bristol et al., 2020). Antecedents or drivers of learner engagement at the institutional level include structural factors (culture, policies, curriculum, assessment) and psychosocial factors (teaching, workload, support) (Trowler et al., 2022). For example, nurse educator competencies in active learning strategies as well as respectful, supportive relationships between instructors and students may support engagement in learning (Bernard, 2015). Inclusive and engaging learning environments and teaching practices are theorized to impact student motivation, self-efficacy, reflectivity, and sense of belonging which are mediators of learner engagement (Trowler et al., 2022). Given the relevance of student engagement to nursing education, understanding the drivers or pathways to student engagement is of critical importance to nurse educators. There have been several recent reviews of learner engagement and related academic and clinical educational interventions applied in the context of nursing and other health care professions. Findings of effective strategies for enhancing student engagement generally fall into four areas: (1) student-centered, inclusive course design (Crookes et al., 2013; Czerkawski & Lymann, 2016; Gaston & Lynch, 2019); (2) active instructional methods (Crookes et al., 2013; Ghasemi et al., 2020; Jeppesen et al., 2017; Kassab et al., 2022; Phillips & Young, 2018); (3) technology-enhanced learning (Crookes et al., 2013; Ghasemi et al., 2020); and (4) partnership-based learning (Kassab et al., 2022). Student-centered, inclusive course design can be met by creating a shared classroom purpose modeled around student voice and choice, shifting the responsibility of learning away from the teacher and toward the learner (Abualhaija, 2019). Active instructional methods are those where students can directly apply their knowledge to a task or situation; Chapter 8, *Strategies for Active and Authentic Learning* discusses this in more detail. Technology-enhanced learning is not using technology for technology's sake; it is the use of technology to support the learning process (Koehler et al., 2017). Partnership-based learning is collaborating with a range of individuals outside of a traditional classroom (e.g., community); Chapter 13, *Service-Learning* discusses different opportunities for student partnerships. Our focus in this chapter is on what we as nurse educators (as influencers on institutional level drivers) might do to enhance learner engagement through planning and structuring learning environments and instructional practices that mediate motivation, self-efficacy, reflectivity, and feelings of belonging for all students (Frazer et al., 2021; Gay, 2015; Trowler et al., 2022).

In the following section, we briefly describe and then apply educational design principles and collaborative learning components for instructors to intentionally develop an inclusive and engaging learning environment. We describe current best practices aimed at institutional-level factors including (1) the structural factors (culture, policies, curriculum, assessment) through the principles of Universal Design for Learning (UDL) (CAST, 2011) and (2) psychosocial factors (teaching, workload, support) using the Community of Inquiry (CoI) Framework (Garrison et al., 2000). The focus of the following sections is on evidence-based practices for course structure and development of learning activities to support academic and clinical engagement.

FRAMEWORKS AND APPLICATION TO ENHANCE ENGAGEMENT IN HEALTH SCIENCES

Hudson (2015) notes that it is vital for nursing instructors to understand and know how to apply a range of different engagement activities for the array of student learning environments (e.g., classroom, labs, clinical). To enhance learner engagement, many educators use different frameworks to guide their teaching practices and the selection of engaging learning activities. Focusing on two major frameworks—Universal Design for Learning (UDL) and Community of Inquiry (CoI)—we explain each framework's purpose and provide teaching examples of how these look in practice.

Universal Design for Learning (UDL)

Universal Design for Learning (UDL) Guidelines are a set of design principles that can be used to help create equitable, inclusive, and accessible learning experiences for all students. Using three primary principles, UDL helps create "flexible goals, methods, materials, and assessments that empower educators to meet these varied needs" (CAST, 2011, p. 4). Founded on neuroscience research, the three principles focus on providing multiple means of (1) engagement, (2) representation, and (3) action and expression. Multiple means are important in UDL as the framework views "inflexible, 'one-size-fits-all' curricula" as the primary barrier to inclusive learning environments (CAST, 2011, p. 4). For a more comprehensive look at the history and theoretical background of UDL, please refer to Chapter 5, *Creating Inclusive Learning Environments*.

Specific to nursing education, Davis et al. (2021) stated that while UDL concepts are not often found in the literature, the UDL "approach is consistent with nursing education initiatives to prepare a more diverse and inclusive workforce" (p. 134). To help prepare this future workforce, we must first prepare our nursing instructors in creating a "learning environment that is conducive to all learners" (Frazer et al., 2021, p. 277). The goal of education from the UDL perspective means creating learners who are (1) resourceful and knowledgeable, (2) strategic and goal-directed, and (3) purposeful and motivated (CAST, 2011).

Organized by principle, the UDL guidelines are arranged from "principle (least detail) to guideline to checkpoint (most detail)" (CAST, 2011, p. 12). Importantly, the UDL guidelines are not meant to be prescriptive, but descriptive as means to "serve as the basis for building in the options and the flexibility that are necessary to maximize learning opportunities" (CAST, 2011, p. 12). Next, we will break down each principle with its definition, its benefit to learners, and an example in practice.

Provide Multiple Means of Engagement

The Multiple Means of Engagement Principle explains how there is not one way to engage all learners in all contexts at once. Instructors must be able to provide different ways to help learners connect with or be motivated to learn the content. CAST (2011) explains, "Some learners are highly engaged by spontaneity and novelty while others are disengaged, even frightened, by those aspects, preferring strict routine" (CAST, 2018, para. 1).

A range of engagement dimensions can be captured using the Multiple Means of Engagement Principle. For example, emotional engagement aligns with the creation of a low-stakes environment, helping influence learners to complete the work at hand (Hudson, 2015). Next, when students are learning new materials that are directly aligned with their own goals, intrinsic satisfaction and cognitive engagement develop (Hudson, 2015).

TABLE 6.2

Multiple Means of Engagement

Engagement Principle: Guidelines & Checkpoints	Definition	Example
Recruiting interest 1. Optimize individual choice and autonomy 2. Optimize relevance, value, and authenticity 3. Minimize threats and distractions	The goal of this guideline is to help "spark excitement and curiosity" to concept(s) to aid new knowledge development (CAST, 2018).	Leverage student interest or learning surveys to gather individual preferences, interests, and needs of learners. This information can be used later in selecting course readings, examples, guest speakers, etc. Consider using case-based learning where mistakes can be made in a low-stakes environment or use simulations to assist in providing authenticity.
Sustaining effort & persistence 1. Heighten salience of goals and objectives 2. Vary demands and resources to optimize challenge 3. Foster collaboration and community 4. Increase mastery-orientated feedback	The goal of this guideline is to help hold the interest previously sparked and maintain focus moving forward.	Task value and the promotion of mastery goals help to maintain learner performance (Trowler et al., 2022). Consider using simulations to practice responses to situations and allow for critical reflection.
Self-regulation 1. Promote expectations and beliefs that optimize motivation 2. Facilitate personal coping skills and strategies 3. Develop self-assessment and reflection	The goal of this guideline is to "develop learners' intrinsic abilities to regulate their own emotions and motivations" (i.e., self-regulate; CAST, 2018).	Provide panel discussions with invited guest speakers who are nursing practitioners on how they deal with real-world issues. Consider recording learners (audio or visual) in role-play scenarios to allow for a different type of self-reflection activity.

The socio-cultural dimension of engagement that calls for "a group of individuals who share the same domain of interest, engage in joint activities or discussions through regular interactions, and develop a shared collection of practice to address recurring problems," occurs when creating collaborative communities in classrooms (Kassab et al., 2022, p. 4). The behavioral dimension of engagement demonstrates what the learner is "doing" or what effort they are showing in their own learning. Table 6.2 defines the Engagement Principle guidelines and checkpoints, providing examples to help guide instructors when creating, sustaining, and optimizing engagement with learning content and environments.

Provide Multiple Means of Representation

The Multiple Means of Representation Principle explains how learners perceive and comprehend information differently; due to this, as instructors, we must provide information to learners in a variety of ways (e.g., video, audio, image). The principles in Multiple Means of Representation (Perception, Language and Symbols, and Comprehension) align with all dimensions as the principles and guidelines in this section are very personalized and contextual. For example, language and symbols can vary from environment to environment—meaning what works in one classroom may not work in another. Nurse educators must take into consideration their learner population and provide opportunities for each individual and individual class to engage with their peers and content to determine the engagement dimension that would work best for their learners. Table 6.3 defines the Multiple Means of Representation guidelines and checkpoints, and provides examples of Perception, Language and Symbols, and Comprehension; the three guidelines help educators to consider how to create and present diverse materials to learners.

Provide Multiple Means of Action and Expression

The Multiple Means of Action and Expression principle looks at how students express what they have learned. Specifically, this principle is aimed at having instructors consider learners with challenges for specific tasks (e.g., "learner can express themselves well in written text but not speech, and vice versa"; CAST, 2018). The engagement dimensions change depending on the guidelines within the Action and Expression category. As behavioral engagement includes "participation, important for positive academic outcomes and preventing students from dropping out," nurse educators must ensure that learners can interact and have access to all learning materials available (Hudson, 2015, p. 45). This is important when looking at physical action and how learners engage with the course materials. In Expression and Communication as well as Executive Functions, behavioral and cognitive dimensions of engagement are both represented. First, behavioral engagement refers to academic and social participation which could be based on how the learners' own goals are developed, or cognitive engagement (Hudson, 2015). Second, as learners demonstrate mastery of course materials (regardless of *how* they demonstrate their understanding), cognitive investment or reflection is required (cognitive engagement dimension). Table 6.4 defines the Multiple Means of Action and Expression guidelines and checkpoints, and provides examples of Physical Action, Expression and Communication, and Executive Functions; these three guidelines help instructors to consider how different methods can be used for learner assessment.

In this section, we covered a range of instructional strategies that could be used to help engage learners using UDL. There are a number of articles that focus on specific strategies and techniques to engage nursing students (see Crookes et al., 2013; Ghasemi et al., 2020).

Community of Inquiry Framework (CoI)

Specific to online learning environments, the Community of Inquiry (CoI) Framework is one of the most highly cited and widely used frameworks for building online

TABLE 6.3

Multiple Means of Representation

Representation Principle Guidelines and Checkpoints	Definition	Example
Perception 1. Offer ways of customizing the display of information 2. Offer alternatives for auditory information 3. Offer alternatives for visual information	The goal of this guideline is to "provide [the] same information in a range of modalities that doesn't depend on a single sense like sight, hearing, movement, or touch" (CAST, 2018). "Such multiple representations not only ensure that information is accessible to learners with particular sensory and perceptual disabilities, but also easier to access and comprehend for many others."	Provide different media of the same topic/lesson. For example, provide a job aid (nonmotion visual), video (motion visual), and text-based instructions or steps for how to administer Narcan nasal spray.
Language and symbols 1. Clarify vocabulary and symbols 2. Clarify syntax and structure 3. Support decoding of text, mathematical notation, and symbols 4. Promote understanding across languages 5. Illustrate through multiple media	The goal of this guideline is to "ensure that alternative representations are provided not only for accessibility, but for clarity and comprehensibility across all learners" (CAST, 2018).	Explain all abbreviations or shorthand to learners to ensure a common language among learners (e.g., ROM means 'range of motion'; TF means 'tube feeding'). Provide or have learners develop a course terminology page to clarify course vocabulary/understanding.
Comprehension 1. Activate or supply background knowledge 2. Highlight patterns, critical features, big ideas, and relationships 3. Guide information processing and visualization	The goal of this guideline is to "teach learners how to transform accessible information into useable knowledge" (CAST, 2018). Both cognitive engagement and critical engagement are met by providing options for comprehension, specifically to help learners with "'information processing skills' like selective attending, integrating new information with prior knowledge, strategic categorization, and active memorization" (CAST, 2018).	Utilize case-based, problem-based, or other situational-based learning activities. For example, development of a patient care plan or concept map based on an authentic scenario.

communities among instructors and learners. Developed by Garrison et al. (2000), the CoI Framework is grounded in Dewey's educational view of practical inquiry and is "a collaborative-constructivist process model that describes the essential elements of a successful online higher education learning experience" (Castellanos-Reyes, 2020). The CoI Framework includes three elements called presences: cognitive presence, social

TABLE 6.4

Multiple Means of Action and Expression

Action and Expression Principle Guidelines and Checkpoints	Definition	Example
Physical action 1. Vary the methods for response and navigation 2. Optimize access to tools and assistive technologies	The goal of this guideline is to "provide materials with which all learners can interact" (i.e., accessibility; CAST, 2018).	Utilize low-stakes environments such as virtual clinicals, labs, simulations, scenarios, games, etc., to provide time and space to practice skills.
Expression and communication 1. Use multiple media for communication 2. Use multiple tools for construction and composition 3. Build fluencies with graduated levels of support for practice and performance	The goal of this guideline is to provide materials that give learners options in how they present what they have learned.	Allow for learner choice (i.e., provide options) when demonstrating mastery of skills or knowledge. When presenting a clinical case, for example, students can select presentation style to meet learning outcomes (e.g., audio, video, text).
Executive functions 1. Guide appropriate goal setting 2. Support planning and strategy development 3. Facilitate managing information and resources 4. Enhance capacity for monitoring progress	The goal of this guideline is to assist learners as they monitor their own learning and work on both long-term goals and strategy development.	Have learners set their own learning goals at beginning of course (based on course objectives, their prior experience, and professional progression or interests); reflect on progress and plan for ongoing educational development at the end of course (i.e., long-term goals).

presence, and teaching presence, which are interdependent and work together to create a meaningful educational experience.

The CoI Framework, although intentionally developed for online learning environments, has concepts that can be adapted to any classroom modality. One of the core goals of the CoI Framework is the creation of a community of learners. The concept of a learning community can extend and has advantages with both hybrid and traditional classroom environments (Warner, 2016). Interaction between members of an online learning environment is important to student success (Fiock, 2020). When exploring how to enhance nursing students' learning experiences, Torbjørnsen et al.'s (2021) literature review found peer learning and student-centered learning approaches as important factors in enhancing students' perceived experiences. As such, the CoI Framework can assist nurse educators and designers in developing meaningful and successful learning environments for learners.

Social Presence

Social presence is the way a person is portrayed and perceived as "real" in online learning environments (Garrison et al., 2000). More importantly, social presence "refers to the extent to which a person feels connected with others, both socially and emotionally"—a concept that expands all types of learning environments (Choy & Quek, 2016, p. 107). Specific to online courses, research has "shown [social presence] to impact student motivation and participation, actual and perceived learning, course and instructor satisfaction, and retention" (Richardson et al., 2017, p. 1). There are three categories that make up social presence: emotional (affective) expression, open communication, and group cohesion (Garrison & Arbaugh, 2007). Plante & Asselin (2014) explain that "caring has been a dominant theme in shaping nursing programs" and that overlapping themes exist between "caring" and "social presence" concepts. This chapter hopes to answer their call for "ways to advance social presence and caring in the online environment" (p. 222).

All three social presence categories (emotional-affective expression, open communication, and group cohesion) align with the affective domain, specifically emotional engagement which "refers to emotional reactions to classroom, school, or teachers such as enjoyment, interest, boredom, anxiety, happiness, and sadness" (Kassab et al., 2022, p. 7). Specific to sadness and moral conflict, Wros et al. (2021) explain the importance for instructors to provide "students with safe spaces to make sense of clinical situations and consider responses and actions" (p. 1092). Allowing for open communication during these emotional situations can help to build group cohesion and creates areas where students can hear from others with "similar experiences and feelings and engaged in planning next steps for themselves" (p. 1092). Furthermore, Garrison & Arbaugh (2007) note that while socio-emotional communication is important, communication rules must be defined in academic terms and educational contexts for both instructors and learners. Table 6.5 defines and provides examples of Social Presence and its categories: emotional-affective expression, open communication, and group cohesion.

Teaching Presence

Focusing on the categories of instructional design and organization, facilitating discourse, and direct instruction, teaching presence "is considered a key element in the establishment of online community" (Fiock et al., 2021, p. 56). The three categories, however, do have implications outside of online classrooms as instructors and peers must work together to meet the educational learning goals of the course (Choy & Quek, 2016). Specific to nursing education, Smadi et al. (2021) found that novice nurse educators failed to adopt teaching presence strategies because of scarce resources and a lack of understanding of the framework and the presence as a whole. This may be due to nurse educators "designing their courses without formal education and they rely on their teaching experience to guide their design techniques" (p. 7). Supporting faculty development, as discussed in Chapter 4, is key to a quality educational experience.

Garrison (2017) explains that teaching presence is "not possible without the expertise of [a] pedagogically experienced and knowledgeable teacher" (p. 76); therefore, nurse educators need to understand how different types of engagement (socio-cultural, behavioral, emotional, and cognitive) should be utilized for different learners when developing and creating course content. For Teaching Presence specifically, all dimensions of engagement should be considered. Nursing instructors should keep in mind that teaching presence is not only between instructor and student but between student and

TABLE 6.5		
Social Presence		
Social Presence Categories	**Definition**	**Example**
Emotional (affective) expression	Emotional (affective) expression is "where learners share personal expressions and values" with other students and instructors in the course (Fiock, 2020, p. 138).	Use video/audio for online discussions. Allow the use of emoticons, emojis, or gifs in online discussions.
Open communication	Helping to create "mutual awareness," open communication is the "reciprocal and respectful exchanges" among participants (Garrison et al., 2000, p. 100).	Create a shared set of rules for discussion. These should encourage open communication and multiple perspectives but should be respectful. Share personal and professional stories/experiences with students to help students feel comfortable communicating with you (and each other).
Group cohesion	"A sense of belonging is important for sharing personal meaning;" therefore, group cohesion is important as it is "exemplified by activities that build and sustain a sense of group commitment" (Garrison et al., 2000, p. 101).	For collaborative experiences (e.g., team-based learning, problem-based learning, collaborative learning), have learners work together to create a group contract where expectations are discussed and allow for opportunities to build teamworking skills (i.e., cooperation, collaboration).

student; therefore, strategies can be varied to increase learner engagement. Table 6.6 defines and provides examples of Teaching Presence and its categories: instructional design and organization, facilitating discourse, and direct instruction. Additional examples can be found in other chapters in this text. A sample course map, integral to facilitating instructional design, can be found in Chapter 7. Chapter 8 provides additional examples of active learning strategies.

Cognitive Presence

Closely associated with critical thinking, cognitive presence is "the ability to construct and confirm meaning through sustained reflection" (Fiock, 2020, p. 137). According to Garrison et al. (2000), cognitive presence is "most basic to success in higher education" because it is a vital element in critical thinking and requires "high degrees of commitment and participation" among participants (p. 89). As demonstrated through the Practical Inquiry Model (PIM), cognitive presence "refers to the progress of students' thinking through the Practical Inquiry phases (ranged from the 'triggering event' phase; to the 'exploration phase' then 'integration' until reaching the 'resolution phase' of the problem)" (Smadi et al., 2021, p. 2). Case-based learning, specifically case-based

	TABLE 6.6	

Teaching Presence

Teaching Presence Categories	Definition	Example
Instructional design and organization	Instructional design and organization are "the design, structure, process, interaction, and evaluative elements of an online course" (Fiock et al., 2021, p. 57).	Develop a course map to share with students (showing alignment of course objectives, unit objectives, assessment, activities, and learning materials). Clearly communicate purpose and expectations for interactions (student-faculty; student-student; student-content)
Facilitating discourse	Facilitating discourse is "the methods or means instructors use to help students engage with course materials" (Fiock et al., 2021, p. 57).	Monitor and guide (as needed) discussions, summarize, and connect student contributions to learning objectives. Consider using primary sources, case study scenarios, games, visualizations, interactive videos, among others to spark student interest and engagement.
Direct instruction	Direct instruction is the "sharing of subject matter knowledge or expertise with students" (Fiock et al., 2021, p. 57).	Design case discussion(s) using the Practical Inquiry Model to promote critical-thinking skills in learners. Allow opportunities for on-site training (e.g., placements, observations, clinicals, labs) where students can gain real-world experience from professionals in the field.

discussions, is a great way of showing delineation between the PIM categories. First, learners engage in solving authentic problems from the case (triggering event) through analysis of the issues (triggering event and exploration), consideration of underlying principles (exploration), development of solutions (integration), and reflection on the problem-solving process (resolution; Sadaf & Olesova, 2017).

Two engagement dimensions work closely within Cognitive Presence—cognitive and sociocultural dimensions. Hudson (2015) describes the cognitive dimension as "the psychological investment in learning, concentration, and completing work," all of which are also critical pieces in Cognitive Presence (p. 45). Additionally, the socio-cultural dimension of engagement supports Cognitive Presence as it "offers an umbrella for understanding student engagement through partnerships" or in this case, the partnership between course content and the learners individually (Kassab et al., 2022, p. 4). Table 6.7 defines and provides examples of Cognitive Presence and its categories: triggering event, exploration, integration, and resolution.

In this section, we covered a range of instructional strategies that could be used to help engage learners using the CoI framework. Refer to Fiock's (2020) article for

TABLE 6.7		
Cognitive Presence		
Cognitive Presence—PIM Categories	**Definition**	**Example**
Triggering event	A triggering event is a "state of dissonance or feeling of unease resulting from an experience" (Garrison et al., 2000, p. 98).	Small group problem-based learning activities based on four phases of PIM. Using low-stakes environments such as virtual clinicals, labs, avatars, scenarios, games, etc., allows a no-risk opportunity for learners to experience a triggering event.
Exploration	Exploration is "a search for information, knowledge and alternatives that might help to make sense of the situation or problem" (Garrison et al., 2000, p. 98).	Provide learners opportunities where they can complete tasks or assignments using a range of information sources (e.g., interviews, simulations, service learning and fieldwork, resources, peers, etc.). Allow areas in the course where students can share resources with each other helping to create a learning community among their peers.
Integration	Integration is when a "coherent idea or concept" has been developed from "integrating the information and knowledge" (Garrison et al., 2000, p. 98).	Consider using role-play or have learners serve as subject matter experts when demonstrating their understanding of newly learned concepts (e.g., in-class presentations, explaining medication instructions to a patient).
Resolution	After an "idea or hypothesis" has been created, the resolution phase determines if further exploration is warranted (Garrison et al., 2000, p. 99).	Consider using reflective practice where learners "look at a situation with an awareness of own beliefs, values, and practice enabling nurses to learn from experiences, incorporate that learning in improving patient care outcomes" (Patel & Metersky, 2022, p. 180).

guidance on instructional strategies and a more exhaustive list of these strategies and how to use them for each presence.

Quality Matters

While also addressed in Chapter 7, *Backward Design: Aligning Outcomes, Assessments, and Activities* and Chapter 9, *Best Practices in Online Education*, Quality Matters (QM) is a peer review process that helps to create and ensure the quality of online courses and online components. Gaston and Lynch (2019) found students in courses developed with the QM rubric were more active in online discussions, engaged with the content more often, and perceived value in the courses. Additionally, research when QM standards are used in course design, students reported having positive learning and engagement experiences (Sadaf et al., 2019). Standard 4 (Instructional Materials) and Standard 5 (Course Activities & Learner Interaction) were found to be "the most important standard(s) to impact student learning and engagement" (p. 229). When looking at creating means of engagement in *any* course, a few of the standards (Standards 4, 5, and 8) should be considered.

Standard 4 focuses on instructional materials and how they are used to help support and meet the course objectives. Instructional materials can be in a variety of formats that may include but are not limited to textbooks, multimedia, and websites. When selecting course instructional materials, consider the input of your learner population, especially as it pertains to their own learning. For example, Kassab et al. (2022) explain engagement through their own learning where "engagement in individual learning activities in the classroom, laboratory, clinical sites, homework, or self-study" helps to increase learner engagement with instructional materials (p. 4). Standard 5 focuses on creating learning activities to facilitate and support learners. Aligned with course objectives, learning activities should be created with learner interaction and engagement in mind. Crookes et al. (2013) reviewed nursing literature specific to strategies and techniques reported as effective in engaging nursing students. Techniques identified for achieving active participation as well as the practical use of information included simulation, gaming, narrative, whether problem-based or scenario-based, and reflection. Lastly, Standard 8 focuses on accessibility; specifically, a commitment that learners can navigate, access, and use all course content and activities (QM Higher Education Rubric, Sixth Edition, 2018). Not only is this standard assumed to be best practice (i.e., designing for accessibility will not only help people with disabilities but also people without disabilities), but also aligned with Interprofessional Education Global Health Competency—Domain 11: Strategic analysis, or systems thinking to shape global health trends (Phillips & Young, 2018). If you are new to accessibility, we suggest following the four main guiding principles of accessibility known by the acronym POUR for perceivable (content is viewable), operable (content can be navigated and works), understandable (consistent and predictable design is used), and robust (users with assistive technologies can use and access content (CUNY Office of Library Services, 2023).

Seven Principles for Good Practice in Undergraduate Education

> These principles … rest on 50 years of research on the way teachers teach and students learn, how students work and play with one another, and how students and faculty talk to each other (Chickering & Gamson, 1987, para. 6).

Chickering & Gamson (1987) created seven guidelines for good practice in undergraduate education and are "perhaps the best known set of [student] engagement indicators" (Kuh, 2001, p. 1). These guidelines are (1) Encourages contact between students and faculty; (2) Develops reciprocity and cooperation among students; (3) Encourages active learning; (4) Gives prompt feedback; (5) Emphasizes time on task; (6) Communicates high expectations; and (7) Respects diverse talents and ways of learning (Chickering & Gamson, 1987, para. 4). See Table 6.8: Seven Principles for Good Practice in Undergraduate Education Examples.

Applying to a range of learning environments (e.g., online, hybrid, face-to-face), these guidelines have been "positively related to student satisfaction and achievement on a variety of [student engagement] dimensions" (Kuh, 2001, p. 1). Cruce et al. (2006) conducted a multivariate longitudinal analysis on Chickering & Gamson's seven guidelines

---

TABLE 6.8

Seven Principles for Good Practice in Undergraduate Education

Principle	Example
Encourages contact between students and faculty	Create an open, warm, and welcoming environment in the classroom. Outside of the classroom, consider holding office hours where students can interact with faculty outside of class.
Develops reciprocity and cooperation among students	Provide opportunities for group work or cooperative learning communities. Encourage students from different backgrounds to share their viewpoints on topics shared in class.
Encourages active learning	Provide low-stakes, experiential, or scenario-based learning activities. Consider having students select topics or bring readings to class.
Gives prompt feedback	Provide students with ongoing formative feedback, connecting the feedback to specific learning objectives. Additionally, feedback needs to be timely in order for it to be useful (Fiock & Garcia, 2019).
Emphasizes time on task	Time on task is the time a student is actively involved in the learning process—whether that is reading, discussing, active listening, presenting, etc. Consider using a similar schedule for each course with a range of different instructional strategies to maintain student engagement. Consider progressive assignments (i.e., each task builds on previous task).
Communicates high expectations	Provide a syllabus with expectations (e.g., class policies, assignment descriptions, grading scale, schedule, etc.). Ensure clarity in objectives, content, and criteria for success for the course.
Respects diverse talents and ways of learning	Allow for learner choice (i.e., provide options). Learner choice can be in how students demonstrate their mastery or how the information is presented to them (e.g., reading, video, image).

and found that at 18 institutions, all guidelines have been related to a number of first-year learners' outcomes such as cognitive development (e.g., comprehension, critical thinking skills) and other orientations to learning (e.g., openness, self-understanding, attitude).

CHAPTER SUMMARY

In preparing prelicense and new nurses to practice and lead in the field, nurse educators must consider the different dimensions of student engagement when creating meaningful learning experiences, using engaging teaching practices for our learners. As nursing students bring diversity (e.g., language, cultural identities, prior knowledge, skills, lived experience, etc.), it is vital nurse educators leverage effective strategies to enhance and engage learners. With "a dynamic, iterative process of investment, participation, and commitment to learning," this chapter reviewed student engagement through three dimensions: behavioral, affective, and cognitive (Noone, 2022, p. 18). Focused on two major frameworks—Universal Design for Learning (UDL) and Community of

Inquiry (CoI)—we explained each framework's purpose and demonstrated example teaching strategies for engagement practices. Jeppesen et al. (2017) note a gap in teaching strategies that directly help to integrate classroom and clinical practice; the tables presented in this paper hope to provide nurse educators guidance and inspiration for filling this void. Specifically, we provided tangible ways to apply UDL and the CoI frameworks through the use of different engagement activities (across different dimensions) for a variety of learning environments (e.g., classroom, labs, clinical) our students may face.

References

Abualhaija, N. (2019). Using constructivism and student-centered learning approaches in nursing education. *International Journal of Nursing and Healthcare Research*, 7, 93. https://doi.org/10.29011/IJNHR-093.100093

Benner, P., Sutphen, M., Leonard, V., & Day, L. (2010). *Educating nurses: A call for radical transformation* (Vol. 15). John Wiley & Sons.

Bernard, J. S. (2015). Student engagement: A Principle-based concept analysis. *International Journal of Nursing Education Scholarship*, 12(1), 111–121. https://doi.org/10.1515/ijnes-2014-0058

Bristol, T., Brett, A., Alejandro, J., Colin, J., Murray, T., Wangerin, V., Linck, R., & Walton, D. (2020). Nursing faculty readiness for student diversity. *Teaching and Learning in Nursing*, 15, 104–108. https://doi.org/10.1016/j.teln.2019.09.0011

CAST. (2011). *Universal design for learning guidelines version 2.0.*

CAST. (2018). *Universal design for learning guidelines version 2.2 [graphic organizer].* Retrieved from https://udlguidelines.cast.org/more/downloads

Castellanos-Reyes, D. (2020). 20 years of the Community of Inquiry framework. *TechTrends*, 64, 557–560. https://doi.org/10.1007/s11528-020-00491-7

Chickering, A. W., & Gamson, Z. F. (1987). Seven principles for good practice in undergraduate education. *The Wingspread Journal*, 9, 1–10.

Choy, J. L. F., & Quek, C. L. (2016). Modelling relationships between students' academic achievement and community of inquiry in an online learning environment for a blended course. *Australasian Journal of Educational Technology*, 32(4). https://doi.org/10.14742/ajet.2500

Clynes, M., Sheridan, A., & Frazer, K. (2020). Student engagement in higher education: A cross-sectional study of nursing students' participation in college-based education in the republic of Ireland. *Nurse Education Today*, 93, 1–7. https://doi.org/10.1016/j.nedt.2020.104529

Crookes, K., Crookes, P. A., & Walsh, K. (2013). Meaningful and engaging teaching techniques for student nurses: a literature review. *Nurse Education in Practice*, 13(4), 239–243. https://doi.org/10.1016/j.nepr.2013.04.008

Cruce, T. M., Wolniak, G. C., Seifert, T. A., & Pascarella, E. T. (2006). Impacts of good practices on cognitive development, learning orientations, and graduate degree plans during the first year of college. *Journal of College Student Development*, 47(4), 365–383. https://doi.org/10.1353/csd.2006.0042

CUNY Office of Library Services. (2023). *Accessibility toolkit for open educational resources (OER): Accessibility principles.* CUNY Library Services. https://guides.cuny.edu/accessibility/whyitmatters#:~:text=There%20are%20four%20main%20guiding,%2C%20operable%2C%20understandable%20and%20robust.

Czerkawski, B., & Lymann, E. W., III (2016). An instructional design framework for fostering student engagement in online learning environments. *TechTrends*, 60, 532–539. https://doi.org/10.1007/s11528-016-0110-z

Davis, D., McLaughlin, M. K., & Anderson, K. M. (2021). Universal design for learning: A Framework for blended learning in nursing education. *Nurse Educator*, 47(3), 133–138. https://doi.org/10.1097/NNE.0000000000001116

Fiock, H. (2020). Designing a Community of Inquiry in online courses. *The International Review of Research in Open and Distributed Learning, 21*(1), 135–153. https://doi.org/10.19173/irrodl.v20i5.3985

Fiock, H., & Garcia, H. (2019, November). *How to give your students better feedback with technology*. The Chronicle of Higher Education. https://www.chronicle.com/article/how-to-give-your-students-better-feedback-with-technology/

Fiock, H., Maeda, Y., & Richardson, J. C. (2021). Instructor impact on differences in teaching presence scores in online courses. *The International Review of Research in Open and Distributed Learning, 22*(3), 55–76. https://doi.org/10.19173/irrodl.v22i3.5456

Frazer, C., Reilly, C. A., & Squellati, R. E. (2021). Instructional strategies: Teaching nursing in today's diverse and inclusive landscape. *Teaching and Learning in Nursing, 16*(3), 276–280. https://doi.org/10.1016/j.teln.2021.01.005

Garrison, D. R. (2017). *E-Learning in the 21st Century: A community of inquiry framework for research and practice*. Routledge. https://doi.org/10.4324/9781315667263

Garrison, D. R., & Arbaugh, J. B. (2007). Researching the community of inquiry framework: Review, issues, and future directions. *The Internet and Higher Education, 10*, 157–172. https://doi.org/10.1016/j.iheduc.2007.04.001

Garrison, D. R., Anderson, T., & Archer, W. (2000). Critical inquiry in a text-based environment: Computer conferencing in higher education. *The Internet and Higher Education, 2*(2–3), 87–105. https://doi.org/10.1016/S1096-7516(00)00016-6

Gaston, T., & Lynch, S. (2019). Does using a course design framework better engage our online nursing students? *Teaching and Learning in Nursing, 14*(1), 69–71. https://doi.org/10.1016/j.teln.2018.11.001

Gay, G. (2015). The what, why, and how of culturally responsive teaching: international mandates, challenges, and opportunities. *Multicultural Education Review, 7*(3), 123–139. https://doi.org/10.1080/2005615X.2015.1072079.

Ghasemi, M. R., Moonaghi, H. K., & Heydari, A. (2020). Strategies for sustaining and enhancing nursing students' engagement in academic and clinical settings: a narrative review. *Korean Journal of Medical Education, 32*(2), 103–117. https://doi.org/10.3946/kjme.2020.159

Groccia, J. E. (2018). What is student engagement? *New Directions for Teaching and Learning, 154*, 11–20. https://doi.org/10.1002/tl.20287

Hudson, K. F. (2015). Nursing student engagement: Student, classroom, and clinical engagement. *International Journal of Nursing, 4*(1), 44–52. https://www.ijnonline.com/index.php/ijn/article/view/195

Jeppesen, K. H., Christiansen, S., & Frederiksen, K. (2017). Education of student nurses— A systematic literature review. *Nurse Education Today, 55*, 112–121. https://doi.org/10.1016/j.nedt.2017.05.005

Johnson, K. Z. (2015). *Student engagement in nursing school: A secondary analysis of the National Survey of Student Engagement data*. [Unpublished doctoral dissertation]. University of Kansas. https://kuscholarworks.ku.edu/bitstream/handle/1808/19449/Johnson_ku_0099D_14023_DATA_1.pdf

Kassab, S. E., Taylor, D., & Hamdy, H. (2022). Student engagement in health professions education: AMEE Guide No. 152. *Medical Teacher*, 1–17. https://doi.org/10.1080/0142159X.2022.2137018

Koehler, A. A., Newby, T. J., & Ertmer, P. A. (2017). Examining the role of web 2.0 tools in supporting problem solving during case-based instruction. *Journal of Research on Technology in Education, 49*(3–4), 182–197. https://doi.org/10.1080/15391523.2017.1338167

Kuh, G. D. (2001). *The National Survey of Student Engagement: Conceptual framework and overview of psychometric properties*. Center for Postsecondary Research, Indiana University. Retrieved from http://nsse.iub.edu/pdf/conceptual_framework_2003.pdf

National League for Nursing. (2023). *NLN Hallmarks of Excellence*. Hallmarks of Excellence. https://www.nln.org/home

National Survey of Student Engagement. (2018). *Engagement indicators &*

high-impact practices. Retrieved from https://irds.iupui.edu/students/student-surveys/nsse/2018.html

Noone, J. (2022). Engaged students: Essential to achieve distinction in nursing education. In M. Adams, & T. Valiga (Eds.). *Achieving Distinction in Nursing Education*. National League for Nursing.

Patel, K. M., & Metersky, K. (2022). Reflective practice in nursing: A concept analysis. *International Journal of Nursing Knowledge, 33*(3), 180–187. https://doi.org/10.1111/2047-3095.12350

Pedler, M., Yeigh, T., & Hudson, S. (2020). The teachers' role in student engagement: A review. *Australian Journal of Teacher Education, 45*(3), 4. https://doi.org/10.14221/ajte.2020v45n3.4

Pentaraki, A., & Burkholder, G. (2017). Emerging evidence regarding the roles of emotional, behavioural, and cognitive aspects of student engagement in the online classroom. *European Journal of Open, Distance and E-Learning, 20*(1), 1–21. https://doi.org/10.1515/eurodl-2017-0001

Phillips, J. M., & Young, J. A. (2018). Strategies for Integrating Global Awareness and Engagement Into Clinical Practice. *Journal of Continuing Education in Nursing, 49*(5), 203–205. https://doi.org/10.3928/00220124-20180417-04

Plante, K., & Asselin, M. E. (2014). Best practices for creating social presence and caring behaviors online. *Nursing Education Perspectives, 35*(4), 219–223. https://doi.org/10.5480/13-1094.1

Popkess, A. M., & McDaniel, A. (2011). Are nursing students engaged in learning? A secondary analysis of data from the National Survey of Student Engagement. *Nursing Education Perspectives, 32*(2), 89–94. https://doi.org/10.5480/1536-5026-32.2.89

QM Higher Education Rubric, Sixth Edition, 2018. Quality Matters. Used under license. All rights reserved. Retrieved from MyQM.

Richardson, J. C., Maeda, Y., Lv, J., & Caskurlu, S. (2017). Social presence in relation to students' satisfaction and learning in the online environment: A meta-analysis. *Computers in Human Behavior, 71*, 402–417. https://doi.org/10.1016/j.chb.2017.02.001

Sadaf, A., Martin, F., & Ahlgrim-Delzell, L. (2019). Student perceptions of the impact of quality matters-certified online courses on their learning and engagement. *Online Learning, 23*(4), 214–233. https://doi.org/10.24059/olj.v23i4.2009

Sadaf, A., & Olesova, L. (2017). Enhancing cognitive presence in online case discussions with questions based on the Practical Inquiry Model. *American Journal of Distance Education, 31*(1), 56–69. https://doi.org/10.1080/08923647.2017.1267525

Smadi, O., Chamberlain, D., Shifaza, F., & Hamiduzzaman, M. (2021). Factors affecting the adoption of the Community of Inquiry Framework in Australian online nursing education: A transition theory perspective. *Nurse Education in Practice, 55*, 103166. https://doi.org/10.1016/j.nepr.2021.103166

Torbjørnsen, A., Hessevaagbakke, E., Grov, E. K., & Bjørnnes, A. K. (2021). Enhancing students learning experiences in nursing programmes: An integrated review. *Nurse Education in Practice, 52*, 103038. https://doi.org/10.1016/j.nepr.2021.103038

Trowler, V., Allan, R., Bryk, J., & Din, R. (2022). Pathways to student engagement: beyond triggers and mechanisms at the engagement interface. *Higher Education, 84*, 761–777. https://doi.org/10.1007/s10734-021-00798-1

U.S. Census Bureau. (2021, Aug 20). *2020 U.S. Population More Racially and Ethnically Diverse Than Measured in 2010*. Retrieved from https://www.census.gov/library/stories/2021/08/2020-united-states-population-more-racially-ethnically-diverse-than-2010.html

Warner, A. G. (2016). Developing a Community of Inquiry in a face-to-face class. *Journal of Management Education, 40*(4), 432–452. https://doi.org/10.1177/1052562916629515

Wros, P. L., Mathews, L. R., Beiers-Jones, K., & Warkentin, P. (2021). Moral distress in public health practice: Case studies from nursing education. *Public Health Nursing, 38*, 1088–1094. https://doi.org/10.1111/phn.12948

<h1>7</h1>

Backward Design: Aligning Outcomes, Assessments, and Activities

Joanne Noone, PhD, RN, CNE, FAAN, ANEF

CHAPTER OVERVIEW

This chapter focuses on intentional course design and concepts of backward design. Backward design emphasizes the importance of learning alignment which involves first identifying learning outcomes, then determining how they will be assessed, and finally developing the learning activities to facilitate the achievement of learning outcomes. Topics addressed in this chapter include writing measurable learning outcomes; models used to develop significant learning experiences, such as the six facets of understanding; and Fink's taxonomy for significant learning. Tools such as design templates and course maps used to apply backward design and alignment concepts when developing a unit of instruction are presented. Examples of backward design in action in a variety of higher education curricula are described.

BACKWARD DESIGN DEFINED

"Backward design" is the term developed by Grant Wiggins and Jay McTighe, noted educators, as they developed their Understanding by Design (UbD®) framework, a purposeful educational approach to designing curriculum, assessments, and activities to facilitate understanding and learning. Often, educators who are about to design an instructional unit or course begin to develop learning activities or assignments in thinking about what they want to teach in this unit or course. I would say this described me as a novice educator who looked for learning activities from peers, texts, or articles without explicitly linking them to what outcomes I wanted my learners to achieve. Backward design reverses this process; Wiggins and McTighe (2005) define backward design as "[a]n approach to designing a curriculum or unit that begins with the end in mind and designs towards that end . . . starting with the end (the desired results) and then identifying the evidence necessary to determine that the results have been achieved (assessments)" (p. 338). Once these have been identified, learning activities can be designed to develop learner knowledge, skills, and abilities to meet the desired results.

Best practices and educational standards such as Quality Matters© emphasize the importance of alignment of outcomes, assessments, and activities as key to quality instruction. Quality Matters (2018, p. 48) defines alignment as "critical course elements working together to ensure that learners achieve the desired learning outcomes." Three of the eight standards identified by Quality Matters in assessing quality of online and blended classrooms evaluate whether the learning assessments, instructional materials, and learning activities all align to promote the achievement of measurable learning outcomes. In this chapter, we will look at best practices in instructional design, whether you are designing an academic course or continuing education program, or a unit or module within a course or program.

THE STAGES OF BACKWARD DESIGN

Wiggins and McTighe (2005) describe three stages of backward design:

> In Stage 1, the desired results are identified.
> In Stage 2, the assessments are identified that will inform whether the results have been met.
> In Stage 3, learning activities are designed to facilitate achievement of the desired results.

Stage 1

Desired learning results are usually written in the form of learning outcomes. We will review how to write measurable learning outcomes in a later section of this chapter. Outcomes, which may also be referred to as competencies or objectives, specify what the learners will be able to know and do as a result of participating in the planned learning experience. For consistency of language, the term "outcomes" will be used throughout this chapter (Hansen, 2011). Wiggins and McTighe (2005) recommend that the faculty designer explore the following questions as they determine the desired results:

> What should students know, understand, and be able to do?
> What standards need to be met?
> What are the priorities for content?
> What content is important for understanding?
> What enduring or long-term understandings are desired?

Faculty designers should consider what standards this unit or course addresses and links to. Academic courses and programs of study are grounded in state and national accreditation standards, such as state board of nursing educational standards; national nursing accreditation organizations, such as the Commission on Collegiate Nursing Education (CCNE) or Accreditation Commission for Education in Nursing (ACEN); or regional accrediting bodies that accredit higher education colleges and universities. National educational competencies may also guide curriculum development. For example, the Quality and Safety Education for Nurses (QSEN, 2020) has identified quality and safety knowledge, skills, and abilities for prelicensure and graduate students and developed related competencies. For graduate practice programs, educational standards may also be set by their specialty organizations; for example, the Council on Accreditation of Nurse Anesthesia Educational Programs (COA) accredits nurse anesthesia programs. Programs, colleges, and universities may have identified core competencies for graduates or student learning outcomes to be achieved by the end of the program. Continuing education programs may link to practice standards or competencies developed by specialty organizations, such as the American Association of Critical Care Nurses or Quality and Safety Education for Nurses.

It is also essential when developing the desired results to consider who are the learners and what prerequisite knowledge they are expected to have and to anticipate what course content they may likely struggle with (Hansen, 2011). For an academic course, consider where this unit or course fits into the curriculum. Aligning the desired results to the level of the learners is also important. For example, how a designer might approach a unit on respiratory assessment might be very different if the learners are first-year prelicensure nursing students as compared to new registered nursing graduates. Considering the learners' prerequisite knowledge is helpful to meeting the learners where they are. For example, if the faculty designer is developing a unit of instruction of respiratory assessment for first-year prelicensure nursing students, they may decide that prerequisite knowledge includes an understanding of respiratory anatomy, physiology, and pathophysiology; concepts of gas exchange and acid-base balance; use of equipment to perform the assessments; knowledge of how to approach and position patients for assessments; and, basic patient safety measures.

Stage 2

In Stage 2, designers select and/or develop learning assessments that provide evidence that learners have met the desired outcomes. Questions that designers can ask at this stage are (Wiggins & McTighe, 2005; Emory, 2014):

> How do I know if students have achieved the desired outcomes and met standards?

> How will the students show what they know?

> How can I determine whether students have attained the desired understanding?

> What evidence is acceptable/needed to document and validate student achievement of the desired understanding and proficiency?

> Does the evidence align with the outcome?

Wiggins and McTighe (2005) emphasize the importance of designing practice opportunities, or formative assessments, of authentic performance tasks to allow learners to rehearse, receive feedback on, and refine performance in order to then demonstrate competency in meeting the learning outcomes through summative assessments. Rubrics ideally should be developed to provide feedback for both formative and summative purposes. Authentic performance tasks situate learners into learning experiences within a social context that aligns with and approximates what happens in actual clinical practice (Kennedy, 2017). Such contextualized learning can provide rich learning that closes the theory-practice gap, integrating classroom and clinical learning. We will explore how to enrich the planning of learning experiences later in this chapter and how to build assessments later in this book.

Stage 3

The learning plan is designed in Stage 3, in which teachers then intentionally select teaching strategies that link to the assessments and learning outcomes. According to Emory (2014, p. 124), "Learning strategies should be selected with intentionality and should lead to the identified methods of assessment and desired outcomes. Educators should use a variety of strategies to address student needs for opportunity to learn with understanding." The authentic performance tasks identified in Stage 2 become the foundation for learning activities in Stage 3 (Hansen, 2011). Questions Wiggins and McTighe (2005) recommend the designer ask at this stage include:

> What knowledge and skills will students need to achieve the desired outcomes?
> What authentic activities will equip students with the needed knowledge and skills?
> What will need to be taught and coached?
> What's the best way to teach it?

It is recommended to sequence learning activities developmentally (Hansen, 2011; Kennedy, 2017) and create a scaffold to support learning. Hansen recommends breaking down large performance tasks into more manageable, smaller "building blocks" that occur throughout the course and building upon the knowledge and skills acquired throughout the course. Breaking down a large assignment such as a paper into parts completed and reviewed over the course rather than being due at the end of the term can allow for enhanced understanding and skill development For example, a learning activity such as writing an evidence-based paper can be broken down to having the learners submit their clinical question and literature search strategy first to receive feedback before proceeding to write the paper. Papers and similar assignments can be submitted in sections, providing feedback with an aim to achieve progressive improvement, rather than one submission at the end of the term. In practice settings, similarly breaking down learning into smaller units and reviewing prerequisite knowledge can assist learners to develop additional skills and abilities.

Nursing, like many professions, is a vast discipline with knowledge growth continually occurring. Instead of focusing on "covering the content" which can lead to an overwhelming amount of information for learners to process and may impact the development of thinking skills (Ironside, 2004). Weimer (2002) advises that we "uncover" the content to make it accessible for learners. Because of time constraints, priorities for content within the allotted time of the unit or course need to be established. Since it is likely impossible to teach everything about a topic within a given time frame, think about what is worthy to know, important to know, and "enduring" understandings. As nurse author Dr. Jan Emory states, "The BD (Backward Design) framework processes serve to strengthen and improve curricular implementation to meet the challenges faced by the content squeeze and saturation present in nursing education. This is accomplished through a clear focus on learner-centered outcomes to prioritize content and concepts and create meaningful understanding for transfer to

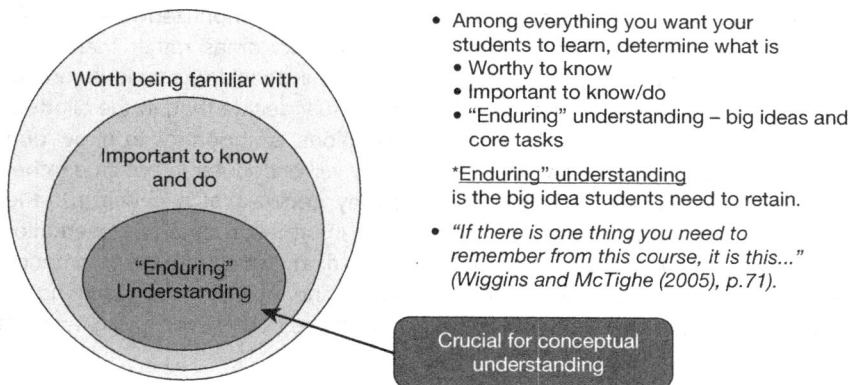

FIGURE 7.1 Identifying Content Priorities. (Adapted from Wiggins & McTighe [2005]; Hansen [2011].)

practice (p. 123). Wiggins and McTighe (2005) recommend separating out and clarifying content priorities into three areas (see Fig. 7.1):

➤ **What is worthy of being familiar with?** As seen in Figure 7.1, this is the outermost circle of content priority which is content that is least critical for learners to know although it is worthy of learners being familiar with. This is content that a designer may review if they have additional time or provide learners access to resources for further learning.

➤ **What is important to know and do** is high-priority content to ensure is included in the learning experience. This may relate to curriculum trends or high priority focus areas or highly prevalent conditions.

➤ **What are the enduring understandings?** Enduring understandings emanate from delineating the unit or course's big ideas and core tasks to focus on. Big ideas refer to the major core concepts of the unit or course and core tasks are essential skills and abilities. For example, in a unit of instruction on pediatric diabetic ketoacidosis, the associated big ideas may be acid-base balance, glucose regulation, development approaches, and fluid-electrolyte balance, to name a few. Associated core tasks may be the ability to develop rapport with a pediatric client, physical assessment skills, clinical reasoning skills in addition to the associated technical skills of intravenous line maintenance, fluid and electrolyte replacement therapy, and medication administration. Enduring understandings are the key understandings the designer wants learners to be able to retain long after the program is over. Hansen (2011) calls these enduring understandings "crucial for conceptual understanding." For example, a clinical educator may be preparing a unit of instruction on pediatric diabetic ketoacidosis and develops the following enduring understandings:

  ➤ Children are sometimes initially misdiagnosed with a respiratory issue because of Kussmaul respirations, so pediatric clients who present with rapid respirations, have a level of suspicion that this may be Kussmaul's respirations related to pediatric diabetic ketoacidosis.

  ➤ Children are more at risk for cerebral edema from rapid fluid resuscitation than adults. While fluid resuscitation is critical, it must also be cautiously administered.

While it may be an inexact science of what content is prioritized where, this intentional focus can facilitate deep learning of high-priority areas rather than superficial learning of scattered, related content. For example, in teaching a module on sexually transmitted infections (STIs), the faculty designer may decide that, in the allotted time, a focus on nationally and locally prevalent infections is important to know and provides for deep learning for what the student likely will encounter in practice rather than superficial learning of all STIs. The designer may decide that it is worth the learner being familiar with how to access resources for information on STI presentation and current treatment recommendations to further learning as treatment recommendations are updated (Noone, 2009). After the implementation and evaluation of a learning activity, the designer may decide to reprioritize content to move from "worth being familiar with" to "important to know and do."

WRITING LEARNING OUTCOMES

Learning outcomes come in various names: goals, objectives, outcomes, and competencies. In this discussion, the term learning outcomes will be used for clarity and consistency. Essentially, learning outcomes are what you anticipate your learners will be able to know and do as a result of participating in your planned learning experience. Learning outcomes are written from the learner's point of view so while my outcome may be that I want to teach students about the elements of backward design, a correctly written learning outcome from the learner's point of view is that: "After this presentation, the learner will be able to write a measurable learning outcome that correctly aligns to an authentic assessment and learning activity."

Learning Taxonomy and Domains of Learning

Educational psychologist Benjamin Bloom and colleagues (Bloom et al., 1956) created a taxonomy of educational objectives in the cognitive domain, which was later updated by Anderson and Krathwohl (2001). Other colleagues contributed additional psychomotor and affective domains of learning (Dave, 1970; Krathwohl et al., 1964). This taxonomy is a hierarchical classification of learning with more complex thinking and doing occurring at higher levels in the taxonomy. The cognitive domain focuses on understanding, thinking, or knowledge; the psychomotor domain on acting or doing; and the affective domain emphasizes feelings, motivation, values, and attitudes. While there are several derivations of the psychomotor domain, the taxonomy developed by Dave (1970) appears to be the taxonomy most commonly referenced in nursing (Schechel, 2020; Oermann & Gaberson, 2021). A description of each of the domains' hierarchy ordered from lowest to highest levels and sample measurable verbs can be found in Tables 7.1 to 7.3.

Principles for Well-Written Learning Outcomes

Use a Framework for Writing Outcomes

Using a framework can help to write clear outcomes. One such framework uses the mnemonic SMART: S is for specific, M is for measurable, A is for achievable, R is for

TABLE 7.1

The Cognitive Domain Hierarchy and Associated Verbs

Level	Description	Sample Verbs	Example
Remembering	Recalling or remembering facts, terms, basic concepts, and answers	Define, identify, recall, state, list, name	After this lesson, the learner will be able to recall the three main coronary arteries.
Understanding	Demonstrates understanding with ability to explain ideas or concepts	Describe, discuss, explain, compare, contrast	After this lesson, the learner will be able to describe the normal blood flow through the heart.
Applying	Using information in new ways or situations to solve problems	Complete, employ, prepare, use, write	At the end of this unit, the learner will be able to use a level of evidence table to identify the level of evidence for a given research article.
Analyzing	Break down information to examine and distinguish different parts	Appraise, classify, differentiate, distinguish, plan	At the end of this unit, the learner will be able to differentiate well-constructed from poorly constructed multiple-choice test items.
Evaluating	Assess or judge against a set of criteria	Argue, assess, defend, evaluate, justify	At the end of this course, the learner will be able to evaluate peers' teaching demonstration according to the assignment rubric.
Creating	Propose new solutions, products, ideas, points of view	Collaborate, construct, create, design	At the end of this unit, the learner will be able to create a teaching plan for a postoperative mastectomy client being discharged with a closed suction drain.

relevant, and T is for time-bound. A specific outcome clearly describes what the learner will be able to know or do after the learning experience. In an example from Table 7.1, the outcome "At the end of this unit, the learner will be able to create a teaching plan for a postoperative mastectomy client being discharged with a surgical drain", specifies the expectation that the learner should be able to achieve after participating in the unit of instruction. Especially for developing course and program outcomes, it is best to avoid interpreting "specific" to mean "narrow" such as in the example from Table 7.1, "After this lesson, the learner will be able to recall the three main coronary arteries." While it was used as an example for the cognitive level of "remembering", a low level of thinking, writing too narrow an outcome usually results in too many needing to be written. We will discuss this more in the section on using higher-ordered outcomes. Use measurable verbs, such as shown in Tables 7.1 to 7.3, which are written from the learner's point of view, and avoid vague verbs that really can't be measured, such as "know,"

TABLE 7.2

The Psychomotor Domain Hierarchy and Associated Verbs

Level	Description	Sample Verbs	Example
Imitation	Ability to imitate a skill or behavior after observing it performed	Repeat, follow, imitate, show, copy	After observing the instructor, the learner will be able to repeat the steps of handwashing.
Manipulation	Ability to perform a skill or behavior from memory or written instructions	Assemble, carry out, perform, manipulate	After this lesson, the learner will be able to assemble the equipment and supplies needed to insert a urinary catheter.
Precision	Ability to perform a skill accurately and independently	Demonstrate, conduct, perform, respond	At the end of this unit, the learner will be able to demonstrate an accurate, focused cardiac assessment of a pediatric client.
Articulation	Ability to perform in a coordinated manner within a reasonable time and under various new or problem situations	Adapt, alter, modify, organize	At the end of this unit, the learner will be able to adapt bathing techniques for a client with dementia.
Naturalization	Performance of skill is second nature and integrated within client care	Integrate, combine, design	At the end of orientation, the learner will be able to integrate a focused assessment while communicating with the client.

"appreciate," "learn," or "understand." Consider if the outcome is achievable within the period given to be completed. Relevant outcomes relate to the scope of practice of the learner. To make an outcome time-bound, consider beginning the outcome with the phrase, "After this course, presentation, unit, etc."

Another framework to consider is the mnemonic ABCD (for actor, behavior, condition, and degree of mastery). The actor is the intended audience or learners. Outcomes should always be from the learner's perspective and what they will be able to do differently. It should not be written from the perspective of what the teacher or course will teach. For example:

Correctly written outcome from the learner's perspective: At the end of this unit, the learner will be able to demonstrate an accurate, focused cardiac assessment on a pediatric client.

Incorrectly written outcome from a teacher or course perspective: This unit will teach cardiac assessment on a pediatric client.

The behavior is the measurable action verb selected to describe what the learner will do differently after the learning experience. The condition is similar to the time-bound

TABLE 7.3

The Affective Domain Hierarchy and Associated Verbs

Level	Description	Sample Verbs	Example
Receiving	Awareness of and receptivity to values, beliefs, and attitudes	Choose, express, ask, acknowledge	After this presentation, the learner expresses an awareness of the Nurses' Code of Ethics.
Responding	Actively participates and engages by reacting to a situation	Share, discuss, clarify, participate	At the end of the clinical experience, the learner will discuss ethical issues observed in client care.
Valuing	Accepts and commits to value; internalizes value	Justify, propose, recognize, commit	At the end of this unit, the learner will commit to supporting client confidentiality.
Organization	Orders and prioritizes values	Arrange, formulate, compare, defend	At the end of this learning activity, the learner will compare the ethical dilemmas of veracity versus withholding information.
Characterization by a value	Lives and practices by a worldview	Act consistently, display, practice, propose	At the end of the program of study, the learner will act consistently to promote client rights.

aspect of SMART and identifies under what condition or when you expect this outcome to be achieved. The degree of mastery is the expected standard. In the example "At the end of this unit, the learner will be able to create a teaching plan for a postoperative mastectomy client being discharged with a surgical drain", the expectation is that the teaching plan will be on this type of postoperative client.

Use One Verb per Outcome

Each outcome should only have one verb to facilitate clear assessment. For example, the following outcome contains two separate outcomes, "assemble" and "demonstrate": "After this lesson, the learner will be able to assemble the equipment and supplies needed to insert a urinary catheter and demonstrate accurate insertion of a urinary catheter in a female client using aseptic technique." The problems with using more than one verb are wordiness, which can cause confusion, and also the dilemma if a learner meets one outcome and not the other. Kennedy (2017) recommends using the higher-order outcome (in this case, "demonstrate"), as assembling the correct supplies and equipment is a necessary component of correct insertion of the catheter.

Develop Unit or Module Outcomes

For academic and larger continuing education courses, chunking the topics presented into units of instruction or modules and developing learning outcomes for these units are considered part of a quality course design (Quality Matters, 2018). These unit outcomes are usually more specific and can be helpful for learners to chart their progress and self-evaluate their achievement in readiness for performance assessments. For example, in a health promotion course, there may be the following topics or units: health promotion concepts, communication, health history, health promotion in the pediatric population, and health promotion in the adult population. As the designer for the communication unit, an educator develops the following unit outcomes. The learner will be able to:

➤ Assess influential factors related to a person's motivation for health behavior change.

➤ Demonstrate basic motivational interviewing strategies with peers related to a health behavior change.

➤ Demonstrate therapeutic communication techniques based on a case study.

➤ Compare use of two methods of interview questions to obtain an accurate assessment.

Align Outcomes Across Units, Courses, and Programs

Most, if not all, academic programs have program or university outcomes that they expect learners to achieve by the end of the program, which are sometimes referred to as student learning outcomes. These are helpful to think about as courses and unit outcomes are developed to see where and how they fit in to help achieve these program outcomes. Making this explicit in the course syllabus or, in another place on the course site, helps learners understand the rationale and see the relevance of doing a learning activity (later we will talk about creating a course map that aligns outcomes, assessments, and learning activities). See Table 7.4 for an example of aligning outcomes across a master's in nursing education program and a course on learner assessment.

Use Higher-Ordered Outcomes

Nursing is a complex discipline that demands critical thinking and clinical reasoning and judgment for safe, effective practice. It is recommended to structure learning outcomes, those in particular for courses and end-of-program, which are on the higher end of Bloom's taxonomy. This is particularly true for courses later in a program of study and for graduate-level courses. Higher-ordered outcomes will integrate many aspects of lower-ordered outcomes. For example, consider these two outcomes:

Higher-ordered outcome: At the end of this unit, the learner will be able to create a teaching plan for a postoperative mastectomy client being discharged with a closed suction drain.

Lower-order outcome: At the end of this unit, the learner will be able to list the steps to empty a closed suction drain.

In this example, in order for the higher-ordered outcome to be attained, to be able to create a teaching plan for this client, the lower one, explaining how to empty a closed

TABLE 7.4		
Sample Alignment of Outcomes Across Program, Course, and Unit		
Program Outcome	**Course Outcome**	**Sample Unit Outcomes**
Determine competencies for selected learner groups, written at appropriate level of achievement and relevant for the specialty.	Design assessments to evaluate student attainment of selected nursing competencies.	Create a three-level rubric to assess a learning outcome. Create multiple-choice test questions that assess a learning outcome.
Integrate consideration of individual variations in learning styles and cultural understanding into assessment and instructional planning.	Evaluate selected assessment tools for use in a formative and summative evaluation of student learning related to the purposes, strengths, and limitations of different assessment approaches.	Compare elements of fair testing with high-stakes testing. Identify facilitators and barriers to effective assessment. Apply principles of effective item writing to revise multiple-choice assessments.
Participate in curriculum development, program evaluation, and improvement initiatives.	Discuss methods of course and program evaluation.	Discuss components of course and program evaluation. Evaluate course strengths and weaknesses, providing recommendations for improvement.

suction drain, also needs to be met. The higher-ordered outcome incorporates multiple other necessary components to be achieved, which may include assessing the client's literacy, explaining signs and symptoms of complications, etc. Higher-ordered outcomes incorporate multiple components and more authentically replicate the complexities of current nursing practice.

DESIGNING FOR RICH, SIGNIFICANT LEARNING

In this section, we will review ways to enhance the design of learning activities to more authentically replicate what students will encounter in clinical practice. As you design learning activities, considering one or more of these frameworks can assist with developing rich learning experiences. Some authors (Fink, 2013; Hansen, 2011) suggest using the facets of understanding or Fink's taxonomy as an alternative to Bloom's taxonomy.

Six Facets of Understanding

Wiggins and McTighe (2005) describe understanding as multidimensional and that for complete understanding to occur students need to be able to explain, interpret, apply, perceive, empathize, and self-evaluate. Figure 7.2 provides a description of each facet. While it might be unrealistic to incorporate all six facets of understanding into every unit of instruction, expanding opportunities to add learning outcomes and activities that incorporate the understanding of perspective, empathy, and self-knowledge can enrich

Explain	• Uses guidelines or principles to make connections • Provides a justification based on knowledge
Interpret	• Uses narratives, metaphors, images to provide meaning • Offers meaningful translation and inferences
Apply	• Uses a concept or skill in a new situation • Effectively adapts in diverse contexts
Perspective	• Shows insightful points of view • Analyzes different interpretations or explanations
Empathy	• Able to understand a situation from another viewpoint • Able to "walk in another's shoes"
Self-Knowledge	• Able to identify gaps in one's knowledge • Understands what biases and beliefs influence one's viewpoint

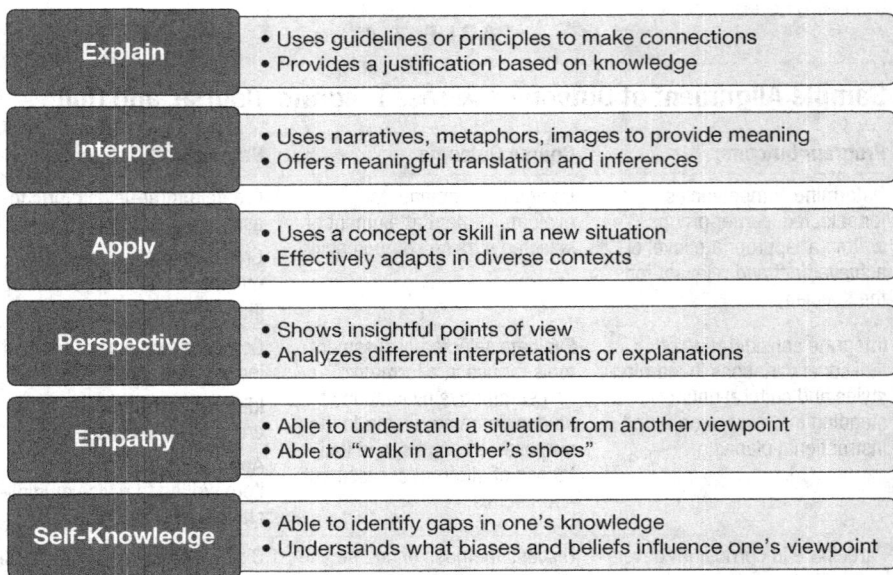

FIGURE 7.2 Six facets of understanding. (Adapted from Wiggins & McTighe [2005].)

units of instruction in nursing that typically rely on explaining, interpreting, and applying. This can facilitate deeper understanding and knowledge transfer and more authentically reflect actual nursing practice. For example, a nurse educator is preparing a unit of instruction on blood administration that includes classroom and lab instruction on the topic. In reviewing the unit outcomes and activities, all center on the understanding of explanation, interpretation, and application. The educator adds in the following learning outcome "Manage client situations related to blood transfusion refusal" and adds a role play where students take on the role of the client and the nurse in a situation where the client is refusing a transfusion. Debriefing through discussion or reflection to focus on different explanations and viewpoints can enrich the unit of instruction through consideration of the additional understanding of perspective and empathy.

The Three Apprenticeships for Professional Practice

Patricia Benner and colleagues (Benner et al., 2010) in their groundbreaking study on nursing education called attention to how learners in a professional practice learn during their education that encompasses the breadth and depth of clinical practice and refer to three apprenticeships of professional education. They caution that the term "apprenticeship of learning" does not refer to an apprenticeship model of learning or "on-the-job" training but is situated within a community of practice. Benner (2021) describes the three apprenticeships for professional practice necessary to develop students' professional identity as a nurse to include:

> The cognitive (or intellectual) apprenticeship focuses on attainment of the conceptual and theoretical knowledge of the practice of nursing. This is what has been traditionally emphasized in classroom learning in nursing education.

> The practice (or skill-based) Apprenticeship refers to the development of what Benner refers to as "skilled know-how" or the development of clinical judgment or reasoning. This apprenticeship is traditionally emphasized in the laboratory, simulation, or clinical settings in nursing education with a focus on acquiring competency in skills and tasks needed for clinical practice.

> The ethical comportment (or professional formation) Apprenticeship refers to learning how to practice within the ethical standards of the profession.

Incorporating these three apprenticeships into units of instruction can simulate an authentic practice world that allows students to rehearse thinking and acting ethically, like professional nurses. It can reduce the disconnect between classroom and clinical learning. The result can be rich, significant learning that can occur within classroom, simulation, or clinical settings. I had the opportunity to hear Dr. Benner speak on this topic right as I was asked to be a guest speaker on the topic of Sexually Transmitted Infections. Prior to attending this presentation, I likely would have focused my unit of classroom teaching on the cognitive apprenticeship but, as I applied what I learned, a richer experience developed (Noone, 2009; Sideras et al., 2013). Case studies were developed that focused on identification of risk factors, diagnosis, and locating current treatment recommendations; and attention was paid to the practice and ethical apprenticeships. A simulation with standardized patients was developed to allow learners to gain skill in taking a sexual history, communicating with clients about sexuality in a professional manner, and counseling for risk reductions for STI development. Classroom activities were incorporated that focused on reflection on biases that may interfere with the care of clients and minors and case studies on confidentiality issues, reporting laws, partner notification, and treatment of minors.

Fink's Taxonomy of Significant Learning

Noted educational consultant L. Dee Fink (2013) proposed his taxonomy of significant learning in part as a response to perceived limitations of Bloom's taxonomy, with its dominant focus on the cognitive domain of learning. Fink identified six significant tax-onomies of learning that are interactive in nature; he terms "significant" as leading to lasting change within the learner that is important within the context of what they are learning. The six areas he identified are:

> Foundational learning—understanding and remembering information and ideas, which is the basis for other kinds of learning.

> Application—engaging in new intellectual, physical, or social action that allows other types of learning to become useful. Examples include learning communication skills, being able to think creatively or practically, and being able to manage projects.

> Integration—making connections between ideas, learning experiences, and realms of life (such as school and work) adds to the learner's intellectual power.

> Human dimension—learning about self and others that allows learners to understand the human significance of what they are learning.

> Caring—developing new feelings, interests, and values to integrate knowledge and stimulate further learning.

➤ Learning how to learn—becoming a self-directed learner allows students to become more effective learners.

Nursing education is ideally situated to interweave Fink's taxonomy of significant learning since nursing practice entails all of these dimensions in a life-long practice. One exemplar of this approach is the Oregon Consortium for Nursing Education's program competencies which identify that a competent nurse (Oregon Consortium for Nursing Education, 2020):

1. Bases personal and professional actions on a set of shared core nursing values
2. Uses reflection, self-analysis, and self-care to develop insight
3. Engages in intentional learning
4. Demonstrates leadership in nursing and health care
5. Collaborates as part of a health care team
6. Is able to practice within, utilize, and contribute to all health care systems
7. Practices a relationship-centered approach
8. Communicates effectively
9. Makes sound clinical judgments
10. Locates, evaluates, and uses the best available evidence

While many nursing programs or courses will typically use the taxonomies of foundational knowledge, application, integration, caring, and perhaps the human dimension of knowing others, this program of study also focuses on knowledge of self and becoming a self-directed learner, which is critical for lifelong learning in a practice-based profession.

Fink also proposes course design that is similar to Backward Design in that he encourages designers to ask, "What do I want students to get out of this course?" and "What can be done to promote lasting and significant learning?" As such, he developed an integrated course design plan that promotes alignment of learning goals, assessments, and activities, and encourages active learning strategies and a student-centered approach. Incorporation of significant learning and integrated course design methods was found to have improved academic success in dental students (Uribe Cantalejo & Pardo, 2020) and improved confidence in clinical reasoning skills in physical therapy students (Stickley, 2019). Mokel (2021) describes a course design of an RN-BSN research course incorporating learning outcomes, assessments, and activities that address all six taxonomies, which resulted in a creative opportunity for significant learning for students. Marrocco (2014) redesigned a graduate course on aging for a nurse practitioner program using Backward Design and significant learning concepts. This redesign resulted in an enriched, interactive course that focused on significant, long-term learning linked authentically to clinical practice.

RECOMMENDATIONS RELATED TO BACKWARD DESIGN

In this section, we will look at the experiences of educators from various disciplines who have used backward design approaches to learn what they perceived as the benefits to students and educators, their recommendations, and cautions.

Learner-Centered Approach

Nursing and other practice discipline authors noted that the use of backward design, with its emphasis on learning outcomes and identification of the desired results as the starting point for instructional design, facilitates a learner-centered design (Emory, 2014; Marrocco, 2014; Slavych, 2020). Marrocco (p. 179) notes "This approach incorporates the principles of adult learning and shifts the focus from faculty as the center of all knowledge to the student as an active participant in learning." Slavych noted that this may be particularly important and of benefit to a program of study, such as practice disciplines in which certain competencies, skills, and knowledge need to be achieved prior to completion of the program and are necessary for practice. These authors also noted that this learning-outcome approach with a focus on identifying authentic performance task assessments resulted in rich, significant, innovative learning activities that more closely reflected and facilitated knowledge transfer to the clinical environment.

The focus on learners and facilitating organized and aligned instructional design can maximize the potential for learning for diverse groups of students. Intentional consideration of diverse contexts for learning, such as incorporating the six facets of understanding or Fink's taxonomy of learning, can broaden and enrich opportunities for learning.

Improved Teaching and Scholarship

The intentional approach that accompanies backward design can result in improved teaching since purposeful learning activities are developed that contribute to a quality learning experience (Carlson & Marshall, 2009; Emory, 2014). Slavych (2020) noted that student satisfaction improved after implementation of backward design with positive comments related to course organization and engagement in learning. Carlson and Marshall also identified that teacher satisfaction and increased enjoyment with teaching occurred in addition to improved student satisfaction. This approach could be especially useful to support faculty who are new to teaching and may not have received pedagogical training in their education (Carlson & Marshall, 2009; Michael & Libarkin, 2016). Tornwall (2017) recommended that this method could be transferable to other aspects of faculty life, such as manuscript preparation and research career planning.

Opportunities for Collaboration

Numerous authors described collaborative opportunities to work on backward design projects that occurred across courses and programs and with community stakeholders. Fox and Doherty (2012) describe an Information Literacy backward design project that included the collaboration of a librarian faculty member, instructional designer, and graphics designer to create teaching modules to meet graduate-level information literacy outcomes. Mills et al. (2019) describe a collaboration between librarians and English department faculty to enhance the implementation of information literacy outcomes in an undergraduate first-year writing course. Feedback from this project by writing faculty and review of assignments completed by students demonstrated the success of this project. Backward design approaches can also be used with community partners to design service-learning projects as Jozwik et al. (2017) describe in developing service-learning projects for a special education teacher program. They reported that the principles of backward design aligned with the principles of service learning and facilitated clear goal setting to meet both community and course needs.

Collaboration also provided opportunities for mentored learning for faculty new to teaching or pedagogical concepts. Michael & Libarkin (2016) describe the collaborative mentorship of using backward design to support the mentoring of a new faculty by a more experienced one. They describe the benefits to both individuals: the obvious benefit to a new faculty to receive support and guidance in pedagogical development as well as cementing and verifying knowledge and skill in the more experienced faculty along with the personal satisfaction of mentoring a colleague. The opportunity for peer support and professional dialogue in a collaboration of education faculty working on backward design resulted in improved course design and delivery (Brown et al., 2013).

Cautions

While the benefits of backward design are numerous, several authors noted some cautions. Michael and Libarkin (2016) noted that learning outcomes do need to be situated within a course and a program of study which may limit the breadth and depth of faculty innovation in developing or modifying learning outcomes for a course. Both Tornwall (2017) and Slavych (2020) note a potential hazard of teaching to the test if learning activities are built from the assessments although they provided no specific examples of this happening and its impact. Slavych (2020) also identified that ongoing course evaluation and improvement are still necessary components of good instruction even with backward design. Both Brown et al. (2013) and Fox and Doherty (2012) noted that collaborative efforts to adopt backward design implementation may result in an increased investment of time.

COURSE DESIGN TOOLS

There are a variety of tools available to support backward course design and alignment of learning outcomes, assessments, and activities. In this section we will focus on describing two: the Unit of Design Template and a course map, with examples. Wiggins and McTighe (2005) developed an Understanding by Design (UbD®) or Unit of Design template that faculty designers can use to develop a unit of instruction that follows the three phases of backward design: (1) identifying results; (2) determining acceptable evidence; and (3) developing learning activities or a learning plan. My colleague and I, Dr. Seiko Izumi, adapted this template for the graduate course we teach on Best Practices in Teaching Nursing. See Tables 7.5 and 7.6 for a blank template with instructions specific to nursing education and a completed example. This template can be helpful to apply the concepts of backwards design whether initially developing or modifying a unit of instruction. This sample template adapted for nursing education is linked to Hansen's (2011) explanations of backward design since it is focused on college-level instructional planning. Our modifications linked the learning outcomes to the facets of understanding and encourage use of a minimum of three facets of understanding, one of which being perspective-taking empathy, or self-knowledge. McGlynn (2015) suggested modifications in Stage 2 to incorporate where to consider providing feedback and to

TABLE 7.5

Modified Unit of Instruction Template for Nursing Education

STAGE 1—Identify Desired Results

Unit Title:_____

Directions are provided in brackets—you can delete these directions when you type in your responses.

Context, learners, and topic. [Describe the context for the unit/course—is it part of an undergraduate or graduate program? What course might that be and what is the purpose of that course? Or is it related to a practice standard in your clinical facility? Describe the learner—what you know about them, what they are likely to already understand about your topic or concept. What would be related prerequisite courses and/or knowledge you would expect learners to have? Describe the topic or concept that you plan to teach to your students.]

What are the big ideas? [What are the important concepts you want to teach in this unit? These are often characterized in one- or two-word terms (Hansen, 2011, pp. 30–36).]

Enduring understandings: [An enduring understanding is a more specific statement(s) of the big idea(s) learners need to retain. For example, a potential enduring understanding about dehydration could be that "Early signs and symptoms of dehydration are subtle and non-specific so identifying and monitoring clients at increased risk is important." There may be other enduring understandings. Enduring understandings should not be bullet points but complete sentences of the key learnings that students will retain years after this class is over (Hansen, 2011, pp. 36–38).]

Learning outcomes (SMART): [Learning outcomes are predictive statements describing the specific outcomes that a training session is intended to achieve; they are a benchmark by which to measure progress towards the achievement of larger goals. Identify the facet(s) of understanding each outcome aligns with.

Learning outcomes [Use a framework such as SMART or ABCD to write clear, measurable outcomes.]	**Facet(s) of understanding:** Try to use a minimum of three facets of understanding, one of which must be perspective-taking, empathy, or self-knowledge. [See Hansen, 2011, pp. 41–42.]

(continued)

TABLE 7.5

Modified Unit of Instruction Template for Nursing Education *(Continued)*

What is the link to academic or professional standards or competencies (provide reference)?
[Where possible, competencies should reflect local, state, or national standards—e.g., consider student learning outcomes, state board of nursing or national nursing education accreditation standards for academic courses or standards of practice, or professional nursing organization core competencies for continuing education units of instruction.]

STAGE 2—Determine Acceptable Evidence (See Hansen, 2011, Chapter 8)

What are the performance tasks?	**Related learning outcome**
[What are the performance tasks you will have the student complete to provide the best evidence that the learner has met the learning outcomes?]	[Link each task to the related learning outcomes.]

Feedback: How will students get feedback on their performance?

STAGE 3—Learning Plan

Summary of learning activities for a unit: [Describe pre-assessment and active learning strategies you will use to support student learning about your unit. Consider how you are going to allocate time for each activity. Link each activity with what outcome it meets.]

Pre-assessment: [What pre-assessments will you use to check students' prior knowledge and abilities and potential misconceptions?]

What are the learning activities?	**Related learning outcome**
[List learning activities, including preparatory work. Allocate time for each activity.]	[Link each activity to the related learning outcomes.]

Progress monitoring: [How will you monitor for student understanding during a unit of instruction?]

Adapted from Wiggins & McTighe, 2005.

TABLE 7.6

Sample Unit of Instruction for Nursing Education

STAGE 1—Identify Desired Results

Unit Title: <u>Health Promotion and Assessment of the Adolescent and Young Adult</u>

Directions are provided in brackets—you can delete these directions when you type in your responses.

Context, learners, and topic. [Describe the context for the unit/course—is it part of an undergraduate or graduate program? What course might that be and what is the purpose of that course? Or is it related to a practice standard in your clinical facility? Describe the learner—what you know about them, what they are likely to already understand about your topic or concept. What would be related prerequisite courses and/or knowledge you would expect learners to have? Describe the topic or concept that you plan to teach to your students.]

This is a unit of instruction within the first course in an undergraduate program of nursing. The course is a combined didactic and clinical course Health Promotion and Assessment. This course reviews health promotion concepts and health assessment throughout the life span. The learners all have personal experience as adolescents and young adults and may have experience in their personal and professional lives in caring for or working with this population. Learners will have taken prerequisite courses in anatomy and physiology and developmental psychology. Prerequisite knowledge that occurred earlier in the term included general health promotion concepts and patient education techniques. This unit of instruction focuses on health promotion concepts and health assessments for the adolescent and young adult with a focus on anticipatory guidance and risk reduction. This unit of instruction will occur over four 120-minute class periods (100 minutes each class after breaks) and a four-hour simulation.

What are the big ideas? [What are the important concepts you want to teach in this unit? These are often characterized in one- or two-word terms. (Hansen, 2011, pp. 30–36)]

➤ Health promotion
➤ Communication
➤ Confidentiality
➤ Risk reduction
➤ Health history and assessment

Enduring understandings: [An enduring understanding is a more specific statement(s) of the big idea(s) learners need to retain. For example, a potential enduring understanding about dehydration could be that "Early signs and symptoms of dehydration are subtle and non-specific so identifying and monitoring clients at increased risk is important." There may be other enduring understandings. Enduring understandings should not be bullet points but complete sentences of the key learnings that students will retain years after this class is over (Hansen, 2011, pp. 36–38).]

1. Key components of providing person-centered care are the ability to develop rapport and trust and to be nonjudgmental.
2. Providers need to have current knowledge of minor consent and state public health reporting laws in order to balance the best interests of the individual and the community.
3. Counseling for risk reduction should encourage self-management of health promotion needs.

Learning outcomes (SMART): [Learning outcomes are predictive statements describing the specific outcomes that a training session is intended to achieve; they are a benchmark by which to measure progress towards the achievement of larger goals. Identify the facet(s) of understanding each outcome aligns with.]

(continued)

TABLE 7.6

Sample Unit of Instruction for Nursing Education *(Continued)*

Learning outcomes [Use a framework such as SMART or ABCD to write clear, measurable outcomes.]	Facet(s) of understanding: Try to use a minimum of three facets of understanding, one of which must be perspective-taking, empathy, or self-knowledge. [See Hansen, 2011, pp. 41–42.]
1. Apply developmental concepts for adolescents and young adults into health history and assessment techniques.	1. Application
2. Integrate identification of unique health needs of adolescents and young adults into counseling for risk reduction.	2. Interpretation, application
3. Discuss personal biases and beliefs that need to be considered in care of this population.	3. Self-knowledge
4. Explain legal and ethical issues related to confidentiality in the treatment of minors and public health reporting.	4. Explanation
5. Demonstrate professional communication techniques in completing a health history on an adolescent client.	5. Application, empathy
6. Develop and implement an evidenced-based birth control teaching plan for a young adult.	6. Application, interpretation

What is the link to academic or professional standards or competencies (provide reference)? [Where possible, competencies should reflect local, state, or national standards—e.g., consider student learning outcomes, state board of nursing or national nursing education accreditation standards for academic courses or standards of practice, or professional nursing organization core competencies for continuing education units of instruction.]

This unit links to three of the 10 core competencies for professional nursing education (American Association of Colleges of Nursing, 2021), including:

Essential 2: Person-Centered Care

2.1 Engage with the individual in establishing a caring relationship.

2.2 Communicate effectively with individuals.

2.3 Integrate assessment skills in practice.

2.4 Diagnose actual or potential health problems and needs.

2.5 Develop a plan of care

Essential 4: Scholarship for the Nursing Discipline

4.2 Integrate best evidence into nursing practice.

Essential 9: Professionalism

9.1 Demonstrate an ethical comportment in one's practice reflective of nursing's mission to society.

9.2 Employ a participatory approach to nursing care.

9.3 Demonstrate accountability to the individual, society, and the profession

9.4 Comply with relevant laws, policies, and regulations.

TABLE 7.6

Sample Unit of Instruction for Nursing Education *(Continued)*

STAGE 2—Determine Acceptable Evidence (See Hansen, 2011, Chapter 8)

What are the performance tasks?	Related learning outcome
[What are the performance tasks you will have the student complete to provide the best evidence that the learner has met the learning outcomes?]	[Link each task to the related learning outcomes.]
1. Completion of pretest	Outcomes 1 and 2
2. Forum posts and in-class discussion	Outcome 3
3. Simulation: Adolescent Health History and Risk Reduction Counseling	Outcomes 1, 2, 4, and 5
4. Written birth control teaching plan	Outcomes 1, 2, 5, and 6
5. In-class Jigsaw teaching demonstration	Outcomes 1, 2, 5, and 6
6. Unit exam	Outcomes 1, 2, 4, 5, and 6

Feedback: How will students get feedback on their performance?
1. Students will receive automatic feedback on pretest submission.
2. Students will receive feedback on their forum posts.
3. Simulation will be debriefed during the last 30 minutes of the simulation with faculty and peer feedback.
4. Written feedback on submitted written teaching plan
5. Peer feedback on in-class teaching demonstration
6. Students will be able to review test scores and rationales upon submission of exam.

STAGE 3—Learning Plan

Summary of learning activities for a unit: [Describe pre-assessment and active learning strategies you will use to support student learning about your unit. Consider how you are going to allocate time for each activity). Link each activity with what outcome it meets.]

Pre-assessment: [What pre-assessments will you use to check students' prior knowledge and abilities and potential misconceptions?]

A pretest will be used to assess knowledge and gaps in understanding particularly focused on developmental prerequisite knowledge for these age groups.

What are the learning activities?	Related learning outcome
[List learning activities, including preparatory work). Allocate time for each activity.]	[Link each activity to the related learning outcomes.]

Preparatory work:

Read Edelman & Kudzma, Chapters 21 and 22 (Health Promotion of Adolescent and Young Adult)	Readings link to all outcomes
Giddens, Chapters 20 and 21 (Reproduction and Sexuality)	
Clinical Guidelines for Care of LGBT Patients	
Clinical Transgender Risk Assessment	
Read: Minors' Rights and Access to Health Care: https://www.oregon.gov/oha/PH/HEALTHYPEOPLEFAMILIES/YOUTH/Documents/minor-rights.pdf	
Complete pretest before class 1	Pretest links to outcome 1

(continued)

TABLE 7.6

Sample Unit of Instruction for Nursing Education *(Continued)*

Week 1
Class 1

Review learning plan for a two-week period. Review birth control teach plan.—10 minutes	All outcomes
Review pretest—10 minutes	Outcome 1
Mini-lecture: Health Promotion and Assessment of Adolescent—30 minutes	Outcomes 1, 2, 4, and 5
Four Corners Value Clarification Activity—20 minutes Explore beliefs, opinions, and potential biases	Outcomes 3 and 4
Adolescent Unfolding Case Study—30 minutes	Outcomes 1, 2, 4, and 5
After class forum discussion: guided reflection and discussion: "When you've seen a health care provider and had to discuss something of an intimate nature, what were the provider's behaviors that put you at ease? What were behaviors that blocked communication or disclosure?" "How comfortable are you talking about sexuality and counseling about sexual issues? How do you see yourself becoming more comfortable talking about these issues?"	Outcomes 3 and 5
Simulation with adolescent standardized patient: This is a four-hour simulation with prebriefing, health history of an adolescent standardized patient, and debriefing. Students practice communication techniques, risk assessment, and counseling and apply concepts of confidentiality and legal limitations in the context of assessment of adolescents.	Outcomes 1–5

Class 2

In-class discussion related to after-class forum discussion—10 minutes	Outcomes 3 and 5
Mini-lecture: Health Promotion and Assessment of Young Adult—30 minutes	Outcomes 1, 2, and 6
Young adult case study—30 minutes	Outcomes 1, 2, and 6
Kahoot review of concepts—20 minutes	All outcomes
Terminology crossword completion—10 minutes	All outcomes

Week 2
Class 3

In-class group to develop a birth control teaching plan with instructor consultation. Students are assigned a case scenario of a client needing birth control instruction in groups of four to prepare a teaching plan about the assigned birth control and come prepared to present this teaching plan in class 4.	Outcomes 1, 2, and 6

Class 4

Birth control teaching demonstration. This occurs in two rounds. During the first round, two people from each group will stay at their table to teach about this method and two will visit other tables to learn about other methods. The people who stay at their table to teach will rotate teaching about this method with each person teaching at least once. Then students flip in round 2. This session concludes with clarification of concepts.	Outcomes 1, 2, and 6

TABLE 7.6

Sample Unit of Instruction for Nursing Education *(Continued)*

Progress monitoring: [How will you monitor for student understanding during a unit of instruction?]
1. Monitoring pretest, Kahoot, and test results
2. Forum post discussion and written teaching plan feedback
3. Assessment during simulation
4. Assessment during teaching plan

American Association of College of Nursing (2021). *The Essentials: Core competencies for professional nursing education.* Retrieved from https://www.aacnnursing.org/Portals/42/AcademicNursing/pdf/Essentials-2021.pdf

---

consider preassessments and monitoring for understanding when developing the learning plan in Stage 3.

A course map is another helpful tool for both faculty and students recommended by Quality Matters (2018). It is a visual representation of the alignment of unit outcomes with assessments and learning activities. Such a tool can be helpful for faculty as they can link the unit outcomes to the course outcomes and improve the alignment of assessments and learning activities with the overall purpose of the course. This map can also be communicated to learners to demonstrate the rationale for selected learning activities. The Digital Learning Hub in the Teaching + Learning Commons at the University of California at San Diego (2019) developed a learning site to develop course maps that provide a useful template and description of one version to a course map (see Box 7.1). Box 7.2 demonstrates another version of a course map for a nursing graduate course.

CHAPTER SUMMARY

Backward design is a recommended strategy for instructional design of a program, course, or unit of instruction that includes three phases: (1) identifying results; (2) determining acceptable evidence; and (3) developing learning activities or a learning plan. This approach can have multiple benefits for teachers and diverse learners through improved organization, a relevant curriculum intentionally linked to educational standards, and the development of authentic learning experiences that closely represent clinical practice. Examples of a framework to first develop clear and measurable learning outcomes include the SMART approach (S is for specific, M is for measurable, A is for achievable, R is for relevant, and T is for time-bound) or ABCD framework (actor, behavior, condition, and degree of mastery). There are several options available to support the development of significant, rich learning experiences that can be used to frame learning outcomes. Wiggins & McTighe's six facets of understanding comprise explanation, interpretation, application, perspective-taking, empathy, and self-knowledge. Fink's taxonomy for significant learning experiences is a second approach that includes foundational learning, application, integration, human dimension, caring, and learning how to learn. A third method incorporates the three apprenticeships for professional education as described by Benner and colleagues as a cognitive (or intellectual) apprenticeship, a practice- or skill-based apprenticeship, and an ethical comportment

BOX 7.1

Course Map Template

Course Map (The Online Course Map Guide, 2019)

Course Name:	
Instructor Name:	**Date:** [Last saved]
Designer Name:	**Version:** [Draft 1, Draft 2, Final]

Program Outcomes Addressed: [Optional]

Course Learning Outcomes:

I.

II.

III.

Course Materials

Textbooks:

Resources:

Module # and Title	Course Learning Outcomes (CLOs)	Module Learning Outcomes (MLOs)	Assessments and Rubrics	Activities: Learner Interaction & Engagement	Instructional Materials
The title should be **short, yet descriptive** and **specific** to content being explored.	List all course learning outcomes addressed in the module by their Roman numerals.	State the module's intended **_measurable_** learning outcomes. MLOs must describe student performance in specific, observable terms. Use suggested action verbs from Bloom's Taxonomy. In parentheses, include the course learning outcomes (CLOs) that align with each MLO.	Specify all assessments that will be used to **measure the stated module learning outcomes.** List the name of rubric (if applicable) that provides descriptive and specific evaluation criteria for the assessment. Also, list the MLO(s) that align with each assessment. If assessment does not count towards the student's grade they should be marked "Not graded" in place of the	List all learning activities that **promote achievement of the stated module learning outcomes and align with assessments.** Learning activities may also be listed in the assessment column if they are graded. In parentheses, include the MLOs that are being met with each activity.	List all instructional materials and technology/media used during the module that **promote achievement of the stated module learning outcome.** This may include readings, web resources, videos, podcasts, audio, etc. In parentheses, include the MLO(s) that align with the materials. If a learning material does not have an aligned MLO, mark it as supplemental or optional.

	After successful completion of the module, the student will be able to:	Discussion	Discussion	Read
Module 1: Introduction to Modern Physics	**After successful completion of the module, the student will be able to:**	**Discussion**	**Discussion**	**Read**
VII	1.1 Recall/employ the main concepts and equations of classical mechanics (kinetic energy, momentum, and vector addition). **(CLO VII)**	▸ Discussion rubric	Intro to Modern Physics **(MLOs 1.3 & 1.4)**	Chapter 1 of Krane **(MLOs 1.1–1.4)**
VIII	1.2 Recall/employ the fundamental concepts and equations of electricity and magnetism. Illustrate the kinetic theory of matter. **(CLO VII)**	▸ **MLOs 1.3 & 1.4**	**Simulation**	Module 1 Exploration **(MLO 1.1)**
IX	1.3 Summarize the failures of classical physics in terms of time, space, velocity, and particle statistics. **(CLOs VII, VIII, & IX)**	**Homework** Problems involve concepts of space & time; classical physics & molecular energies **(MLOs 1.1, 1.2, & 1.4)**	Normal Modes http://phet. colorado.edu/en/simulation/ normal-modes **(MLO 1.1)**	
	1.4 Differentiate between classical physics theories and modern physics theories. **(CLOs VII, VIII, & IX)**			
Module 2				
Module 3				
Module 4				
Module 5				
Module 6				
Module 7				

The Online Course Mapping Guide Course Map Template is licensed under a Creative Commons Attribution 4.0 International License.

BOX 7.2

Sample Course Map

NURS 559 Understanding Social Determinants of Health Course Map

Course Objectives

1. Describe local, regional, and national health disparities.
2. Identify factors that contribute to health disparities and vulnerability and interventions to mitigate them.
3. Select and evaluate resources and tools on health disparities and social determinants of health for different target audiences.
4. Design health disparity educational presentations for target audiences.
5. Examine how to integrate concepts related to vulnerable populations and health disparities into teaching, practice, and/or policy development.
6. Analyze literature related to topics pertinent to vulnerable populations and health disparities.

This course map is a visual representation that lists the components of your course and alignment of the components with your learning objectives.

Books and Resources:

Barr, D. A. (2019). *Health disparities in the United States.* (3rd ed.). The Johns Hopkins University Press.

IHI Open School Modules on Triple Aim for Population Health

Harvard Implicit Bias Website

Unit	Unit Objectives	Assessments	Learning Materials	Activities
Weeks 1–3: Concepts of Health Disparities, Health Equity, and Social Determinants of Health	1. Meet peers enrolled in this course (all course objectives or COs) 2. Identify ways to facilitate respectful conversations about topics of a sensitive nature (All course objectives) 3. Identify selected concepts related to health disparities (CO 2)	▶ Completion of IHI modules (5% each) ▶ **Weeks 2–3:** Forum posts– 4 points (forums are 25% of grade). (See Online Forum Grading Criteria for Forum Discussions in Assignments and Rubrics)	▶ Barr (2019) Chapters 1–5 ▶ Institute for Health Care Improvement (IHI) TA 101 Introduction Triple Aim for Populations and TA 102: Improving Health Equity	▶ Post your picture and name pronunciation in your profile and introduction ▶ Group norms wiki post ▶ Attend or watch recorded orientation ▶ Set up IHI Account ▶ Complete tutorial on Echo 360 ▶ Set up an appointment with librarian to review how to do literature search (optional) ▶ **Weeks 2–3:** Initial and re-

Topic/Weeks	Learning Objectives	Assignments/Assessments	Readings	Activities
Weeks 4–5: Health disparities for selected populations	1. Identify a population of interest and potential related health disparities. (COs 1 and 2) 2. Identify an evidenced-based strategy to reduce health disparities (CO 2) 3. Evaluate an educational resource on health disparities (CO 3) 4. Appraise peers' educational resource review against given criteria (CO 3)	► Educational Resource Review (10%). See instructions and grading criteria in Assignments and Rubrics ► Peer Review–4 points (forums are 30% of grade). See criteria in Online Forum Grading Criteria for Peer Evaluation in Assignments and Rubrics ► **Weeks 4–5:** Forum post–4 points	► Barr (2019) Chapters 6–7	► Complete Educational Resource Review 1 ► Complete peer review of two peers' educational resource review 1 ► **Weeks 4–5:** Book forum initial and response forum post
Weeks 6–7: Understanding implicit bias	1. Discuss the role implicit bias plays in health disparities (COs 1 and 2) 2. Describe strategies to mitigate implicit bias (COs 1 and 2)	► **Weeks 6–7:** Forum post–4 points (forums are 25% of grade) ► Completion of IHI Modules (5%)	► Barr, Chapter 9 ► Bertrand, M., & Mullainathan, S. (2004). Are Emily and Greg more employable than Lakisha and Jamal? A field experiment on labor market discrimination. *The American Economic Review, 94*(4), 991–1013. ► Hall, W. J., Chapman, M. V., Lee, K. M., Merino, Y. M., Thomas, T. W., Payne, B. K., ... Coyne-Beasley, T. (2015). Implicit racial/ethnic bias among health care professionals and its influence on health care outcomes: A systematic review. *American Journal of Public Health, 105*(12), e60–e76. ► Noone, J., & Najjar, R. (2021). Minimizing Unconscious Bias in Admission to Nursing School. *Journal of Nursing Education, 60*(6), 317–324.	► Watch the Ted Talk on Immaculate Perception ► Take the Harvard Project Implicit Bias test. Take the Race (Black-White) IAT and another of your choice. Or complete the Patient-Provider or Health Educator Implicit Bias Self-Evaluation ► Watch the webinar by the Campaign for Action on Diversity and Inclusion: Promotion of Health Equity By Understanding Unconscious Bias ► **Weeks 6–7:** Forum initial and response forum post

(continued)

BOX 7.2

Sample Course Map *(Continued)*

Unit	Unit Objectives	Assessments	Learning Materials	Activities
			▶ Quillian, L., Pager, D., Hexel, O., & Midtboen, A. H. (2017). Meta-analysis of field experiments show no change in racial discrimination in hiring over time. *PNAS, 114*(41), 10870–10875. ▶ Institute for Health Care Improvement (IHI) TA 104: Building Skills for Anti-Racism Work: Supporting the Journey of Hearts, Minds, and Action.	
Weeks 8–9: Interventions to Address Health Disparities	1. Discuss frameworks and interventions to reduce health disparities (COs 2, 5, and 6). 2. Evaluate an educational resource on interventions to eliminate health disparities (CO 3) 3. Appraise peers' educational resource review against given criteria (CO 3)	▶ Educational Resource Review (10%). See instructions and grading criteria in Assignments and Rubrics ▶ Peer review—4 points (forums are 25% of grade). See criteria in Online Forum Grading Criteria for Peer Evaluation in Assignments and Rubrics ▶ **Weeks 8–9:** Forum posts—4% (see Online Forum Grading Criteria for Forum Discussions in Assignments and Rubrics)	▶ Barr, Chapters 10 and 11 ▶ National CLAS standards ▶ Read one of the following (feel free to read both): ▶ Drevdahl, D. J. (2018). Cultural shifts: From Cultural to Structural Theorizing in Nursing. *Nursing Research, 67*(2), 146–160. ▶ Metzl, J. M., & Hansen, H. (2014). Structural competency: Theorizing a new medical engagement with stigma and inequality. *Social Science & Medicine, 103*, 126–133.	▶ Complete Educational Resource Review 2 ▶ View webinar on Improving Student Wellness by Understanding Microaggressions by the Campaign for Action ▶ Complete peer review of 2 peers' Educational Resource Review 2 ▶ **Weeks 8–9:** Forum initial and response forum post

| **Weeks 10–11:** Educational Presentations of Selected Health Disparities | 1. Design an educational presentation on selected health disparities appropriate to a given audience (CO 4)
2. Utilize evidence-based resources to identify potential resolutions to the health disparities discussed (COs 2, 5, and 6)
3. Use appropriate technology to deliver the educational presentation electronically (CO 4)
4. Summarize self-learning related to the purpose of the course (all COs)
5. Evaluate course strengths and weaknesses, providing recommendations for improvement | ▶ Educational presentation (40%)
▶ Peer review—4 points | ▶ Complete educational presentation
▶ Complete peer review of two peers' educational presentations
▶ Complete course evaluation
▶ Complete self-evaluation learning audit wiki |

(or professional formation) apprenticeship. Course tools, such as the Understanding by Design (UbD®) template or a course map, can facilitate the alignment of learning outcomes, assessments, and activities.

References

Anderson, L. W., & Krathwohl, D. R. (Eds.). (2001). *A taxonomy for learning, teaching, and assessing: A revision of Bloom's taxonomy of educational objectives*. Longman.

Benner, P. (2021). *The Three Universal Professional Apprenticeships: The Ethical Comportment and Formation Apprenticeship featuring Dr. Sarah Shannon*. www.educatingnurses.com

Benner, P., Sutphen, M., Leonard, V., & Day, L. (2010). *Educating nurses: A call for radical transformation*. Jossey-Bass.

Bloom, B. S., Englehart, M. D., Furst, E. J., Hill, W. H., & Krathwohl, D. R. (1956). *Taxonomy of educational objectives: The classification of educational goals. Handbook I: Cognitive domain*. Longman.

Brown, B., Eaton, S., Jacobsen, D., Roy, S., & Friesen, S. (2013). Instructional design collaboration: A professional learning and growth experience. *Journal of Online Learning and Teaching, 9*(3), 439. http://hdl.handle.net/1880/109272

Carlson, D. L., & Marshall, P. A. (2009). Learning the science of research, learning the art of teaching: Planning backwards in a college genetics course. *Bioscience Education, 13*(1), 1–9. https://doi.org/10.3108/beej.13.4

Dave, R. H. (1970). Psychomotor levels. In R. J. Armstrong (Ed.), *Developing and writing behavioral objectives*. Educational Innovators.

Emory, J. (2014). Understanding backward design to strengthen curricular models. *Nurse Educator, 39*(3), 122–125. https://doi.org/10.1097/NNE.0000000000000034

Fink, D. (2013). *Creating significant learning experiences: An integrated approach to designing college courses* (2nd ed.). Jossey-Bass.

Fox, B. E., & Doherty, J. J. (2012). Design to learn, learn to design: Using backward design for information literacy instruction. *Communications in Information Literacy, 5*(2), 144–155.

Hansen, E. J. (2011). *Idea-based learning: A course design process to promote conceptual understanding*. Stylus Publishing.

Ironside, P. M. (2004). "Covering content" and teaching thinking: deconstructing the additive curriculum. *The Journal of Nursing Education, 43*(1), 5–12. https://doi.org/10.3928/01484834-20040101-02

Jozwik, S., Lin, M., & Cuenca-Carlino, Y. (2017). Using backward design to develop service-learning projects in teacher preparation. *New Waves-Educational Research and Development Journal, 20*(2), 35–49.

Kennedy, S. (2017). *Designing and teaching online courses in nursing*. Springer Publishing Company.

Krathwohl, D., Bloom, B., & Masia, B. (1964). *Taxonomy of educational objectives. Handbook II: Affective domain*. Longman.

Marrocco, G. F. (2014). Fostering significant learning in graduate nursing education. *Journal of Nursing Education, 53*(3), 177–179. https://doi.org/10.3928/01484834-20140223-02

McGlynn, L. (2015). *Information literacy by design: Creating a teaching and training template for developing library instructors*. [Unpublished manuscript]. School of Information and Library Science, University of North Carolina at Chapel Hill. https://cdr.lib.unc.edu/concern/masters_papers/sj139578w

Michael, N. A., & Libarkin, J. C. (2016). Understanding by design: Mentored implementation of backward design methodology at the university level. *Bioscene: Journal of College Biology Teaching, 42*(2), 44–52.

Mills, J., Wiley, C., & Williams, J. (2019). "This is what learning looks like!": Backward design and the framework in first year writing. *Libraries and the Academy, 19*(1), 155–175.

Mokel, M. J. (2021). A course design format to facilitate teaching research online to RN–BSN students. *Teaching and Learning in Nursing, 16*(2), 143–148.

Noone, J. (2009). Teaching to the three apprenticeships: Designing learning activities for professional practice in an undergraduate curriculum. *Journal of Nursing Education, 48*(8), 468–471.

Oermann, M. H., & Gaberson, K. B. (2021). *Evaluation and testing in nursing education* (6th ed.). Springer Publishing Company.

Oregon Consortium for Nursing Education. (2020). *Curriculum.* https://www.ocne.org/curriculum/

Quality and Safety Education for Nurses. (2020). *QSEN Competencies.* Retrieved from https://qsen.org/competencies/pre-licensure-ksas/

Quality Matters. (2018). *Higher education rubric workbook: Standards for course design* (6th ed.). MarylandOnline.

Schechel, M. (2020). Designing courses and learning experiences. In D. M. Billings, & J. A. Halstead (Eds.), *Teaching in nursing: A guide for faculty* (6th ed.). Elsevier.

Sideras, S., McKenzie, G., Noone, J., Markle, D., Frazier, M., & Sullivan, M. (2013). Making simulation come alive: Standardized patient in undergraduate education. *Nursing Education Perspectives, 34*(6), 421–425.

Slavych, B. K. (2020). Designing courses in communication sciences and disorders using backward design. *Perspectives of the ASHA Special Interest Groups, 5*(6), 1530–1541. https://doi.org/10.1044/2020_PERSP-20-00053

Stickley, L. (2019). Creating significant learning experiences for clinical Reasoning by Physical Therapist students. *Internet Journal of Allied Health Sciences & Practice, 17*(1), 1–11. https://doi.org/10.46743/1540-580X/2019.1828

Tornwall, J. (2017). Backward design toward a meaningful legacy. *Nurse Education Today, 56*, 13–15. https://doi.org/10.1016/j.nedt.2017.05.018

University of California at San Diego. (2019). The online course mapping guide. Retrieved from https://www.coursemapguide.com/

Uribe Cantalejo, J. C., & Pardo, M. I. (2020). Fink's integrated course design and taxonomy: The impact of their use in a "Basics of Dental Anatomy" course. *Journal of Dental Education, 84*(9), 964–973. https://doi.org/10.1002/jdd.12183

Weimer, M. E. (2002). *Learner-centered teaching: Five key changes to practice.* Jossy-Bass.

Wiggins, G., & McTighe, J. (2005). *Understanding by design* (2nd ed.). Association for Supervision and Curriculum Development.

8

Strategies for Active and Authentic Learning

Seiko Izumi, PhD, RN, FPCN

CHAPTER OVERVIEW

This chapter will review common active learning strategies that engage students and close the theory-practice gap. Recommended implementation of the flipped classroom approach will be reviewed. Concepts including situated learning, unfolding cases, and common active learning strategies in nursing will be highlighted. Best practices in discussion as a teaching technique to facilitate learning will be reviewed, including engaging students through questioning; creating groups that facilitate discussion; and avoiding common pitfalls in discussions, such as student silence and domination of certain voices.

WHY ACTIVE LEARNING IN NURSING EDUCATION?

The traditional teaching methods in nursing and many other fields have been lectures where educators on the stage deliver information and knowledge and students listen and absorb (Waltz et al., 2014). In a classroom setting, nursing students are typically presented with information about physiology, diseases, interventions, and outcomes as taxonomies to memorize, not how to use such taxonomies in actual patient care (Benner et al., 2010). The implicit assumption is that, if the students have this information, they should be able to apply and integrate it in their practice. From the nursing student standpoint, they feel like they are expected to do two types of learning: "classroom" or "theory" learning which mostly relies on lectures and memorizing what is presented, and "clinical" learning where they are expected to apply theories and concepts in real life practice or how to act like a nurse (Benner et al., 2010). Students feel they are learning two different things and there is not much opportunity to integrate or connect them, thus a theory-practice gap in nursing education exists.

Complex and high-stakes practice, such as nursing, requires knowledge beyond factual information stored in short-term memory. As described in more detail in Chapter 3, *The Science of Learning*, long-term learning requires the creation of neuronal connections to encode and store a piece of information in a network of long-term memory and strengthening of neuronal networks to retain and retrieve the memory when needed. Practitioners, such as nurses, are not only able to store all relevant knowledge but also discern and retrieve knowledge that is relevant and needed in a given situation from their memory using these strengthened neural networks. Nurses apply knowledge to new settings or situations by connecting concepts, patterns, and what is salient in the specific situation to make decisions about appropriate interventions for the particular patient (Benner et al., 2009). Nurses who practice lifelong learning keep building and strengthening the neuronal connections as they practice, and their recognition of patterns, retrieval of needed knowledge, and clinical judgment become faster and more fluid.

In nursing programs, learners need to practice (1) how to encode, store, and retrieve relevant information, (2) how to connect and apply this information to the situation in front of them, and (3) how to start building the neuronal network to think like a nurse (Tanner, 2006). This type of learning does not happen by being a passive recipient of knowledge. Rather it requires active engagement and effortful higher-order thinking that learners need to grapple with by themselves. The educator's role is to intentionally use strategies to promote this type of learning; guide learners to practice, build, and strengthen their neuronal network; and create a safe environment that challenges and stimulates learners to practice and learn from it.

As strategies to engage learners in authentic learning while integrating theory and clinical practice, active learning is gaining momentum in nursing education (Waltz et al., 2014). The concept of active learning emerged from the field of higher education and was popularized by Bonwell and Eison (1991). Based on constructivist theory, the underlying principles of the active learning concept is that, in order to learn, students need to engage with the content in activities beyond just listening (such as reading, discussing, or writing), involve higher-order thinking (analysis, synthesis, and evaluation), think deeply about what they are doing, and be the knowledge creator rather than recipients or consumer of knowledge (Bonwell & Eison, 1991; Cattaneo, 2017; Hyun et al., 2017). An increasing body of literature demonstrates that many strategies promoting active learning are comparable to lectures in the mastery of content but overall superior to lectures in promoting the development of students' skills in thinking (Adkins, 2018; Bristol et al., 2019; Shatto et al., 2019; Thomas & Schuessler, 2016; Waltz et al., 2014). Active learning strategies are associated with higher grades and a lower likelihood of failure across majors and class sizes in science, technology, engineering, and mathematics (STEM) courses (Freeman et al., 2014). Studies show that active learning strategies also narrow the achievement gap for minoritized students and increase students' self-efficacy and perceptions of inclusiveness in the classroom (Ballen et al., 2017; Lumpkin et al., 2015; Theobald et al., 2020). As such, active learning strategies hold much potential as equitable learning strategies for diverse learners that can help to prepare safe practitioners and lifelong learners.

KEY TENETS OF ACTIVE LEARNING

Although there is no clear and agreed-upon definition of active learning, there are a few tenets that characterize active learning strategies: learner-centered, activity-oriented, and authentic experiences that are close to real practice.

Learner-Centered

In contrast to traditional teaching centered on teachers who are the subject expert and handing down their knowledge to learners, learners are the center and focus of active learning (Cattaneo, 2017). The educator's role is not to be the content expert teaching the content to students, but rather a facilitator creating a space for learners to exercise their learning. Educators using active learning strategies consider how their learners learn and how to best guide them to develop skills for learning and apply them in real-life practice (Owens & Tanner, 2017).

Learners in nursing education are adults; thus, it is important to understand how adult learners learn and tailor activities to engage them. Adult learning theory was developed by Malcolm Knowles in the 1960s (Knowles, 1968) that describes how adults learn differently from children. Adult learning theory describes five characteristics of adult learners: they (1) are self-directed; (2) have experiences from which they can draw resources for learning; (3) are ready to learn when there is a reason, such as tasks or social roles expected for them; (4) are oriented to immediate application and problem-solving at hand rather than general learning about the subject; and (5) want to learn for their own reasons (Knowles, 1984). Given these characteristics, ideal learner-centered active learning strategies for nursing students would be problem-oriented that have immediate relevance to their job (i.e., nursing), encourage learners to use and build on their own experiences, and involve them in planning and evaluating their learning. Instructions for adult learners should be activity-oriented instead of memorization because they learn from doing rather than listening and memorizing. For them to be motivated and engaged in the learning, there is a need to explain why they need to learn specific concepts (e.g., physiology, treatments, social determinants of health, interventions, outcomes) in relation to their reasons (e.g., their reason is to become a competent nurse).

Activity Oriented

Although some educators assume that all learning is inherently active and students are actively involved while listening to lectures in the classroom, Bonwell and Eison assert "students must do more than just listen. They must read, write, discuss, or be engaged in solving problems. . . . . To be actively involved, students must engage in such higher-order thinking tasks such as analysis, synthesis, and evaluation" (Bonwell & Eison, 1991, p. 5). Some examples of activities that facilitate student engagement in higher-order thinking include think-pair-share, 1-minute writing, classroom discussions or debates, and peer-teaching. In these activities, learners have to engage their brains to make sense of and connect information, terminologies, and concepts they are learning or retrieving from stored memories, and form their own knowledge to solve the problem, answer questions, or explain it to others in discussion or writing. By engaging in these activities, learners build and strengthen the neuronal network to think like a nurse. Without doing these activities, the neurons in their brain are not connected to adequately store and retrieve knowledge when it is needed.

Adult learners may have rich and relevant past experiences, and so they tend to learn more readily when they can connect new learning to what they already know to strengthen the connections (Ambrose et al., 2010). Learners use prior learning experiences to make sense of new learning and strengthen the connection to retrieve the information when needed (Brown et al., 2014). Some learners may have limited past experiences in building the neuronal network or effectively activating prior knowledge. Educators need to be aware that building and connecting the network takes time; learners need guidance and repetitive practice. To transform their teaching into active learning, educators need to examine how much and what type of learning activities are included in their teaching compared to the amount of time lecturing, and how to increase the opportunities where learners can practice their own higher-order thinking with guidance. To increase the opportunities for guided but learner-centered activities, flipping the classroom may be a consideration. Using a flipped classroom model, learners spend the majority of classroom time engaged in activities where they practice higher-order thinking and build their neuronal network guided by instructors (Harvard University, 2023).

Authentic Experiences

Given that students in nursing education are adult learners who are motivated to solve real-life problems in their expected role (i.e., a nurse), they learn best from authentic experiences where they are situated in close-to-real life settings and addressing real-life problems. Real-life situations where nurses practice are complex, demanding, and ever-changing. For learners to learn how to think and act as a nurse in such complex situations, they also need to engage in authentic learning activities that mimic the complex real professional world (Ndawo, 2022). When learners are situated in an activity that engages them to solve an authentic problem, their brain starts learning what they need to pay attention to and focus on to solve the problem in the situation at hand (Eyler, 2018). Authentic learning links conceptual knowledge to the specific context and enables learners to experience how to apply the knowledge in the context of real-life situations (Brown et al., 1989). The use of high-fidelity simulation is an example of an authentic learning experience where a mannequin mimics physiological changes and actors and the room setting create an authentic environment and situation where learners experience the role of a nurse. Unfolding cases and role-plays are other examples of creating an environment where it is similar to real-life practice for authentic learning experiences.

Although they may be motivated and best learn from real-life situations, the complexity of real-life practice and the amount of knowledge needed to incorporate into nurses' clinical judgment could be overwhelming for novice learners. Strategies of scaffolding, where assignments or concepts are broken down into smaller units and learners are guided to build on these units to achieve more complex problem-solving, would be a useful approach (Coombs, 2018; Herrington & Schneidereith, 2017). In this video (Educating Nurses, 2014), Dr. McKenzie demonstrates how to break down an assignment (a role-play activity in a classroom) into smaller units and guides students through how to build on these units to address complex issues of mental health with an adolescent patient. Scaffolding from addressing simple or smaller units to more complex and comprehensive (thus realistic and authentic) situations can be done at an assignment level as well as a course or curriculum level. While active learning should aim for authentic context and tasks (Huang-Saad et al., 2021), levels of complexity should be considered and modified based on the learners' past experiences and readiness for effective learning experiences.

EXAMPLES OF ACTIVE LEARNING STRATEGIES

As briefly described before, the flipped classroom approach is a useful framework for how to implement active learning strategies into classroom learning. A concrete example of how to flip the classroom in nursing education and descriptions of commonly used activities to promote active learning will follow.

Flipped Classroom

The definition of a flipped classroom originated from a work by Lage and colleagues "Inverting the Classroom" (2000). Flipped learning is described as "a pedagogical approach in which direct instruction moves from the group learning space to the individual learning space, and the resulting group space is transformed into a dynamic, interactive learning environment where the educator guides students as they apply concepts and engage creatively in the subject matter" (Teach Thought, 2014). In the flipped classroom model, learners engage in activities aiming for lower-order learning objectives (e.g., reading, listening, watching lectures) in the pre-class work by themselves and at their own pace. In the classroom, learners engage in activities aiming for higher-order learning objectives such as application, analysis, synthesis, and evaluation in the group (Long et al., 2017).

Table 8.1 is an example of a flipped classroom in a nursing program. This is a 120-minute class as part of a chronic illness management course that is offered to second-year prelicensure nursing students. Specific content in this class is the management of diabetes mellitus. Students have either completed or are concurrently taking pathophysiology and pharmacology courses during the last term or the same term where they learn about the pathophysiology of type II diabetes mellitus (T2DM) and medical treatments for patients with T2DM.

Pre-Class Activities

In the flipped classroom, the majority of in-class time is used to engage learners to exercise how to connect and apply knowledge to nursing practice. Information and concepts they need to have to engage in classroom activities (e.g., knowledge about T2DM and chronic condition management) are presented as pre-class activities. Given that the learners already have knowledge about pathophysiology and various medications for diabetes mellitus from other courses, the instructor does not need to deliver a full lecture about them in the pre-class video. Instead, this pre-class video lecture should focus on how to use this knowledge to plan for care scaffolding on the knowledge the learners already have or reminding them where to look for this knowledge.

Although video-recorded lectures give learners the flexibility to review at their own time and pace, lengthy recorded lectures are often not effective. Learners' attention spans are short, typically 7–8 minutes in a lecture among college students. It is more

TABLE 8.1

Example of Flipping a Traditional Classroom

	Traditional Classroom	Flipped Classroom

Pre-class activities	▸ Read assigned materials (e.g., textbook, articles) (total 60–100 pages)
	▸ Completion of homework from last class (e.g., case study, developing care plan for other chronic condition)
		▸ Learning new content by
		  1. Reading assigned materials (max 20 pages)
		  2. Watching video (instructor recorded lecture, less than 20 min)
		  3. Searching stories/narratives by person living with T2DM from internet

In-class activities	▸ Checking homework from last week (10 min) ▸ Lecture about T2DM and care for patients living with T2DM (60 min) ▸ Break (10 min) ▸ Case study and development of a care plan (40 min)	▸ Ungraded pop quizzes related pre-class activities #1 and #2, and classroom discussion to clarify and elaborate on the materials (15 min) ▸ Think-pair-share about what they learned about patient experience living with T2DM from #3 pre-class activities (15 min) ▸ Unfolding case study about a patient with T2DM facilitated by the instructor (20 min) ▸ Break (10 min) ▸ Small group work to develop a care plan for the case (each group is assigned for a portion to do) (10 min) ▸ Fishbowl role play to deliver care planned by each small group and debriefing (30 min) ▸ Write a care plan for the case by integrating learning from pre-class learning, unfolding case, and fishbowl role play (individual activity; 5 min) ▸ Share and discuss about care plan developed (10 min) ▸ One-minute paper about one take-away learning and muddiest points remaining (5 min)
Post-class activities	▸ Complete care plan for the case (group or solo)	▸ Optional to complete their care plan if it was not completed in the class or modify it based on what was discussed. ▸ Instructor to review submitted 1-minute paper and follow up as needed

effective to deliver a short and focused lecture highlighting learning goals (what they need to know and be able to do) and why it is important to learn in order to situate and motivate learners to come to the class to learn. In addition, using the concepts of Universal Design for Learning presented in Chapter 6, having the video available with closed captioning or a transcript, and having a podcast available is recommended to accommodate different learning styles. Similarly, the number of reading assignments also should be reasonable given that amount of knowledge learners can retain by reading is limited. Instructing learners to do their own search and learn from what they find (e.g., patient's experience with T2DM) is a more learner-directed activity where they can determine how to search and what patient stories they feel more connected to or learn most from.

In-Class Activities

At the beginning of in-class time, a quick assessment of learners' knowledge and readiness for the in-class activities is useful. In the example in Table 8.1, the instructor uses an ungraded pop quiz to assess learners' knowledge based on the pre-class activities. The intention behind this pop quiz is to assist learners to recall knowledge from pre-class activities in their short-term memory and build a connection to long-term learning and how to use it in nursing practice in the classroom activities that follow. The instructor may use a classroom polling response system such as Poll Everywhere or Kahoot! to facilitate learner discussion and interaction not only on what the right answer is but also their thought process for their choices. Sometimes learners are required to bring some materials to the class as "a ticket to the class" to show their engagement in the pre-class activities and readiness for class. In the Table 8.1 example, learners are asked to search for patient stories and bring them to the class to share with their classmates. By doing this activity, learners exercise higher-order thinking skills to understand patient experiences by analyzing, synthesizing, and evaluating the information they search on the internet and articulating it to their classmates. The learners are accountable to bring their ticket to the class to contribute to their classmates' learning. Adult learners are often motivated to keep that level of accountability.

The rest of the in-class time includes various activities. The instructor's main role is to facilitate learning rather than lecturing. Depending on where learners are in the program, the instructor designs the classroom activities intentionally to scaffold the knowledge they already have. The instructor designs activities spiraling from simple and basic to more complex and holistic thinking, connecting, and building neuronal networks, and giving multiple opportunities to practice how to apply concepts in nursing care. Each learner has a different learning style and experience. The instructor should consider using multiple strategies to meet different learning styles. Teaching or explaining things to someone is often the best way to learn about the subject. The instructor does not need to be the one who teaches everything all the time. Peer teaching is an effective learning strategy that can be embedded in classroom activities, and classmates can teach and learn from each other.

How nurses think and use knowledge in a specific situation and make clinical judgments, however, is unique to the nursing profession and new to most of the learners in the nursing program. Therefore, learners need guidance to develop this higher-order thinking skill to think like a nurse. Unfolding cases, role-play, and simulations are some examples of activities to give opportunities to learn and practice to build the circuit to think like a nurse. To create these guided learning opportunities, instructors need to be intentional to plan these activities to be authentic while it is appropriate for the learners' readiness and not overwhelming. Assigned activities should be authentic, i.e., an authentic problem real nurses face and need to solve in a real-life situation. In order to guide learners through the complexity inherent in real-life practice without overwhelming them, the assignment may need to be broken down into smaller units, with instructors assisting learners to build the thinking process expected of nurses.

Again, given the learners' attention span and different learning styles, it is considered to be more effective to include multiple activities with relatively short time frames and provide multiple opportunities to practice in different formats. Having multiple fast-paced activities packed into a classroom session, learners may feel bewildered or unclear about what they learned. It is recommended to give learners time to reflect and consolidate what they practiced and learned in this classroom session (Bonwell & Eison, 1991). Debriefing after the simulation or role-play, giving a brief time for learners to stop and reflect on what they just did/thought, and writing down or talking about their key take-away learning are useful exercises to reflect and solidify their learning at the end of an in-class session.

Post-Class Activities

Unlike traditional classroom teaching where learners are expected to do homework after the class period to connect content learned in the classroom to nursing practice (e.g., completing a case study, writing a care plan) outside of the classroom individually or in a small group, homework or after-class activities are usually not expected in active learning because the guided learning to connect concepts to practice is done in the classroom. Learners may be encouraged to reflect on and practice more on the activities they have done in the classroom to enhance their learning if they did not have enough time for debriefing or reflection. Learners' main focus after class should be on pre-class activities for the next class. If it is designed well for scaffolding, learners are expected to use and build on what they learned in the prior class to solve new or more complex problems in the following class.

The more important post-class activity is for the instructors to review and reflect on one-minute papers or any other feedback from learners. It is important to assess what is working and where some learners are struggling to achieve the learning objectives. Then instructors can follow up on this feedback to add more explanations to clarify the muddiest points or modify activities in the following class to supplement or better tailor their learning experiences.

EXAMPLES OF ACTIVITIES PROMOTING ACTIVE LEARNING

The following are some examples of activities that are commonly used as active learning strategies. They can be combined or modified to suit learners' needs and the teaching environment, such as class size, time limitations, or learning objectives for the specific module of instruction. Some activities are already mentioned in the flipped classroom example above. Role play will be described below as a simulated learning activity, but more detailed descriptions of simulation learning are discussed in Chapter 12, *Best Practices in Simulation Learning*.

Think-Pair-Share

A think-pair-share is a useful activity that is easy to adopt in varied-size classrooms and engages learners in active discussion. Instructors pose a question, and learners consider the question for a minute or so, then pair up with a person sitting near them and share their thoughts about the given question. Finally, learners share what they discussed with their partners with the entire class and discuss (Lightner & Tomaswick, 2017). It could be a 5-minute activity or 30 minutes in-depth discussion. Learners get time to think critically, practice how to communicate and share their thoughts with others and learn from others. It is useful to create opportunities to hear thoughts from many students including those who tend not to speak up in the classroom. The key to a successful think-pair-share is the question posed. The question should be open-ended (thus no one right answer), closely and clearly align with the learning objectives, and authentic. The question posed in the Table 8.1 example was "What did you learn about the patient experience living with T2DM from the stories you found on the internet for pre-class activities?" After 5 minutes of both partners sharing their response to this question, learners are prompted to report to the class on behalf of their partner. This activity stimulates not only higher-order thinking skills to analyze and synthesize but also the skills of active listening and communication which are critical for nursing. This activity is also considered a culturally responsive pedagogy as it allows learners with different learning styles time to reflect before talking and those who may be more introverted a less stressful environment to rehearse before speaking in a larger group (Chavez et al., 2016; Seaman et al., 2021).

One-Minute Paper

This is a commonly used classroom assessment technique, but it could be used as a tool for learners to take a pause, reflect, and consolidate what they have just learned. At the end of class or at the end of any topic discussion or activity, ask learners to write down responses to questions such as "What are three key things you learned in today's class?," "In your own words, tell me what you understand about XYZ," or "What was most confusing or muddiest point in today's class?" Depending on the questions asked, this activity can last more than one minute, but it should not be a lengthy essay. This is a quick way to assess class comprehension of the materials and identify areas learners still struggle with or gaps in their knowledge. The instructors can respond to this in a subsequent class or class communication (Saltise, 2023). The one-minute paper also provides an opportunity for learners to take time to review what they just learned and self-assess their understanding. This pause is important to build the neuronal connection for long-term learning.

Unfolding Cases

Unlike a traditional case study that is static and all relevant information is presented initially to learners, an unfolding case is incomplete, and the learners need to actively explore and seek information to understand the condition and situation (Englund, 2020). Unfolding cases evolve over time as learners ask more questions (McKenzie et al., 2016). Learners need to interact with the case to collect information, assess the situation, and make judgments about what they need to do similar to authentic nursing practice (Kaylor & Strickland, 2015). Instructors can start by providing basic information about a patient that is similar to the information nurses would have when they first encounter the patient (e.g., age, sex, race, chief complaints, and vital signs). Then learners are asked what they want to know about this patient in order to provide care. This mimics the exchange between nurses when they are handing off a patient during the shift change. The instructors guide learners to think about what they need to know, how to get this information, and what they should anticipate, are concerned about, or need to prepare for. As the situation evolves, the instructor guides the learners to think through what action they should take (or not take) using this information. In unfolding cases, the learners go through the process of information gathering, assessment, identifying problems, clinical judgment, intervention, and planning how to evaluate the outcomes of the case. An unfolding case is most effective when the case is authentic. To make unfolding cases authentic and valuable learning experiences, including issues of social determinants of health that impact the care of the patient and their family is recommended. By guiding learners to consider these issues, instructors help learners examine their positionality as a nurse and patients' experiences that are structured not only by disease or illness but the structure existing in society (Altman et al., 2021). By going through unfolding cases, the learners strengthen the neuronal network in their brains to process and connect related concepts to the specific situation. A key to conducting effective unfolding cases is for instructors to be patient and allow learners to explore what information they need and find their own way to connect concepts and situations and think through what they need to do as a nurse.

Reverse Case

An alternative format for an unfolding case is the reverse case study. In this activity, learners are provided with limited information about the case, such as a list of medications and presenting signs and symptoms (Smallheer, 2016). Students then work in groups to create a case study of a potential client and their associated story, health trajectory with expected lab and diagnostic test results, possible illness course, and expected treatment. Learners can use a concept map, discussed next, to organize their case (Beyer, 2011).

Concept Mapping

Concept mapping is an activity to organize and visualize relationships between concepts. Concept mapping helps learners see how various concepts relate to each other (e.g., sub-concept, causal relationship), synthesize information, and see a larger picture (Tomaswick & Marcinkiewicz, 2018). Concept mapping requires learners to use their higher-order thinking to analyze, synthesize, and evaluate and assists them to understand multifaceted factors affecting patient health and what nurses need to consider to effectively care for the patient. Concept mapping could be about a subject (e.g., T2DM), a domain (e.g., chronic illness management), a problem (e.g., pain), or a case. Learners create a visual depiction of several factors about the topic. Concept mapping can be used before or after a case study (unfolding or traditional) to organize the concepts and facts related to the case and have a holistic picture of the patient. Concept mapping can be used at the end of the class to summarize and synthesize what students have learned in the class about the subject. It can be used as an individual activity to then share and discuss with classmates. Alternately, it can be a small group exercise, or the map can be created with the entire class engaged. Web-based resources for electronic concept mapping are also available (Educational Technology and Mobile Learning, 2023).

Role Play/Fishbowl

Role play gives learners the opportunity to assume the role of the nurse or other roles in a care team and act out in a given situation. Scenarios for role play should be similar to a real-life situation with complexity and challenges to create an authentic learning experience. The learners need to connect the concepts and apply them to actions as a nurse. A role-play activity could be designed as a brief skit to experience a narrowly focused action (e.g., have an advance care planning conversation), or it could be an elaborate scenario including a high-fidelity simulation. Regardless of the scale of the role play, thoughtful preparation is key to making the role-play activity effective learning. Instructors need to identify the purpose and learning outcomes of the role play; decide the scenario, tasks, and roles; decide on logistic aspects of activities (scale, time, resource); prepare how to facilitate and evaluate the learning through role play; and plan how to prepare learners to participate (King's College London, 2019). Learners need to be prepared to have the knowledge to act the role in the given scenario with clear descriptions and instructions about the situation, and time to think through what they are going to do in the role play. In role play, learners not only go through the motion as an actor but experience and examine personal feelings toward others and their circumstances (Bonwell & Eison, 1991). It is a powerful activity to experience and learn about perspective-taking and the affective side of practice that is a critical aspect of professional nursing (King's College London, 2019). When it is designed well to make it an authentic situation, even in a brief role play, learners can feel what it is like to be a nurse in the situation and sense the ownership of their comportment as a nurse. Debriefing after the role play is critical to allow the learners to reflect on that experience and feeling to encode it into their neuronal network to think and act like a nurse. Sometimes, we ask learners to play other roles in the scenario such as a patient or patient family members. Taking the perspectives of a patient or family member are also meaningful learning experiences. It is effective to ask these learners how they felt and what they were thinking when they encountered and received care from "the nurse" acted by their classmate during the debriefing to expand their clinical imagination to the patient experience.

Because of the highly engaging nature of role play, it could make learners vulnerable. To make the role play a positive and effective learning experience, creating a safe space for learners to be open and vulnerable is a critical task for the instructor. Setting up ground rules of conduct in the role play may be one approach. Asking learners to create the ground rules that work for their group is a strategy to enhance adult learners' engagement with the activity. Instructors and facilitators should set the boundaries of the activity and be prepared to anticipate learners' needs and how to intervene when needed. Cues for debriefing should focus on positive aspects of the learning experiences (e.g., what they have learned from the experience and what they may do differently in the future) rather than critiquing mistakes or what went wrong. Role play could be an emotionally charged experience. It may trigger past traumatic or adverse experiences. Taylor (2018) emphasizes the importance of instructors being able to support learners to navigate through the emotionality and learn from it. It is also critical for the instructors to be prepared to intervene with the notion of trauma-informed care when their learners are experiencing it. Some preventive strategies include informing learners about the role-play scenario ahead of time, alerting them it may include potential triggers (e.g., end-of-life, suicide, abuse), and letting learners know that they are allowed to choose a pass or time out if it is hitting too close to home.

Due to the time restriction and/or classroom arrangement, instructors may choose to incorporate a large-scale role play in a setting similar to a fishbowl discussion. A fishbowl discussion is a strategy where a small group of learners talks about or demonstrates their argument in front of another groups of learners, and other learners observe, discuss, and provide constructive feedback on the argument presented or topic under discussion. This is an effective active learning to engage more learners in higher-order thinking (Barkley et al., 2014). In the context of nursing education, the instructor may break down a scenario for a role play into smaller units or tasks. Each small group is assigned a task and instructed to come up with a plan to address the task in a role play. Then one or two representatives from each group take turns and play the role of the nurse in the scenario executing the task they planned. The rest of the group members as well as other groups observe the role play, then discuss, provide feedback, and learn from that demonstration. Members of the group who planned the task can share the rationale and thinking behind their plan, how their thoughts manifested in action, and what they learned from this process. Learners in other groups who observed the demonstration can also learn not only from observing the role play but hearing how their classmates thought through how to prepare to act as a nurse. By discussing in a large group throughout the role play, learners can learn from each other, what concepts they used, how to integrate various information and concepts into nursing action, and how to break down nursing care into manageable tasks and then put them back together to deliver a coherent and integrated care experience. Because it makes it possible for the entire class to learn from one role play, it is more time effective and could be a rich learning experience. However, the instructors need to be aware of the potential vulnerability associated with role-play activity especially when multiple observers exist and ensure the safety of the learning environment and weigh the risks and benefits of conducting role play using the fishbowl format.

Jigsaw

The jigsaw technique is a peer teaching activity in which learners master a section of a focused subject and then teach it to others in the class, who in turn, teach others about their area of mastery (Barkley et al., 2014). An example of this technique is a Birth Control Teaching Plan learning activity using the jigsaw technique (J. Noone, personal communication, February 20, 2023). Groups of students are assigned to develop a teaching plan for a specific method of birth control with a plan to teach a 10-minute session on their method in an in-class session. Learners are given time and resources to develop their teaching plans in previous classes. Each group has the opportunity to teach their method and then learn about the other methods. The faculty's role in this activity is to monitor for areas for clarification and summarize learning.

CHALLENGES AND PITFALLS IN ACTIVE LEARNING

Being learner-centered, active learning requires educators to be skillful facilitators, assessing different needs and readiness of learners and meeting diverse learning styles. Discussion is the most commonly used strategy embedded in various activities to engage learners and activate their higher-order thinking. However, facilitating discussions as meaningful learning poses challenges for many educators. Educators must be knowledgeable of various techniques and strategies for questioning and facilitation to spark meaningful discussions (Bonwell & Eison, 1991). Adult learners are more engaged in activities if the concept or problem is their direct or immediate interest. Educators need to explain and help the learners to see how the discussion topics relate to their future role as a nurse and why they need to discuss it to achieve their learning goals. The questions or topics of the discussion need to be authentic so that learners can see themselves using them in their future role as a nurse. If the goal of the discussion is to achieve an understanding of complex concepts using higher-order thinking, the educators may plan to ask a series of discussion questions ranging from simple and concrete to more complex instead of asking general questions that are too abstract to tackle. Similar to facilitating unfolding case studies, the educator's role is to guide learners to practice identifying the information they need, connecting this information, applying it to a specific situation through questioning, and soliciting them to verbalize their thoughts.

Some learners may be ready to participate and speak their thoughts or questions in the discussions. Some others may be engaged but not willing to speak up. Small group discussions or think-pair-share are useful techniques to encourage them to share their thoughts with classmates. On the other hand, there may be some learners who dominate or monopolize the discussions. Instructors should plan to create a space where all learners are invited to participate, share their thoughts, and be listened to by setting up ground rules or a culture of respect and professional civility. It may be helpful for instructors to have some reminders or vocabulary to invite learners to speak up such as those shown in Table 8.2. Adding an idea of "step-up-step back" (Meeting Intentions, 2019) as a ground rule from the beginning of the class and reminding them as needed may be a helpful approach.

Another challenge educators may face especially when they transition from more lecture-based teaching to active learning is the learners' resistance or disfavor about new ways of learning. Many learners are accustomed to taking a passive role in the traditional teaching approach and may be comfortable with listening to lectures (Oermann, 2015). Some learners who are accustomed to traditional teaching expect their instructors to give them the right answers. Flipped classroom and active learning techniques direct learners to find their own answer, and many times there is no one right answer. The answer is different depending on the situation and context. Active learning may require that learners change their learning habits and actively engage in "doing." Active learning activities appear to be more effortful, thus the learners who are used to the traditional way of learning may feel more stressed and express disfavor. For instructors who are new to active learning, this initial resistance may result in lower course evaluation by students which can often discourage efforts. But the evidence is clear that effortful active learning is superior and linked to stronger long-term retention and the

TABLE 8.2

Useful Phrases and Techniques for Discussion

Technique	Useful Phrases
To invite learners who have not shared	➤ I also would like to hear from students who have not shared their thoughts. ➤ I have not heard from small groups 3 and 4. Would anybody from that group share what you discussed in your group? ➤ (If it is a small group and have safety and trust) [call out student name], you have a patient with this condition. Would you share what you thought or did with your patient?
To redirect dominant students to step back	➤ Thank you for sharing. Let's give someone else a chance to share. ➤ I want to give those who are sharing a lot a chance to step back and listen and give others a chance to step up and speak. ➤ I want to remind you the ground rule of "step-back and step-up" we discussed at the beginning of the class. Let's take a small break and come back to continue the discussion and listen from students who have not shared their thoughts yet.

ability of higher-order thinking. Sharing this information with learners about how active learning improves their abilities to think like a nurse, connecting theory and practice, is a useful strategy. For instructors who are considering flipping their classroom or adding more active learning strategies, it is recommended to start by incorporating a small activity promoting active learning that they feel comfortable with (Bonwell & Eison, 1991). As they develop more skills to facilitate activities for active learning and more learners experience how active learning works for them, the paradigm shift to acceptance of active learning can happen.

Another challenge in implementing active learning in nursing education is time management. Many learning activities are open-ended and learner-driven. It is difficult to predict how long these activities will take for learners to immerse themselves into and achieve the learning goals. For learners to build their thinking skills takes time and the method to build the skill varies widely by learners. Learners new to this process often struggle not knowing what to look for and may ask tangential questions. Redirecting the course of discussions to focused area takes time and skill. Therefore, managing time to achieve the learning goals in classroom time can be a major challenge. Traditionally, nursing program curricula are packed with content that "is necessary to cover." Instructors are often concerned that they are not able to adequately "cover" all assigned course content in limited class time especially when they think about increasing classroom activities and limiting lecture time. To address this concern, instructors need to reexamine what are the educational or learning goals and objectives of the course and their teaching. The overall goal of nursing education is for their learners to gain the ability to think and act like a nurse (discern needed information for a situation, make decisions and deliver care by using this knowledge, and evaluate their care). Educators need to evaluate what class content and what activities should be prioritized and included in their teaching to reach this goal since it is impossible to teach everything about nursing. For more detailed explanation and steps, see Chapter 7, *Backward Design: Aligning Outcomes, Assessments, and Activities* in this book. Additional resources to support adoption of active learning techniques can be found in Table 8.3.

TABLE 8.3	
Resource List for Active Learning Strategies	
Resource	**Description**
Center for Research on Learning & Teaching University of Michigan	➤ https://crlt.umich.edu/ The Center for Research on Learning & Teaching at University of Michigan offers various resources to support and advance evidence-based learning and teaching
The Derek Bok Center for Teaching and Learning	➤ https://bokcenter.harvard.edu/ The Derek Bok Center for Teaching and Learning creates transformational learning experiences for faculty and students in Harvard's Faculty of Arts and Science. Learning labs and various resources are available in this site.
EducatingNurses	➤ https://www.educatingnurses.com/educating-nurses-a-call-for-radical-transformation/ EducatingNurses.com is a website directed by Dr. Patricia Benner who was the Director of the Carnegie Foundation for Advancement of Teaching National Nursing Education Study. This website contains various nursing education modules, videos, and articles discussing and demonstrating issues to transform and advance nursing education.
Educational technology and mobile learning	➤ https://www.educatorstechnology.com/ This website provides a resource of educational web tools and mobile apps for educators (including K-12)
Flipped learning	➤ https://flippedlearning.org/ Flipped Learning Network (FLN) is the nonprofit online community for educators utilizing or interested in learning about flipped classroom and flipped learning practices.
MedEdPortal	➤ https://www.mededportal.org/ The journal of teaching and learning resources by the Association of American Medical Colleges
MERLOT	➤ https://merlot.org/merlot/ The MERLOT is an international community of educators, learners, and educators providing online learning and support materials and content creation tools.
SALTISE	➤ https://www.saltise.ca/ SALTISE (Supporting Active Learning & Technological Innovations in Studies of Education) is a learning community in Montreal, Canada. This website offers various webinars, tools, and opportunities for peer mentoring.

CHAPTER SUMMARY

Active learning is gaining interest and is gradually being adopted in the field of education, and nursing education is no exception. Based on a constructivist framework, active learning strategies are particularly well-suited for nursing education where learners need to gain higher-order thinking skills to situate their knowledge in specific and complex clinical situations. Active learning is part of the solution to narrow the theory-practice gap in today's nursing education. Yet many challenges exist to implement active learning strategies into nursing education. Three essential tenets of active learning (i.e., learner-centered, activity-oriented, and authentic experiences) are delineated in this chapter. Nurse educators are encouraged to consider how to integrate these tenets into their current teaching and to transform nursing education. Activities to promote active learning described in this chapter are examples to consider adapting into one's teaching techniques. Nurse educators can be creative to mix and modify these and other activities to fit into their own teaching philosophy, setting, and skillset, as well as their learners' needs.

References

Adkins, J. K. (2018). Active learning and formative asserssment in a user-centered design course. *Information Systems Educational Journal, 16*(4), 34–40.

Altman, M. R., Kantrowitz-Gordon, I., Moise, E., Malcolm, K., Vidaković, M., Barrington, W., & de Castro, A. B. (2021). Addressing positionality within case-based learning to mitigate systemic racism in health care. *Nurse Educator, 46*(5), 284–289. https://doi.org/10.1097/nne.0000000000000937

Ambrose, S. A., Brigdges, M. W., DiPietro, M., Lovett, M. C., & Norman, M. K. (2010). *How learning works*. John Wiley & Sons.

Ballen, C. J., Wieman, C., Salehi, S., Searle, J. B., & Zamudio, K. R. (2017). Enhancing diversity in undergraduate science: Self-efficacy drives performance gains with active learning. *CBE Life Sciences Education, 16*(4), ar56. https://doi.org/10.1187/cbe.16-12-0344

Barkley, E. F., Major, C. H., & Cross, K. P. (2014). *Collaborative learning techniques: A handbook for college faculty*. Jossey-Bass.

Benner, P., Sutphen, M., Leonard, V., & Day, L. (2010). *Educating nurses: A call for radical transformation*. Jossey-Bass.

Benner, P., Tanner, C. A., & Chesla, C. A. (2009). *Expertise in nursing practice: Caring, clinical judgment, and ethics* (2nd ed.). Springer Publishing Company.

Beyer, D. A. (2011). Reverse case study: To think like a nurse. *The Journal of Nursing Education, 50*(1), 48–50. https://doi.org/10.3928/01484834-20101029-06

Bonwell, C., & Eison, J. (1991). *Active learning: Creating excitement in the classroom*. Jossey-Bass.

Bristol, T., Hagler, D., McMillian-Bohler, J., Wermers, R., Hatch, D., & Oermann, M. H. (2019). Nurse educators' use of lecture and active learning. *Teaching and Learning in Nursing, 14*(2), 94–96. https://doi.org/10.1016/j.teln.2018.12.003

Brown, J. S., Collins, A., & Duguid, P. (1989). Situated cognition and the culture of learning. *Educational Researcher, 18*(1), 32–42. https://doi.org/10.3102/0013189X018001032

Brown, P. C., Roediger, H. L., & McDaniel, M. A. (2014). *Make it stick: The science of successful learning*. Belknap Press.

Cattaneo, K. H. (2017). Telling active learning pedagogies apart: From theory to practice. *Journal of New Approaches in Educational Research, 6*(2), 144–152.

Chavez, A. F., Longerbeam, S. D., & White, J. L. (2016). *Teaching across cultural strengths: A guide to integrated and individuated cultural framework in college teaching*. Stylus Publishing.

Coombs, N. M. (2018). Educational scaffolding: Back to basics for nursing education in the 21st century. *Nurse Education Today, 68*, 198–200. https://doi.org/10.1016/j.nedt.2018.06.007

Educating Nurses. (2014). *Preview: Situated Coaching & Knowledge Use in a "Flipped" Classoom* [Video]. Retrieved from https://www.educatingnurses.com/situated-coaching-knowledge-use-flipped-classroom/

Educational Technology and Mobile Learning. (2023). Best concept mapping tools for teachers and students. Retrieved from https://www.educatorstechnology.com/2018/01/9-great-concept-mapping-tools-for.html

Englund, H. (2020). Using unfolding case studies to develop critical thinking skills in baccalaureate nursing students: A pilot study. *Nurse Education Today, 93*. https://doi.org/10.1016/j.nedt.2020.104542

Eyler, J. (2018). *How humans learn: The science and stories behind effective college teaching*. West Virginia University Press.

Freeman, S., Eddy, S. L., McDonough, M., Smith, M. K., Okoroafor, N., Jordt, H., & Wenderoth, M. P. (2014). Active learning increases student performance in science, engineering, and mathematics. *Proceedings of the National Academy of Sciences, 111*(23), 8410–8415. https://doi.org/10.1073/pnas.1319030111

Harvard University. (2023). *Flipped Classroom*. Retrieved from https://bokcenter.harvard.edu/flipped-classrooms

Herrington, A., & Schneidereith, T. (2017). Scaffolding and sequencing core concepts to develop a simulation-integrated nursing curriculum. *Nurse Educator, 42*(2), 204–207. https://doi.org/10.1097/NNE.0000000000000358

Huang-Saad, A., Schmedlen, R., Sulewski, R., & Springsteen, K. (2021). Reconceptualizing BME Authentic Learning in the Age of COVID-19 and Remote Learning. *Biomedical Engineering Education, 1*(1), 55–59. https://doi.org/10.1007/s43683-020-00013-0

Hyun, J., Ediger, R., & Lee, D. (2017). Students' satisfaction on their learning process in active learning and traditional classrooms. *International Journal of Teaching and Learning in Higher Education, 29*(1), 108–118. https://www.scopus.com/inward/record.uri?eid=2-s2.0-85056144253&partnerID=40&md5=21f4eba60584630053c6b6f74cb9a31c

Kaylor, S. K., & Strickland, H. P. (2015). Unfolding case studies as a formative teaching methodology for novice nursing students. *The Journal of Nursing Education, 54*(2), 106–110. https://doi.org/10.3928/01484834-20150120-06

King's College London. (2019). *Role-play*. Retrieved from https://blogs.kcl.ac.uk/activelearning/2019/08/20/role-play

Knowles, M. S. (1968). Andragogy, not pedagogy. *Adult Leadership, 16*(10), 350–352, 386.

Knowles, M. S. (1984). *The adult learner: A neglected species* (3rd ed.). Gulf Publishing.

Lage, M. J., Platt, G. J., & Treglia, M. (2000). Inverting the classroom: A gateway to creating an inclusive learning environment. *The Journal of Economic Education, 31*(1), 30–43.

Lightner, J., & Tomaswick, L. (2017). *Active learning—Think, pair, share*. Kent State University Center for Teaching and Learning. Retrieved from https://www.kent.edu/ctl/think-pair-share

Long, T., Cummins, J., & Waugh, M. (2017). Use of the flipped classroom instructional model in higher education: Instructors' perspectives. *Journal of Computing in Higher Education, 29*, 179–200. https://doi.org/10.1007/s12528-016-9119-8

Lumpkin, A. L., Achen, R. M., & Dodd, R. K. (2015). Student perceptions of active learning. *College Student Journal, 49*(1), 121–133.

McKenzie, G., Freiheit, H., Steers, D., & Noone, J. (2016). Veteran and Family health: Building competency with unfolding cases. *Clinical Simulation in Nursing, 12*(3), 79–83. https://doi.org/10.1016/j.ecns.2015.12.011

Meeting Intentions. (2019). *Step up, step back*. Retrieved from https://www.meetingintentions.com/post/step-up-step-back

Ndawo, G. (2022). The development of self skills in an authentic learning environment: A qualitative study. *Curationis, 45*(1), e1–e10. https://doi.org/10.4102/curationis.v45i1.2198

Oermann, M. H. (2015). Techonology and teaching innovations in nursing education: Engaging the student. *Nurse Educator, 40*(2), 55–56.

Owens, M. T., & Tanner, K. D. (2017). Teaching as brain changing: Exploring connections between neuroscience and innovative teaching. *CBE-Life Sciences Education, 16*(2), fe2. https://doi.org/10.1187/cbe.17-01-0005

Saltise. (2023). *Strategies: One minute paper.* Retrieved from https://www.saltise.ca/teaching-resources/strategies/one-minute-paper

Seaman, P., Cowden, C., Copeland, S., & Gao, L. (2021). Teaching with intent: Culturally responsive teaching to library instruction. *Libraries and the Academy, 21*(2), 231–251. https://doi.org/10.1353/pla.2021.0014

Shatto, B., Shagavah, A., Krieger, M., Lutz, L., Duncan, C. E., & Wagner, E. K. (2019). Active learning outcomes on nclex-rn or standardized predictor examinations: An integrative review. *Journal of Nursing Education, 58*(1), 42–46. https://doi.org/10.3928/01484834-20190103-07

Smallheer, B. A. (2016). Reverse case study: A new perspective on an existing teaching strategy. *Nurse Educator, 41*(1), 7–8. https://doi.org/10.1097/NNE.0000000000000186

Tanner, C. A. (2006). Thinking like a nurse: A research-based model of clinical judgment in nursing. *Journal of Nursing Education, 45*(6), 204–211.

Taylor, V. F. (2018). Afraid of the deep: Reflections and analysis of a role-play exercise gone wrong. *Journal of Management Education, 42*(6), 772–782. https://doi.org/10.1177/1052562918802875

Teach Thought. (2014). *4 pillars of flipped learning.* Retrieved from https://www.teach-thought.com/learning/pillars-of-flipped-learning/

Theobald, E. J., Hill, M. J., Tran, E., Agrawal, S., Nicole Arroyo, E., Behling, S., Chambwe, N., Cintrón, D. L., Cooper, J. D., Dunster, G., Grummer, J. A., Hennessey, K., Hsiao, J., Iranon, N., Jones, L., 2nd, Jordt, H., Keller, M., Lacey, M. E., Littlefield, C. E., . . . Freeman, S. (2020). Active learning narrows achievement gaps for underrepresented students in undergraduate science, technology, engineering, and math [Article]. *Proceedings of the National Academy of Sciences of the United States of America, 117*(12), 6476–6483. https://doi.org/10.1073/pnas.1916903117

Thomas, V., & Schuessler, J. B. (2016). Using innovative teaching strategies to improve outcomes in a pharmacology course. *Nursing Education Perspectives, 37*(3), 174–176.

Tomaswick, L., & Marcinkiewicz, J. (2018). *Active learning—Concept maps.* Kent State University Center for Teaching and Learning. Retrieved from https://www-s3-live.kent.edu/s3fs-root/s3fs-public/file/Teaching%20Tools%20In%20a%20Flash%20-%20Concept%20Maps.pdf?VersionId=6zp_lbr4m-dPTV5oaARCWs.pU7ms6RWkk

Waltz, C. F., Jenkins, L. S., & Han, N. (2014). The use and effectiveness of active learning methods in nursing and health professions education: A literature review. *Nursing Education Perspectives, 35*(6), 392–400. https://doi.org/10.5480/13-1168

9

Best Practices in Online Education

Glenise McKenzie, PhD, MN, RN
Heather Hawk, DNP, RN, CCRN-K, CNE

CHAPTER OVERVIEW

This chapter reviews online teaching strategies for nurse educators in the context of collaborative learning environments. Topics include learner-centered course design, intentional integration of educational technology, and development of interactive learning environments to engage diverse learners. Collaborative learning approaches are integrated throughout the chapter, emphasizing the importance of the inclusion of cognitive, social, and teaching presences in online teaching and learning environments. Effective online course design is discussed with attention to equitable access and alignment of learning objectives, assessments, and materials. Best practices for online teaching and learning are reviewed with supporting evidence from nursing and other health care literature.

BACKGROUND/INTRODUCTION

Online learning has become an integral part of contemporary nursing education, from prelicensure through doctoral programs. With rapidly evolving changes in course delivery capabilities, online education gives nurse educators the opportunity to create an engaging learning environment that is accessible to a broad range of learners. The recent global health pandemic increased the profile of online learning; while the hasty pedagogical shift to emergency remote instruction was challenging and not always successful, it underscored potential opportunities for new or modified modes of delivery for education in nursing. While the "new normal" for delivery of nursing education continues to unfold after the pandemic, educators and researchers are trying and testing strategies to improve online teaching and learning for students and faculty (Gazza, 2022). A national survey of undergraduates who experienced unplanned online learning during the first phase of the COVID-19 pandemic highlighted challenges with a sudden shift to remote online learning, including motivation, active learning, collaborating with peers, and barriers related to technology (Means & Neisler, 2020). These challenges were disproportionately reported by Hispanic students. However, this survey demonstrated higher student satisfaction when instructors used quality online teaching practices. Online education presents nurse educators with unique opportunities for continuing transformation in nursing education from instructor-centered to learner-centered approaches (Yilmaz, 2017).

Higher education institutions are rapidly expanding access to nursing education through online courses and programs. The exact number of nursing students enrolled in online courses or programs is not known, but growing numbers of online nursing program offerings indicate steadily increasing numbers of nursing students taking online courses. As of 2022, about 49 percent of entry-level nursing baccalaureate programs, 89 percent of master's and post-master's nursing programs, and 90 percent of doctoral programs deliver at least a portion of their programs online (American Association of Colleges of Nursing [AACN], 2022). Online learning offers the benefits of flexibility, lower cost, and improved accessibility for adult learners who represent various cultural and educational backgrounds and are often balancing multiple responsibilities. In addition to convenience and flexibility, nursing students have reported that online learning strategies increased options for communication with their teachers, improved understanding of content, and increased opportunities for self-directed learning (Bdair, 2021). English as a second language (ESL) nursing students report that online courses allow them the benefit of adequate time to engage with course material, including reading and writing discussion posts (Sailsman et al., 2018).

Developing and delivering high-quality online education is a complex process, and the role of the nurse educator is both congruent with and different from teaching in the in-person classroom. The essential leadership role in designing learning experiences based on adult learning theory and content expertise is consistent across modes of delivery. However, when compared with traditional (in-person) delivery, online teaching and learning brings unique characteristics; one difference is that interaction (student-content, student-faculty, and student-student) occurs at a distance and is taking place at various times (asynchronously). Another difference is the role of technology in mediating interactions for meaningful learning experiences (designing and managing activities online to enhance critical judgment and collaborative problem-solving skills). These differences in space, time, and types of interaction bring challenges and opportunities for instructors related to enhancing student engagement in learning, facilitating a sense of belonging, and maintaining a focus on academic purpose (Garrison, 2017). Because of these differences, faculty cannot promote meaningful learning by simply transitioning in-person learning into an online format; online teaching requires specific design and delivery strategies in order to promote interaction and engage students in the learning process. Indeed, the sudden transition to online teaching in March 2020 was described by academic nurse educators as chaotic, as they lacked the knowledge and resources to shift their learning activities from in-person to online (Gazza, 2022). The focus of this chapter is on the nurse educator's role in developing student-centered, inclusive, and collaborative online learning environments. Following a brief review of the online learning theories and frameworks that inform our work as nurse educators, we recommend a set of best teaching practices focusing on online course design, facilitation, and direct instruction.

INFRASTRUCTURE FOR ONLINE TEACHING AND LEARNING

In the following sections, we provide the "nuts and bolts" of best practices for nurse educators in online course design and teaching practices, including selection and integration of educational technology. However, implementation of these best practices by faculty is only possible when there is an established and solid foundation to build on. Selecting, maintaining, and supporting learning management systems (LMS) and related technology is central to the success and sustainability of online and blended learning (Garrison, 2017). An assumption taken in the writing of this chapter is that the decision to deliver a course in an online, technology-enhanced environment was strategic, appropriately resourced, based on adult learning theory, and aligned with intended program outcomes. In our experience, and supported in the literature, infrastructure to support equitable online learning includes the establishment of (a) personnel and support services (instructional designers, academic support services for helping learners succeed online); (b) organizational policies (teaching load, enrollment criteria, evaluation standards, differential tuition rates); and (c) digital technology support (both hardware and software) (Garrison, 2017). Additionally, the infrastructure related to human resources (teachers trained to support learning online) is outside the scope of this chapter; however, targeted faculty development in online pedagogical and technical skills, designing for equity and accessibility, and ethical use of intellectual property are all vital to a successful online learning experience (for instructor satisfaction and student success) (Tate & Warschauer, 2022). As noted by Garrison (2017), successful design, facilitation, and direction of learning in an online environment is "not possible without the expertise of a pedagogically experienced and knowledgeable teacher" (p. 76).

As technology-enhanced learning has evolved, so has the terminology for delivery methods. The distinctions between various modes of delivery are important, as we consider teaching-learning applications, as well as the ability to compare research findings. Table 9.1 provides the definitions used throughout this chapter.

OVERVIEW OF ONLINE LEARNING THEORIES AND FRAMEWORKS

As noted in the introduction, the context of online teaching and learning requires the educator to teach in different ways when compared to more traditional teaching practices. Online teaching supports a pedagogical shift for both teachers and learners from an instructor-centered paradigm to a student-centered approach, where the learner is a partner and active participant in learning. In the following section, we briefly review learning theories and related frameworks specific to online education. Social-constructivist learning theory, situated cognition theory, collaborative learning, equity and inclusion, the Community of Inquiry (CoI) framework, and Quality Matters© all guide instructional practices in the online setting with a focus on active and authentic learning, engagement, inclusion, interaction, and structured course design. Chapter 6 provides further foundational background on adult learning theory and related constructivist pedagogy, which is relevant to all modes of delivery.

ONLINE LEARNING THEORIES

Effective online pedagogy is based on constructivist learning theories that focus on designing activities that encourage construction of knowledge and understanding (students as active learning makers) through meaningful interaction between and among learners and instructors (collaborative learning) (Alemàn de la Garza et al., 2019; Cope & Kalantzis, 2021; Garrison, 2016). *Social-constructivist learning theory* adds to the psychological focus of constructivism through inclusion of social explanations for learning. Social

TABLE 9.1

Definitions Used in This Chapter

Note that these definitions can be applicable at the course or program level.

Term	Definition
Technology-enhanced learning (also called digital education or e-Learning)	Innovative application of technology to enhance the learning experience
Online	Coursework is primarily designed for asynchronous learning in which the material is delivered to students at variable times and locations. Content is intentionally created to foster student engagement that does not depend on real-time interaction, although some synchronous learning activities might be included.
Remote	Teaching and learning are conducted online, generally through videoconferencing, with student and instructor engagement and interaction occurring simultaneously.
In-person	Teaching-learning takes place in one physical space with learners and instructors physically present. Technology may be used to facilitate learning.
Synchronous	Web-based technologies enable classroom activities to be accessible to learners at remote sites in real time. The faculty can be seen and students and faculty can hear and see each other.
Asynchronous	Teaching, learning, and communication occur at various times, based on learner convenience, with time delays. Audio and visuals may be present.
Blended (also referred to as hybrid)	An intentional combination of online instruction and traditional in-person teaching. Students are expected to participate in both online and in-person learning activities. The purpose and rationale for the delivery method of content should be purposeful and stated explicitly for the learners.
Bichronous	Blending of synchronous and asynchronous online delivery, in which a portion of a course is delivered asynchronously, with other portions delivered online in synchronous sessions (Martin et al., 2020).
HyFlex	Students select from delivery modes (in-person, synchronous, or asynchronous) for each class session, providing student flexibility and choice of when and how they learn (Chicca, 2021).

constructivists argue that we learn through active interaction with others. Students are conceptualized as co-creators of knowledge, which is "constructed and reconstructed through conversation and interaction that is situated in their unique social, cultural, and historical context" (Kennedy, 2017, p. 33). A related social learning theory that is especially relevant in nursing education, *situated cognition theory*, proposes that we think and learn in context and includes five related elements: context, authenticity, activity and participation, community of practice, and shared or distributed cognition (Kennedy, 2017, p. 34). Situated cognition (thinking in context) supports learners' understanding and evaluation

TABLE 9.2

Elements of Situated Cognition Theory with Example Assignment

Elements (Kennedy, 2017)	Application in an Online Assignment for an Evidence-Based Practice Course
Context: The situation in which knowledge exists, with consideration of each component of learning as part of a bigger picture	Present students with specific details of a case scenario: An interprofessional unit-based evidence-based practice (EBP) committee is reviewing readmission rates for patients with heart failure. This has implications related to patient satisfaction, morbidity and mortality, and financial reimbursement. The student is an active member of this committee.
Authenticity: Realistic situations or professional context for application of learning	Present a simulated video of the EBP committee's meeting, including realistic dialog from multiple members of the interprofessional team.
Activity and participation: The dynamic process of communicating ideas, reflecting, and revising viewpoints as a result of engaging with other students and the educational materials	Begin problem solving with an online discussion in which students share ideas for addressing the readmission problem. Continue this discussion as students find relevant research to support their recommendations.
Community of practice: A group with similar roles that coalesce to share thoughts and perspectives in order to provide a sense of meaning	Create groups in which students will address the readmission problem. Groups can meet asynchronously or synchronously to share ideas and complete learning activities.
Shared or distributed cognition: The creation of shared knowledge in order to achieve common goals through active discourse	Guide students to collaboratively create an evidence table and provide a video in which they present their recommendations to the committee. Include structured touchpoints throughout the process, including online discussions.

of situational factors impacting clinical reasoning (Merkebu et al., 2020). See Table 9.2 for further exploration of the elements of situated cognition theory and how an instructor could apply these elements in an online assignment. *Collaborative learning,* which is central to optimal teaching and learning online, is grounded in social constructivist and situated cognition pedagogy. Students are individually responsible for making sense of new concepts and skill development, but learning occurs with support and feedback within a community of learners (peers, mentors, instructors) (Vaughn et al., 2013). Implementing opportunities for collaborative learning are especially relevant to nursing, given the significant role of teamwork and collaboration in improving health-related outcomes.

Equity and Inclusion Frameworks

Inclusive and equitable teaching strategies are shaped by several theoretical frameworks, which we integrate into our recommendations for best teaching practices. The Psychosociocultural framework recognizes the importance of learner choice in promoting collaboration and interdependence (Castellanos & Gloria, 2007). Validation theory, originally developed with low-income, first-generation higher education students, suggests that learners require intentional and proactive affirmation in order to enable them to feel capable of learning and to promote their role in the learning community (Linares & Munoz, 2011). Validation can be applied academically, through learning opportunities that promote student success, and interpersonally, through the cultivation of relationships (Brooks & Grady, 2022). Specific to the online educational setting, Warschauer's (2003) framework proposes that digital inclusion is shaped by physical, human, and social resources. Therefore, attention to access (hardware and internet), individual resources (digital literacy and self-regulation skills), and communities (both inside and outside the classroom) are important to consider when designing and delivering online courses and programs.

Community of Inquiry Framework

The overarching teaching and learning framework applied in this chapter is the Community of Inquiry (CoI), based on social constructivism and developed specifically for the design and delivery of online teaching and learning (Garrison, 2017). The CoI framework supports the core components of meaningful interaction and integrates critical discourse and practical inquiry to build learners' critical thinking and higher-order learning (Hickey, 2022). The elements of the CoI framework (teaching, social and cognitive presence) provide "a map for thinking and learning collaboratively" and provide a sense of connection with the content of the course, the instructor, and with peers (Garrison, 2016, p. 58). The element of teaching presence is "key to a successful and sustained community of inquiry" and "provides the essential leadership dimension that keeps a learning community functioning effectively and efficiently" (Garrison, 2016, p. 61). Social presence compliments both teaching and cognitive presence, functioning "to create an environment for thinking and learning collaboratively that is connected to the academic goals and dynamics of inquiry" (Garrison, 2016, p. 75). The third intersecting component of the CoI framework is cognitive presence, which is characterized as "the academic process that supports sustained critical thinking and discourse, and higher-order knowledge acquisition and application" (Garrison, 2017, p. 50). See Figure 9.1 for a graphic of the CoI Framework.

CoI is a well-established model for the design and facilitation of collaborative learning environments in many disciplines, including nursing. The CoI framework has been utilized successfully by nurse educators for online curricular design and evaluation (Smadi et al., 2021; Waddington & Porter, 2021). Nurse researchers have also utilized the CoI components to review the design of courses and have identified opportunities for educators in strengthening "social and teaching" presences in online nursing courses (Smadi et al., 2021). In a large meta-analysis of 425 studies of computer-supported collaborative learning, collaboration was significantly associated with knowledge gain and skill acquisition (Chen et al., 2018). These findings are also demonstrated within nursing; a systematic review of collaborative learning in online nursing education indicates that collaboration increases knowledge, problem-solving skills, satisfaction, and motivation for learning (Männistö et al., 2020). CoI, therefore, provides nurse educators with a relevant model for building online and hybrid learning environments where learners "collaboratively construct meaning and share understanding through shared discourse and deep, meaningful experiences" (Garrison, 2016, p. 53).

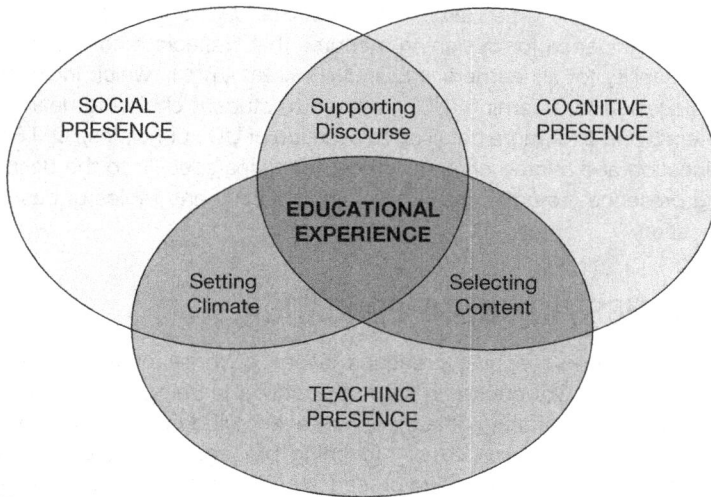

FIGURE 9.1 Community of Inquiry (COI) Framework. From "Online Educators' Recommendations for Teaching Online: Crowdsourcing in Action," by J.C. Dunlap & P.R. Lowenthal, 2018, *Open Praxis, 10*(1), 81. (Use permitted by Creative Commons Attribution 4.0 license.)

Online Course Design Standards

Quality Matters© (QM) is a national organization that sets standards for the design of online and blended courses with a commitment to accessibility and usability for all learners (Quality Matters, 2021). Improved teaching presence, including improvements in course alignment, increased communication with students, and enhanced authentic assessment strategies were themes identified in a review of multiple studies evaluating the impacts of implementing QM standards in online and hybrid courses (Shattuck, 2015). This review also demonstrated student reports of improved learning and motivation. In a comparison of QM-designed online nursing courses with traditionally designed courses, Gaston and Lynch (2019) found higher engagement and variety of teaching and learning activities in the QM-designed courses. The eight QM standards are course overview and introduction, learning objectives (Competencies), assessment and measurement, instructional materials, learning activities and learner interaction, course technology, learner support, and accessibility and usability.

While all eight QM Standards are important when designing any course (online, hybrid, and in-person), in this chapter we focus on only a portion of the standards. To learn more about the QM standards that support the alignment of course outcomes and learning activities, please refer to Chapter 6. The Standards we include relative to the design of collaborative online learning environments are: *Standard 1: Course Overview and Introduction,* defined by QM as designing to "set the tone for the course, let learners know what to expect, and provide other guidance to help learners succeed from the outset" (Quality Matters, 2021, p. 1); *Standard 5: Learning Activities and Learner Interaction,* which focuses the facilitation and support of learner interaction and engagement; *Standard 6: Course Technology*, which highlights the importance of selection of technologies for "enabling the various tools used in course facilitate rather than impede the learning process" (Quality Matters, 2021, p. 28); and *Standard 8: Accessibility and Usability,* which provides guidance for designing a course that "reflects a commitment to accessibility and usability for all learners" (Quality Matters, 2021, p. 34), which includes principles of Universal Design for Learning (UDL), related to student choice for learning activities (see Chapters 5 and 6 for more detail on application of UDL principles). QM Standards for Higher Education and related criteria for best practices specific to the design elements of teaching presence are noted in the following sections and tables of best practices in online education.

BEST PRACTICES IN ONLINE EDUCATION

In the CoI Framework, teaching presence is one of three interdependent elements. *Teaching presence* in CoI creates a student-focused learning experience through the design, facilitation, and sharing of subject matter knowledge and clinical expertise with and between learners (Garrison, 2016). "Teaching presence is key to establishing and maintaining both social and cognitive presence and achieving worthwhile learning outcomes" (Garrison, 2017, p. 161). In a CoI survey of online graduate students, teaching presence was the highest predictor of student satisfaction (Kucuk & Richardson, 2019). Students who completed a semester-long collaborative learning project indicated that teacher-student interaction has a positive influence on active learning (Molinillo et al., 2018). Based on the CoI framework, there are three primary responsibilities of the instructor within the element of teaching presence: *design and organization*; *facilitating discourse*; and *direct instruction* to create meaningful learning experiences. In the CoI model, the element of teaching presence overlaps with both social and cognitive presence, with related teaching responsibilities of *establishing an inclusive learning climate* and *selecting relevant, authentic, and meaningful content* to support meaningful learning. While the focus of this chapter is on the role and best practices for the nurse educator, it is important to keep in mind that the CoI model is designed to include all participants, including students, as having a role in all three presences, including teaching presence. For example, faculty may design a learning activity for meaningful student-student interactions, such as a peer review, which would include student responsibility for the facilitation of discourse and, in some cases, direct instruction (providing formative feedback to peers).

Our recommendations for best practices for teaching presence are organized around the three responsibilities of online educators in building a collaborative and inclusive learning environment: (a) *course design and organization;* (b) *facilitating social presence;* and (c) *facilitating and direct instruction for cognitive presence*. We incorporate our experience in online teaching and learning and evidence from higher education, focusing on nursing education literature. More information and considerations of the nurse educator's responsibilities related to teaching presence are provided in the following sections.

Teaching Presence: Instructional Design and Organization

One of the benefits for learners afforded by online delivery is the anywhere, anytime nature of asynchronous learning. A challenge for faculty is that the increased flexibility for online students means that they are accessing and interacting with course content and peers regardless of when faculty may be present. In the CoI model, the educator's first responsibility in developing and sustaining teaching presence is in the design and organization of the course (Garrison, 2016). Course design provides the architecture to support learners to succeed in an online inquiry-based and collaborative learning environment. As you design your course, consider that the course structure and organization are "setting the stage" for online technology-enhanced collaborative learning that is inclusive and accessible to all learners.

Educational technology brings the potential for new and efficient ways to present, interact, create, and share content (Cope & Kalantzis, 2021) as well as to facilitate active, problem-based, and case-based collaborative learning (Alemàn de la Garza et al., 2019). However, it is also important to "avoid simply layering these digital tools on a deficient educational design (e.g., information transfer model, which only focuses on presentation and organization of content)" (Vaughn et al., 2013, collaboration section). In addition to the positive learning outcomes associated with collaborative learning, Chen and colleagues' (2018) meta-analysis of collaborative learning online demonstrated that technology-based learning activities have a positive impact on knowledge gain, skill acquisition, student perceptions, group task performance, and student interaction. In a qualitative study of culturally and linguistically diverse online learners, 89 percent of the participants reported that technology-enhanced teaching and learning approaches promoted positive educational experiences and achievements (Kumi-Yeboah et al., 2020). Therefore, online course design also requires educators to thoughtfully plan for and select technology to best support the pedagogical goal of social constructivism and achievement of learning objectives (Bower, 2019; Cope & Kalantzis, 2021). To assess a technology-enhanced tool's ability to support learning, consider Anstey and Watson's (2018) rubric for eLearning Tool evaluation, which provides a selection framework focused on support of the three presences of CoI (teaching, social, cognitive) as well as functionality, accessibility, technical requirements, mobile design, privacy, and data protection criteria.

The following best practices for designing and organizing courses to support teaching presence are based on: QM Standard 1: Course Overview and Introduction; QM Standard 5: Learner Activities and Learner Interaction; QM Standard 6: Course Technology; and QM Standard 8: Accessibility and Usability. The QM rubric can be accessed on the QM website: https://www.qualitymatters.org/qa-resources/rubric-standards/higher-ed-rubric. Our recommendations are also informed by adult learning theory, collaborative learning theory, and the authors' online teaching and learning experiences.

Best Practices for Teaching Presence: Instructional Design and Organization

Design a course that is consistent with clear structure. Best practices for online course design and organization include attention to introducing learners to the purpose and structure of the course, establishing clear communication expectations in an online setting, and clear directions on minimum technology requirements and required computer skills. This information should be posted where the learner will easily find it on their first visit to the course site; an eye-catching "start here" link can provide helpful guidance to the learner.

Select course technology to support learning. Selecting course technology to support learners includes recommendations for aligning technology tools with the intended learning objectives, utilizing a variety of technology tools to promote learner engagement, and protecting learner data and privacy.

Design for accessibility and usability for all learners. The final recommended best practice in this section is to design for accessibility and usability for all learners by designing LMS navigation and course multimedia to be easy to use and to meet the needs of diverse learners.

See Table 9.3 for examples of teaching strategies to support best practices for design and organization.

Teaching Presence: Facilitating Social Presence

Online education brings unique challenges related to building trust, feelings of belonging, and a sense of group purpose (Garrison, 2017). A supportive and safe learning environment is foundational to cognitive presence (interaction for purposeful learning) and best supported by teaching strategies aimed to promote affective expression, open communication, and group cohesion (Garrison, 2017). Therefore, a key role of the online educator is to plan for, and then actively facilitate, social presence to create a learning environment where "each student feels welcomed and is given the reassurance that they are part of a purposeful community of learners" (Garrison, 2017, p. 114). In the CoI framework, a sense of belonging and safety is foundational to open communication and for creating group cohesion (Garrison, 2017). In a qualitative study by Grech (2022), nursing students recognized the importance of social presence for their learning; this included affective association, community cohesion, and instructor involvement. Social presence also is linked with knowledge construction, collaboration, and participation in active learning (Garrison, 2016). In a survey of online RN-to-BSN students, student satisfaction was highly associated with social presence (Cobb, 2011). The following best practices for facilitating social presence are based on: QM Standard 1: Course Overview and Introduction and Standard 5: Learner Activities and Learner Interaction. Inclusion and equity frameworks, integrated with adult learning and collaborative learning theories, inform our recommendations, in addition to the authors' combined experience with online education.

Best Practices for Facilitating Social Presence

Facilitate a sense of belonging and trust. A sense of belonging on behalf of the student is a critical component of equitable learning (Brooks & Grady, 2022). Deliberate teaching practices are required to establish trust and thus an equity-focused, socially inclusive learning environment. Best practices for facilitating social presence include designing introductions that are welcoming and encourage a sense of connection; creating

TABLE 9.3

Elements of Teaching Presence: Instructional Design and Organization

Best Practice	Teaching Strategies
Design a course that is consistent with clear structure	➤ Collaborate with subject matter experts and instructional designers when designing the LMS structures, processes, and content (Martin et al., 2019) ➤ Within the LMS, provide a brief course overview, explaining the expectations, purpose, and general navigation of the course (QM [Quality Matters] 1.2) (Lewis, 2021) ➤ Create clear instructions for how to get started and where to find course components (QM 1.1) ➤ Clearly communicate expectations for online discussions, email, and other forms of interaction (QM 1.3), including expectations for learner interaction (QM 5.4) ➤ Develop a Course Map, either graphic or text-based, outlining the layout and alignment of the course objectives, assessments, activities, and learning materials (for example, see Chapter 7, *Backward Design: Aligning Outcomes Assessments, and Activities*) ➤ Structure learning activities (individual and collaborative) to include clear directions, due dates, and assessment processes (Garrison, 2017) ➤ Organize the course by modules or weeks; "chunking" the content allows students to manage the course materials in a way that maximizes content processing (Martin et al., 2019) ➤ Provide a checklist summarizing required work for each week or module, which helps students to organize and focus systematically on the learning materials (Hensley et al., 2021)
Design for accessibility and usability for all learners	➤ Plan course navigation to be easy to use; for example, limit number of "clicks" required to locate information (QM 8.1) ➤ At the onset of the course, use short instructional videos to demonstrate course navigation (for example, using screen-casting technology) ➤ Design for readability and accessibility of text and images in files, LMS pages, and web pages to meet the needs of all learners (QM 8.3) ➤ Provide alternative means of access to multimedia content (for example closed caption for video, and/or transcripts of audio recordings) (QM 8.4) ➤ Use a standardized course template so students have a predictable experience with the LMS as they move from course to course within a program ➤ Plan for appropriate student workload (Billings et al., 2001; Smith et al., 2021) and communicate the expected time commitment for each lesson or module (Martin et al., 2019) ➤ Provide accessible academic support services, such as virtual writing assistance ➤ Provide a neutral source (not the course faculty) for writing support, particularly for ESL (English as a Second Language) students (Sailsman et al., 2018) ➤ Offer technology support and specific directions to obtain needed resources, such as internet hot spots (Morton & Phillips, 2022) ➤ Provide video lectures, learning activities, and course content that can be viewed and conducted offline, so that students do not need to be connected to the internet for all course activities ➤ Consider including a balance of asynchronous and synchronous components, utilizing hyflex or bichronous delivery model, if this is supported by the program

(continued)

TABLE 9.3

Elements of Teaching Presence: Instructional Design and Organization *(Continued)*

Best Practice	Teaching Strategies
Select course technology to support learning	➤ Select technology tools that support learning objectives, assessments, instructional materials, and learning activities (QM 6.1)
	➤ Design course assessment and learning activities to utilize a variety of technology tools to promote learner engagement and active learning (QM 6.2 and 6.3)
	➤ Provide learners with privacy policies and measures for protecting student data for all technology tools used in the course (QM 6.4).
	➤ Apply the eLearning Tool Rubric to evaluate technology tools to support CoI elements (teaching, social, cognitive presence) (Anstey & Watson, 2018)
	➤ Optimize LMS technology to support course design and organization
	➤ Integrate technology for communication and interaction: email, videoconferencing, discussion forums (text/audio), screencasting for mini-lectures, collaboration tools, asynchronous presentation, and feedback tools

activities for learner participation in discussions and other learning activities; encouraging interactive negotiation of online behavioral expectations; and providing informal opportunities for students and instructors to share common experiences and interests. See Box 9.1 for examples of welcoming introduction prompts that promote connection. This could be conducted in a discussion forum or using a digital whiteboard or online noticeboard. Box 9.2 provides an example of collaborative development of online behavioral expectations. Using a collaborative LMS discussion tool would be appropriate to develop shared group norms.

Promote affective expression and open communication. Facilitation of social presence is further supported by frequent and meaningful instructor engagement with learners; planning for active learning with interaction between all community of inquiry participants

BOX 9.1

Welcoming Introduction Prompts

➤ Share your first name and what you prefer to be called
➤ Tell us the story of your name
➤ Share your hopes and/or expectations for the course
➤ Describe how your past experiences connect to the course
➤ Provide a photo (or a collection of photos) that depicts:
　➤ Where you like to study
　➤ Your hobbies or interests
　➤ Something that brings you joy
➤ What motivates your learning?

BOX 9.2

Example Prompt to Collaboratively Establish Online Behavioral Expectations

It can be difficult to interpret tone and meaning in a discussion post, and this is especially true in discussions on sensitive topics. Online discussion should be respectful to everyone and relevant to the topic we are discussing. We may not always agree with one another, but discussion is meant to allow us to hear a variety of viewpoints. This can only happen if we respect each other and our differences. Please post a group norm you have found to be successful in dealing with topics of a sensitive nature. We will post these as group norms for discussions.

(Noone, J., personal communication, February 15, 2023)

(instructors and learners); and modeling caring and appreciation for contribution to the learning community.

Promote group cohesion. The final recommendation in this section on facilitating social presence includes modeling respectful and inquiry-based discourse, focusing discussions on the inquiry process, and promoting opportunities for collaborative learning, such as group projects and peer review.

See Table 9.4 for examples of teaching strategies to support best practices for facilitating social presence.

Teaching Presence: Facilitate Discourse and Directly Instruct for Cognitive Presence

Facilitating and directly instructing to support cognitive presence and learning is the third primary component of teaching presence in the CoI framework, which focuses on the challenge of "engaging learners in purposeful collaborative inquiry" (Garrison, 2017, p. 50). Therefore, the cognitive presence element of CoI focuses on instructional processes and strategies for supporting and sustaining critical thinking, knowledge building, and application of learning through active learning and discourse within a community of learners (Garrison, 2017). Meaningful learning is optimized when learning occurs in context; therefore, it is important to situate active learning activities in authentic, real-world practice situations. In the CoI model, cognitive presence is operationalized by the Practical Inquiry Model (PIM), which is focused on supporting learners in integrating and situating their public (social) and private (psychological) experiences for the purpose of building "discipline-specific, critical-thinking abilities through the process of constructing meaning and confirming understanding" (Garrison, 2017, p. 54). The CoI element of cognitive presence is described by the four phases of the PIM: triggering, in which an authentic problem is identified for further investigation; exploration, in which the learner delves into the issue; integration, where learners construct meaning from ideas; and resolution, in which learners apply knowledge. Our recommendations for best practices for facilitating discourse and directly instructing for cognitive presence are informed by situated cognition theory, collaborative learning theory, and our online teaching and learning experiences.

TABLE 9.4

Elements of Teaching Presence: Facilitating Social Presence

Best Practice	Teaching Strategies
Facilitate a sense of belonging and trust	➤ Get involved early; the beginning of the course is particularly important for the instructor's involvement, to build a sense of belonging and human connection (Martin et al., 2019) ➤ Demonstrate polite, respectful, and encouraging communication (Plante & Asselin, 2014) ➤ Use first names and address students by their preferred name and pronouns ➤ Provide a self-introduction and a welcome from the instructor in the first week of the course (QM 1.8). Share academic and practice qualifications and passions, and personal interests to project your personality and contribute to a welcoming and more relaxed environment (Garrison, 2017; Hensley et al., 2021). ➤ Prompt learners to introduce themselves and share their experience and learning goals related to course content (QM 1.9) ➤ Form students into small groups and ask each group to identify questions they have. For example, as part of an orientation to the course and/or for specific assignments (synchronous, when possible, with recording for students who cannot attend). ➤ Plan for informal student socialization with items like course chat features and informal discussion boards (Jain & Jain, 2015) ➤ Post "netiquette" guidelines and, if relevant, program-level code of conduct expectations ➤ Develop weekly updates for learning activities and include bridges to content from the prior week and upcoming week
Promote affective expression and open communication	➤ "Show up for class" and make your presence known through frequent and supportive engagement in the online classroom (Darby & Lang, 2019). For example, demonstrate presence by posting weekly announcements (text, video, or audio), summarizing discussions, and acknowledging contributions ➤ Communicate your plan for interaction with learners (QM 5.3) that includes a variety of opportunities for public and private teacher-student interaction (asynchronously or synchronously) via discussion boards, virtual office hours, chat, text, phone, and/or video conferencing ➤ Communicate clear expectations for student-student interactions (for example, posting and responding in discussion forums 3 times a week) ➤ Demonstrate caring: Contact students who are not engaging; check in on students' well-being and offer support. When possible, build in flexibility in due dates and provide reasonable extensions and alternative ways to complete assignments. ➤ Include discussion prompts that encourage sharing of feelings and questions related to course content and learning objectives

TABLE 9.4

Elements of Teaching Presence: Facilitating Social Presence *(Continued)*

Best Practice	Teaching Strategies

Promote group cohesion	➤ "Sustain respect and responsibility" between all participants in the online learning community through modeling and facilitation of discourse (Garrison, 2017, p. 112)
	
	 ➤ Focus discussions on shared understandings and connecting of ideas and concepts in relation to course objectives (group purpose)
	
	 ➤ Design learning activities that require interactions and support active learning (QM 5.2). For example, design small group problem-solving activities such as developing a plan of care based on a clinical scenario.
	
	 ➤ Utilize audio and video formats for presenting content and for small group discussions to promote social presence (Delmas, 2017; Kumi-Yeboah et al., 2020; Merriam & Hobba-Glose, 2021; Reyes et al., 2020; Serembus & Murphy, 2020) and to support emotional connection with the instructor (Delmas, 2017) and with other learners (Grech, 2022)
	
	 ➤ Plan for collaborative writing activities to help students engage with each other and the course content (for example Wikis, or Teams) (Kumi-Yeboah et al., 2020)
	
	 ➤ Pre-record a mini-lecture or case study and pose questions in audio/video format, and prompt students to respond to faculty and each other via audio and/or video response tools
	
	 ➤ Scaffold discussions (move from low-stake activities like introductions, to sharing experiences, to active problem-solving)
	
	 ➤ Consider using peers to moderate a discussion, changing the moderator for each lesson
	
	 ➤ Provide opportunities for synchronous small group activities to facilitate interactive learning and group cohesion (Foronda & Lippincott, 2014)
	
	 ➤ Potential synchronous group activities include:
	     ➤ Orientation session with dedicated time for small group discussion (Jain & Jain, 2015; Waddington & Porter, 2021)
	     ➤ Recurrent study sessions throughout the term to explore course material (Foronda & Lippincott, 2014)
	     ➤ Student-led groups focused on a collaborative task, such as having students create behavioral norms for their online classroom

Best Practices for Facilitating Discourse and Directly Instructing for Cognitive Presence

Construct learning activities for authentic learning and inquiry. Within the CoI framework, the selection of relevant, authentic, and meaningful content by an instructor with content expertise provides the overlap between teaching presence and cognitive presence. First, the online educator designs the setting for situated, authentic learning that optimizes learner connections with course content. A systematic review of active learning in health care professions students demonstrated that active student participation in the learning process through inquiry, discussion, and creation promotes higher-order thinking skills and improves student learning outcomes (Harris & Bacon, 2019). In a survey of online RN-to-BSN students from 36 states, use of collaborative assignments was associated with higher learner presence (Olson & Benham-Hutchins, 2020). Online graduate nursing students identified improved critical thinking after participating in course learning teams (Nichols et al., 2016). Active learning strategies include skill-based practice, which reinforces the bridge between theory and clinical learning; game-based learning, which increases learner engagement and attitudes toward learning (van Gaalen et al., 2021); multimedia, which promotes accessible, inclusive, and engaging learning; and collaborative learning, which supports teamwork and the co-construction of knowledge.

Facilitate discourse by integrating the practical inquiry model in discussions. To guide learners' movement through all four phases of the PIM, the instructor needs to do more than pose an isolated question and prompt students to complete a learning activity. Asynchronous discussions allow time for thinking and reflection, which assists in knowledge making, and, through prompts that elicit deliberation of course content, motivates students to stay on track with course readings (Osborne et al., 2018). For the *triggering* stage, the faculty role cannot be overstated. At the foundation of PIM is the creation of well-written, problem-based questions which stimulate thinking and require interaction. In the *exploration* phase, learners are encouraged to discuss assigned instructional materials, bring in additional evidence, and make connections with their attitudes and experiences. In this phase, the educator's role is to observe and monitor the direction of discussion, allowing students to explore and discuss. Too much involvement of the instructor can diminish productive conversation; however, too little can alienate the students (Claywell et al., 2016; Jain & Jain, 2015). In the *integration* and *resolution* phases, the role of the instructor shifts from observer to active participant, through joining discussions and offering prompts for students to: reflect on their learning (e.g., awareness of implicit or explicit bias); examine their ideas in the context of real-world scenarios; and to apply their learning to the clinical setting. The resolution stage is where formative and/or summative assessment is provided by the instructor, and by other learners (e.g., in responses from learners during discussion or in peer review activities).

Provide feedback and guidance to support critical inquiry. By providing effective feedback and assessment, guiding discussions, and summarizing learning, the online educator guides the learning process. The instructor needs to continuously offer additional sources of information, correct misconceptions as they arise, and provide synopses of learning. Instructor-to-student feedback on assignments should be specific and individualized, recognizing this is a primary mode of instruction from the content expert. Using structured and clear rubrics that align with learning outcomes, provide feedback and assessment oriented to the learner's level.

See Table 9.5 for examples of teaching strategies to support best practices for facilitating discourse and directly instructing for cognitive presence.

Best practice for promoting equity and inclusion in online environments. It is a moral imperative that online educators build and deliver courses with a clear focus on equitable and inclusive teaching practices for a diverse group of learners. "Equitable learning

TABLE 9.5

Elements of Teaching Presence: Directly Instructing for Cognitive Presence and Facilitating Discourse

Best Practice	Teaching Strategies
Construct learning activities for authentic learning and inquiry	Plan for situated learning ▶ Clearly explain the importance of student interaction as it relates to collaborative inquiry ▶ Integrate current events and real-life stories related to course content ▶ Integrate examples of personal relevance or experience to support integration of content into the clinical setting (Robb & Spadaro, 2022) ▶ Include time for reflection on the inquiry process (metacognition) ▶ Use small learning groups (Nichols et al., 2016) and consider forming groups based on student-submitted information about clinical interest (Mayne & Wu, 2011) ▶ Assign roles for collaborative projects, and change roles amongst students for different phases of the project, or as assignments change ▶ Incorporate culturally inclusive learning activities Create a variety of active learning opportunities to support authentic learning, including: *Skill-based practice* ▶ Iterative practice scenarios with video recordings (Yeh et al., 2019) ▶ Video-based physical assessment practice (Barnes & Vance, 2022; Webber-Ritchey et al., 2020) ▶ Virtual reality (Bayram & Caliskan, 2019) *Game-based learning* ▶ Gamified quizzes (Nurse-Clarke, 2022; Park et al., 2020) ▶ Polling/audience-response systems ▶ Quest-based games with formative feedback to develop mastery of a particular concept (virtual escape rooms) (Davidson & Candy, 2016) *Multi-media* ▶ Virtual poster sessions, in which students demonstrate their learning (Murphy et al., 2021) ▶ Integrated simulation scenarios with reflection and conceptualization (Stanley et al., 2018) ▶ Video presentations help students connect with the learning content (Kumi-Yeboah et al., 2020) ▶ Students post on Instagram, Twitter, or other social media to facilitate connection with course content (Walker, 2022) ▶ Digital storytelling, in which students use video to share narratives, to enhance learning, particularly about complex or emotional topics while also promoting reflection and collaboration (DeLenardo et al., 2019; Price et al., 2015) ▶ Blogging, as a reflective and knowledge-building interactive tool (Kumi-Yeboah et al., 2020) ▶ Student-led design and facilitation of peer learning activities (Volkert et al., 2021) *Collaborative learning* ▶ Online collaborative spaces for group projects ▶ Collaborative editing applications for writing (Vess, 2022) ▶ Wikis (websites that allow participants the ability to edit) (Trocky & Buckley, 2016) ▶ Video chats

(continued)

TABLE 9.5

Elements of Teaching Presence: Directly Instructing for Cognitive Presence and Facilitating Discourse *(Continued)*

Best Practice	Teaching Strategies
Facilitate discourse by integrating the Practical Inquiry Model into discussions	*Triggering* ➤ Develop realistic scenarios to apply content ➤ Create discussion prompts to encourage students to connect personal experiences or perspectives to course material ➤ Provide provocative, open-ended, critical thinking questions ➤ Develop probing questions based on Socratic questioning techniques *Exploration* ➤ Plan time for learners to engage in question-driven and problem-based learning activities ➤ Create a discussion board with multiple disciplines working on a case, which also meets essential learning related to interprofessional activities (Posey, 2021) ➤ Structure a student debate on a focused topic ➤ Encourage diverse perspectives ➤ Create a role-play discussion, in which learners assume the perspective of a particular discipline or person *Integration* ➤ Create a case-based discussion, which provides an authentic context that reflects the way knowledge will be used in real-life situations (Kuchinski-Donnelly & Krouse, 2020; Moore & Miller, 2022; Scott & Turrise, 2021) ➤ Structure the discussion around an open-ended, realistic problem that students need to solve together *Resolution* ➤ Scaffold the discussion, by asking probing questions throughout the discussion that intentionally moves the discourse to resolution (Darabi et al., 2011) ➤ Prompt students to reflect on application of their learning in the clinical setting
Provide feedback and guidance to support critical inquiry	Provide individualized feedback and assessment of learning that is: ➤ Timely, so that student feedback is provided in close proximity to the learning activity, correcting misconceptions as they arise ➤ Detailed, recognizing this is the primary mode of individual student guidance from the content expert ➤ Respectful (Authement & Dormire, 2020; Sinacori, 2020; Smith et al., 2021; Zajac & Lane, 2020) ➤ Focused on areas for improvement, rather than what they did wrong ➤ Structured and clear, using rubrics ➤ Aligned with learning objectives (Garrison, 2017) ➤ Authentic

TABLE 9.5

Elements of Teaching Presence: Directly Instructing for Cognitive Presence and Facilitating Discourse *(Continued)*

Best Practice	Teaching Strategies
	Guide discussion
	▸ Design discussions with mid-week postings to discourage weekend-only conversations
	▸ Provide a timely response to the first post in a discussion
	▸ Challenge ideas
	▸ Resolve misconceptions, but reserve individual corrections for private instructor-student interactions, rather than on the group discussion board
	▸ Identify areas of agreement and disagreement
	▸ Move the conversation forward, providing encouraging words and phrases to continue the interactive dialog (Waddington & Porter, 2021)
	▸ Assign participants to moderate a discussion, using peer facilitation, to increase metacognitive awareness of the inquiry process
	Summarize learning
	▸ Provide weekly summaries of course content and student learning
	▸ In discussion boards, provide a synopsis of the conversation at the conclusion
	Utilize technology to support feedback, assessment, and guidance
	▸ Screen casting applications
	▸ Asynchronous video chat software

occurs when every learner belongs, contributes, and thrives, regardless of race/ethnicity or socio-economic status" (Tate & Warschauer, 2022, p. 192). Online educators have positional influence to address existing disparities and strengthen the voice of students from historically marginalized communities. Due to flexibility and accessibility, the online classroom can serve a broad range of students with various cultural, geographic, economic, and educational backgrounds. When this diverse group of students shares their experiences, viewpoints, and knowledge in a safe and inclusive environment, all students have an enhanced learning experience. To guide effective teaching strategies, we have integrated elements of teaching presence with concepts derived from educational frameworks that focus on equity and inclusion. However, to specifically promote equity and inclusion, we recommend a focused subset of inclusive teaching strategies to be employed in the online learning environment.

▸ Explicitly express a willingness to support learners with diverse needs (Brooks & Grady, 2022)

▸ Use plain language for course navigation that supports learners from multiple linguistic backgrounds (Brooks & Grady, 2022)

▸ Design instructional materials so that learners with diverse abilities can engage and interact (Lewis, 2021)

> ➤ Select representative instructional materials, including images, guest speakers, and case scenarios, which reflect people of diverse backgrounds (Lewis, 2021)

> ➤ Provide exemplars that allow students to imagine their future successful selves (Brooks & Grady, 2022)

> ➤ Include learning activities that integrate course content with learners' lived experiences (Lewis, 2021)

When assessing a course for equity, we recommend the *Online Equity Rubric*, which educators can use to appraise a course's equity and inclusion principles (Peralta Community College District, 2020). Domains in the tool include technology, student resources and support, UDL, diversity and inclusion, images and representation, human bias, content meaning, and connection and belonging.

SYNCHRONOUS ONLINE ACTIVITIES

While we have focused this chapter primarily on the best practices in asynchronous online teaching, we recognize the prevalence and effectiveness of synchronous online delivery for supporting social and cognitive presence. In hybrid, hyflex, and bichronous delivery, synchronous videoconferencing sessions are a common modality for course delivery; the ability to provide live, spontaneous communication fosters interaction and enjoyment among nursing students (Foronda & Lippincott, 2014). Student use of webcams is often preferred in synchronous sessions to promote a sense of community and interaction, but educators should be cognizant of valid reasons for students to not use a webcam, including hardware limitations, low internet bandwidth, and privacy concerns. Considerations of equity and inclusion must be present when planning webcam-dependent learning activities, and accommodations for students who cannot be on webcam should be provided. Provide an option to submit a prerecorded video for learning activities that require webcams, such as presentations. Other than the visual presence of students through a webcam, there are many non-visual ways to engage students in the online asynchronous classroom. Table 9.6 provides approaches, through effective use of technology, to optimize teaching and learning through synchronous online learning, including specific strategies for teaching in the hyFlex environment, in which the educator might simultaneously have students in the in-person classroom and the remote virtual environment.

CHAPTER SUMMARY

The increase in online programs and courses provides nursing students with increased flexibility and convenience when advancing their education. Teaching online comes with unique challenges and opportunities in applying adult learning theory to stimulate and support student engagement, creativity, and teamwork without in-person interaction. Online nurse educators are instrumental to learner engagement and achievement of learning outcomes. Intentional design, organization, facilitation of discourse, and creation of active, authentic learning experiences are all central to an inclusive, student-centered, collaborative learning environment. Technology-enhanced learning activities offer unique opportunities in the transformation of education from instructor-centered to

TABLE 9.6

Best Practices for Synchronous Online Activities

	Best Practice	Technology to Support Effective Synchronous Delivery
Prior to the synchronous session	Provide explicit directions for learners ➤ Display the complete connection information in the LMS ➤ Notify students in advance if the session will be recorded ➤ Clarify webcam expectations ➤ Provide advanced notice if the learning activity requires a webcam (such as student presentations) Optimize teaching presence ➤ Practice and have a working knowledge of the functionality of the videoconferencing software prior to facilitating a class session ➤ Find a location with good lighting (avoid backlighting) and is quiet with limited background noise ➤ Arrive at least 10 minutes early ➤ Greet students as they enter the virtual space to provide a welcoming presence as well as an audio check ➤ Assure that your name is displayed as you would like to be addressed	➤ Videoconferencing system with institutional support and training for students and faculty ➤ Welcoming slide on view when learners log in to the synchronous session ➤ A window or artificial light source behind the monitor avoids a back-lit appearance ➤ Videoconferencing software that allows name configuration and the ability to display pronouns
During the synchronous session	Webcams ➤ Keep the instructor's webcam on, even during synchronous lectures (Katai & Iclanzan, 2022) ➤ Provide an option to submit a prerecorded video for learning activities that require webcams, such as presentations ➤ For recorded class sessions, pause the recording during discussion time Define expectations for student participation ➤ Engage students in the co-creation of class norms (examples: staying muted unless you are speaking, using webcams during breakout sessions, closing browser windows that are not related to course content, and turning on the camera to say hello at the beginning of class) ➤ Explicitly communicate how students can best indicate that they have a question, and how you would like students to contribute to class conversations, such as through the chat feature or with the microphone	➤ Encourage the use of digital backgrounds if students are concerned about sharing video of their home environment ➤ Student access to and training for video recording software ➤ Digital whiteboards that allow collaborative real-time sharing ➤ Chat feature ➤ Reaction buttons and emoticons

(continued)

TABLE 9.6

Best Practices for Synchronous Online Activities *(Continued)*

	Best Practice	Technology to Support Effective Synchronous Delivery
	Encourage student engagement ➤ Minimize lecture time and focus on collaborative and interactive learning activities ➤ When using breakout rooms, move between the breakout rooms to provide real-time feedback ➤ Assign student roles in breakout rooms	➤ Chat feature ➤ Reaction buttons ➤ On-screen annotations or drawing ➤ Polling ➤ Digital whiteboards ➤ Breakout rooms ➤ Shared documents ➤ Competitive quizzes
During a hyflex session (in-person students and remote online students)	➤ Welcome all learners, both in-person and remote, looking into the camera to greet remote learners ➤ Provide clear communication about expectations for participation, for both in-person and remote learners ➤ Check the chat for questions and comments from remote students ➤ Repeat student questions from the classroom ➤ Utilize web-based meeting software to facilitate break-out rooms that can be shared by in-person and remote students ➤ Design activities that promote interaction between in-person and remote students, such as polling, think-pair-share, and breakout rooms ➤ Create spaces with breakout rooms to provide opportunities for informal social discussion among remote students during break times	➤ Polling ➤ Digital whiteboards ➤ Web-based meeting software, such as Zoom, for both in-person and remote students

(The Columbia Center for Teaching and Learning, n.d.)

student-centered teaching approaches. The CoI framework with its three interdependent elements (teaching, social, and cognitive presences) at the center of a collaborative learning experience offers nurse educators the architecture to develop and implement effective, inclusive, and interactive online learning communities.

References

Alemàn de la Garza, L., Anichini, A., Antal, P., Beaune, A., & Crompton, H. (2019). *Rethinking pedagogy: Exploring the potential of digital technology in achieving quality education*. Mahatma Gandhi Institute of Education for Peace and Sustainable Development.

American Association of Colleges of Nursing. (2022). *2021-2022 enrollment and graduations in baccalaureate and graduate programs in nursing*. American Association of Colleges of Nursing.

Anstey, L. M., & Watson, G. P. (2018). *Rubric for eLearning tool evaluation*. Centre for Teaching and Learning, Western University. Retrieved from https://teaching.uwo.ca/pdf/elearning/Rubric-for-eLearning-Tool-Evaluation.pdf

Authement, R. S., & Dormire, S. L. (2020). Introduction to the online nursing education best practices guide. *SAGE Open Nursing*, 6, 2377960820937290. https://doi.org/10.1177/2377960820937290

Barnes, E. R., & Vance, B. S. (2022). Transitioning a graduate nursing physical examination skills lab to an online learning modality. *Nurse Educator*, 47(6), 322–327. https://doi.org/10.1097/NNE.0000000000001220

Bayram, S. B., & Caliskan, N. (2019). Effect of a game-based virtual reality phone application on tracheostomy care education for nursing students: A randomized controlled trial. *Nurse Education Today*, 79, 25–31. https://doi.org/10.1016/j.nedt.2019.05.010

Bdair, I. A. (2021). Nursing students' and faculty members' perspectives about online learning during COVID-19 pandemic: A qualitative study. *Teaching and Learning in Nursing*, 16(3), 220–226. https://doi.org/10.1016/j.teln.2021.02.008

Billings, D. M., Connors, H. R., & Skiba, D. J. (2001). Benchmarking best practices in web-based nursing courses. *Advances in Nursing Science*, 23(3), 41–52. https://doi.org/10.1097/00012272-200103000-00005

Bower, M. (2019). Technology-mediated learning theory. *British Journal of Educational Technology, 50*(3), 1035–1048. https://doi.org/10.1111/bjet.12771

Brooks, R., & Grady, S. D. (2022). Course design considerations for inclusion and representation. Quality Matters. Retrieved from https://www.qualitymatters.org/sites/default/files/research-docs-pdfs/Course-Design-Considerations-for-Inclusion-and-Representation.pdf

Castellanos, J., & Gloria, A. M. (2007). Research considerations and theoretical application for best practices in higher education: Latina/os achieving success. *Journal of Hispanic Higher Education, 6*(4), 378–396.

Chen, J., Wang, M., Kirschner, P. A., & Tsai, C.-C. (2018). The role of collaboration, computer use, learning environments, and supporting strategies in CSCL: A meta-analysis. *Review of Educational Research*, 88(6), 799–843. https://doi.org/10.3102/0034654318791584

Chicca, J. (2021). Designing courses using the hyflex model. *Nurse Educator*, 46(5), 289–289. https://doi.org/10.1097/NNE.0000000000000991

Claywell, L., Wallace, C., Price, J., Reneau, M., & Carlson, K. (2016). Influence of nursing faculty discussion presence on student learning and satisfaction in online courses. *Nurse Educator, 41*(4), 175–179. https://doi.org/10.1097/NNE.0000000000000252

Cobb, S. C. (2011). Social presence, satisfaction, and perceived learning of RN-to-BSN students in web-based nursing courses. *Nursing Education Perspectives*, 32(2), 115–119. https://doi.org/10.5480/1536-5026-32.2.115

Cope, B., & Kalantzis, M. (2021). Pedagogies for Digital Learning. In M. G. Sindoni, & I. Moschini (Eds.), *Multimodal literacies across digital learning contexts* (1st ed., pp. 34–54). Routledge. https://doi.org/10.4324/9781003134244-3

Darabi, A., Arrastia, M. C., Nelson, D. W., Cornille, T., & Liang, X. (2011). Cognitive presence in asynchronous online learning: A comparison of four discussion strategies: Discussion strategies in online learning. *Journal of Computer Assisted Learning*, 27(3), 216–227. https://doi.org/10.1111/j.1365-2729.2010.00392.x

Darby, F., & Lang, J. M. (2019). *Small teaching online: Applying learning science in online classes* (1st ed.). Jossey-Bass, a Wiley Brand.

Davidson, S. J., & Candy, L. (2016). Teaching EBP using game-based learning: Improving the student experience. *Worldviews on Evidence-Based Nursing*, 13(4), 285–293. https://doi.org/10.1111/wvn.12152

DeLenardo, S., Savory, J., Feiner, F., Cretu, M., & Carnegie, J. (2019). Creation and online use of patient-centered videos, digital storytelling, and interactive self-testing questions for teaching pathophysiology. *Nurse Educator*,

44(6), E1–E5. https://doi.org/10.1097/NNE.0000000000000646

Delmas, P. M. (2017). Using VoiceThread to create community in online learning. *TechTrends*, *61*(6), 595–602. https://doi.org/10.1007/s11528-017-0195-z

Foronda, C., & Lippincott, C. (2014). Graduate nursing students' experience with synchronous, interactive videoconferencing within online courses. *Quarterly Review of Distance Education*, *15*(2), 1–8.

Garrison, D. R. (2016). *Thinking collaboratively: Learning in a community of inquiry.* Routledge.

Garrison, D. R. (2017). *E-Learning in the 21st century: A community of inquiry framework for research and practice* (3rd ed.). Routledge.

Gaston, T., & Lynch, S. (2019). Does using a course design framework better engage our online nursing students? *Teaching and Learning in Nursing*, *14*(1), 69–71. https://doi.org/10.1016/j.teln.2018.11.001

Gazza, E. A. (2022). The experience of being a full-time academic nurse educator during the COVID-19 pandemic. *Nursing Education Perspectives*, *43*(2), 74–79. https://doi.org/10.1097/01.NEP.0000000000000933

Grech, J. (2022). Exploring nursing students' need for social presence and its relevance to their learning preferences. *Nursing Open*, *9*(3), 1643–1652. https://doi.org/10.1002/nop2.1189

Harris, N., & Bacon, C. E. W. (2019). Developing cognitive skills through active learning: A systematic review of health care professions. *Athletic Training Education Journal*, *14*(2), 135–148. https://doi.org/10.4085/1402135

Hensley, A., Hampton, D., Wilson, J. L., Culp-Roche, A., & Wiggins, A. T. (2021). A multicenter study of student engagement and satisfaction in online programs. *Journal of Nursing Education*, *60*(5), 259–264. https://doi.org/10.3928/01484834-20210420-04

Hickey, D. T. (2022). Situative approaches to online engagement, assessment, and equity. *Educational Psychologist*, *57*(3), 221–225. https://doi.org/10.1080/00461520.2022.2079129

Jain, S., & Jain, P. (2015). Designing interactive online nursing courses. *Education*, *136*(2), 179–191.

Katai, Z., & Iclanzan, D. (2022). Impact of instructor on-slide presence in synchronous e-learning. *Education and Information Technologies*, *28*(3), 3089–3115. https://doi.org/10.1007/s10639-022-11306-y

Kennedy, S. (2017). *Designing and teaching online courses in nursing.* Springer Publishing Company, LLC.

Kuchinski-Donnelly, D., & Krouse, A. M. (2020). Predictors of emotional engagement in online graduate nursing students. *Nurse Educator*, *45*(4), 214–219. https://doi.org/10.1097/NNE.0000000000000769

Kucuk, S., & Richardson, J. C. (2019). A structural equation model of predictors of online learners' engagement and satisfaction. *Journal of Asynchronous Learning Networks*, *23*(2), 196.

Kumi-Yeboah, A., Sallar, A., Kiramba, L. K., & Kim, Y. (2020). Exploring the use of digital technologies from the perspective of diverse learners in online learning environments. *Online Learning*, *24*(4). https://doi.org/10.24059/olj.v24i4.2323

Lewis, E. (2021). Best practices for improving the quality of the online course design and learners experience. *The Journal of Continuing Higher Education*, *69*(1), 61–70. https://doi.org/10.1080/07377363.2020.1776558

Linares, L. I. R., & Muñoz, S. M. (2011). Revisiting validation theory: Theoretical foundations, applications, and extensions. *Enrollment Management Journal, 2*(1), 12–33.

Männistö, M., Mikkonen, K., Kuivila, H.-M., Virtanen, M., Kyngäs, H., & Kääriäinen, M. (2020). Digital collaborative learning in nursing education: A systematic review. *Scandinavian Journal of Caring Sciences, 34*(2), 280–292. https://doi.org/10.1111/scs.12743

Martin, F., Polly, D., & Ritzhaupt, A. (2020). Bichronous online learning: Blending asynchronous and synchronous online learning. *Educause Review.* Retrieved from https://er.educause.edu/articles/2020/9/bichronous-online-learning-blending-asynchronous-and-synchronous-online-learning

Martin, F., Ritzhaupt, A., Kumar, S., & Budhrani, K. (2019). Award-winning faculty online teaching practices: Course design, assessment and evaluation, and facilitation. *The Internet and Higher Education, 42,* 34–43. https://doi.org/10.1016/j.iheduc. 2019.04.001

Mayne, L. A., & Wu, Q. (2011). Creating and measuring social presence in online graduate nursing courses. *Nursing Education Perspectives, 32*(2), 110–114. https://doi.org/ 10.5480/1536-5026-32.2.110

Means, B., & Neisler, J.; Langer Research Associates. (2020). *Suddenly online: A national survey of undergraduates during the COVID-19 pandemic*. Digital Promise. Retrieved from https://www.everylearner-everywhere.org/resources/suddenly-online-national-undergraduate-survey

Merkebu, J., Battistone, M., McMains, K., McOwen, K., Witkop, C., Konopasky, A., Torre, D., Holmboe, E., & Durning, S. J. (2020). Situativity: A family of social cognitive theories for understanding clinical reasoning and diagnostic error. *Diagnosis, 7*(3), 169–176. https://doi.org/10.1515/dx-2019-0100

Merriam, D., & Hobba-Glose, J. (2021). Using VoiceThread to build a community of inquiry in blended RN-to-BSN education. *Nursing Education Perspectives, 42*(1), 44–45. https://doi.org/10.1097/01. NEP.0000000000000655

Molinillo, S., Aguilar-Illescas, R., Anaya-Sánchez, R., & Vallespín-Arán, M. (2018). Exploring the impacts of interactions, social presence and emotional engagement on active collaborative learning in a social web-based environment. *Computers & Education, 123,* 41–52. https://doi.org/10.1016/j. compedu.2018.04.012

Moore, R. L., & Miller, C. N. (2022). Fostering cognitive presence in online courses: A systematic review (2008–2020). *Online Learning, 26*(1). https://doi.org/10.24059/ olj.v26i1.3071

Morton, K., & Phillips, B. (2022). Online learning challenges for nursing students in Appalachia. *Nursing Education Perspectives, 43*(6), E103–E105. https://doi. org/10.1097/01.NEP.0000000000001039

Murphy, J., Leggieri, A., & Murphy, G. (2021). Fostering the integration of extrinsic motivation in an online graduate nursing education course. *Nursing Education Perspectives, 42*(6), E63–E65. https://doi.org/10.1097/01. NEP.0000000000000654

Nichols, M. R., Malone, A., & Esden, J. (2016). Learning teams and the online learner. *Nurse Educator, 41*(2), 62–63. https://doi. org/10.1097/NNE.0000000000000209

Nurse-Clarke, N. J. (2022). The research Is right: Gamifying nursing research. *Journal of Nursing Education, 61*(10), 604–604. https://doi.org/10.3928/01484834-20220803-02

Olson, C., & Benham-Hutchins, M. (2020). Exploring online RN-to-BSN student perceptions of learner presence. *Nursing Education Perspectives, 41*(2), 92–96. https:// doi.org/10.1097/01.NEP.0000000000000529

Osborne, D. M., Byrne, J. H., Massey, D. L., & Johnston, A. N. B. (2018). Use of online asynchronous discussion boards to engage students, enhance critical thinking, and foster staff-student/student-student collaboration: A mixed method study. *Nurse Education Today, 70,* 40–46. https://doi.org/ 10.1016/j.nedt.2018.08.014

Park, M., Jeong, M., Lee, M., & Cullen, L. (2020). Web-based experiential learning strategies to enhance the evidence-based-practice competence of undergraduate nursing students. *Nurse Education Today, 91,* 104466. https://doi.org/10.1016/j. nedt.2020.104466

Peralta Community College District. (2020). *Peralta online equity rubric*, version 3.0. https://www.peralta.edu/distance-education/ online-equity-rubric

Plante, K., & Asselin, M. E. (2014). Best practices for creating social presence and caring behaviors online. *Nursing Education Perspectives, 35*(4), 219–223. https://doi.org/ 10.5480/13-1094.1

Posey, K. (2021). Online interprofessional learning environment to prepare doctor of nursing practice students for team-based primary care. *The Nurse Practitioner, 46*(4), 29–32. https://doi.org/10.1097/01. NPR.0000737204.76053.14

Price, D. M., Strodtman, L., Brough, E., Lonn, S., & Luo, A. (2015). Digital storytelling: An innovative technological approach to nursing education. *Nurse Educator, 40*(2), 66–70. https://doi.org/10.1097/NNE.0000000000000094

Quality Matters. (2021). *Standards from the quality matters higher education rubric* (6th ed.). Retrieved from Specific Review Standards from the QM Higher Education Rubric, Sixth Edition.

Reyes, I., Clement, D., Sheridan, T., Abraham, C., & Wright, P. (2020). Connecting with students: Using audio-enhanced discussion boards in a nursing curriculum. *Nurse Educator, 45*(2), 71–72. https://doi.org/10.1097/NNE.0000000000000714

Robb, M., & Spadaro, K. C. (2022). Exploration of online doctor of nursing practice students' perceptions of effective teaching methods using the critical incident technique. *Nurse Educator, 47*(6), 328–331. https://doi.org/10.1097/NNE.0000000000001217

Sailsman, S., Rutherford, M., Tovin, M., & Cianelli, R. (2018). Cultural integration online: The lived experience of English-as-a-second-language RN-BSN nursing students learning in an online environment. *Nursing Education Perspectives, 39*(4), 221–224. https://doi.org/10.1097/01.NEP.0000000000000301

Scott, M., & Turrise, S. L. (2021). Student perspectives: Discussion boards as learning strategies in nline accelerated nursing courses. *The Journal of Nursing Education, 60*(7), 419–421. https://doi.org/10.3928/01484834-20210616-12

Serembus, J. F., & Murphy, J. (2020). Creating an engaging learning environment through video discussions. *Nurse Educator, 45*(2), 68–70. https://doi.org/10.1097/NNE.0000000000000701

Shattuck, K. (2015). *Research inputs and outputs of Quality Matters: Update to 2012 and 2014 versions of what we're learning from QM-focused research*. Quality Matters.

Sinacori, B. C. (2020). How nurse educators perceive the transition from the traditional classroom to the online environment: A qualitative inquiry. *Nursing Education Perspectives, 41*(1), 16–19. https://doi.org/10.1097/01.NEP.0000000000000490

Smadi, O., Chamberlain, D., Shifaza, F., & Hamiduzzaman, M. (2021). A community of inquiry lens into nursing education: The educators' experiences and perspectives from three Australian universities. *Nurse Education in Practice, 54*, 103114–103114. https://doi.org/10.1016/j.nepr.2021.103114

Smith, Y., Chen, Y.-J., & Warner-Stidham, A. (2021). Understanding online teaching effectiveness: Nursing student and faculty perspectives. *Journal of Professional Nursing, 37*(5), 785–794. https://doi.org/10.1016/j.profnurs.2021.05.009

Stanley, M. J., Serratos, J., Matthew, W., Fernandez, D., & Dang, M. (2018). Integrating video simulation scenarios Into online nursing instruction. *The Journal of Nursing Education, 57*(4), 245–249. https://doi.org/10.3928/01484834-20180322-11

Tate, T., & Warschauer, M. (2022). Equity in online learning. *Educational Psychologist, 57*(3), 192–206. https://doi.org/10.1080/00461520.2022.2062597

The Columbia Center for Teaching and Learning. (n.d.). *Five tips for hybrid/hyFlex teaching with all learners in mind*. https://ctl.columbia.edu/resources-and-technology/teaching-with-technology/teaching-online/five-tips-hybrid/

Trocky, N. M., & Buckley, K. M. (2016). Evaluating the impact of wikis on student learning outcomes: An integrative review. *Journal of Professional Nursing, 32*(5), 364–376. https://doi.org/10.1016/j.profnurs.2016.01.007

van Gaalen, A. E. J., Brouwer, J., Schönrock-Adema, J., Bouwkamp-Timmer, T., Jaarsma, A. D. C., & Georgiadis, J. R. (2021). Gamification of health professions education: A systematic review. *Advances in Health Sciences Education: Theory and Practice, 26*(2), 683–711. https://doi.org/10.1007/s10459-020-10000-3

Vaughn, N. D., Cleveland-Innes, M., & Garrison, D. R. (2013). *Teaching in blended learning environments: Creating and sustaining communities of inquiry*. AU Press.

Vess, K. R. (2022). Using online collaborative spaces to build graduate students' success in scholarly writing. *Nurse Educator*, *47*(6), E131. https://doi.org/10.1097/NNE.0000000000001234

Volkert, D., Castleberry, J., Fellows, B. J., Goodreau, M., Hesser, L., & Whitley, C. (2021). Resurrecting philosophers in an online doctoral philosophy course in nursing. *Nursing Education Perspectives*, *42*(6), E54–E56. https://doi.org/10.1097/01.NEP.0000000000000690

Waddington, A. M., & Porter, S. D. (2021). Developing social presence in online learning among nurses: Exploration of the community of inquiry models domain of social using a qualitative descriptive design. *Nurse Education in Practice*, *52*, 103000. https://doi.org/10.1016/j.nepr.2021.103000

Walker, C. (2022). Promoting health and active learning with social media. *Nurse Educator*, *47*(6), E144. https://doi.org/10.1097/NNE.0000000000001230

Warschauer, M. (2003). *Technology and social inclusion: Rethinking the digital divide*. MIT Press.

Webber-Ritchey, K. J., Badowski, D., & Gibbons, L. (2020). An online asynchronous physical assessment lab (OAPAL) for graduate nursing students using low-fidelity simulation with peer feedback. *Nursing Education Perspectives*, *41*(6), 378–379. https://doi.org/10.1097/01.NEP.0000000000000677

Yeh, V. J.-H., Sherwood, G., Durham, C. F., Kardong-Edgren, S., Schwartz, T. A., & Beeber, L. S. (2019). Designing and implementing asynchronous online deliberate practice to develop interprofessional communication competency. *Nurse Education in Practice*, *35*, 21–26. https://doi.org/10.1016/j.nepr.2018.12.011

Yilmaz, R. (2017). Exploring the role of e-learning readiness on student satisfaction and motivation in flipped classroom. *Computers in Human Behavior*, *70*, 251–260. https://doi.org/10.1016/j.chb.2016.12.085

Zajac, L. K., & Lane, A. J. (2020). Student perceptions of faculty presence and caring in accelerated Online courses. *Quarterly Review of Distance Education*, *21*(2).

10

Current Concepts in Clinical Education

Paula Gubrud, EdD, RN, CHSE, FAAN, ANEF

CHAPTER OVERVIEW

This chapter provides an overview of current and emerging models of clinical education in nursing. Topics include the Oregon Consortium for Nursing Education's clinical model and application of pedagogies that support each element of the model. The use of dedicated education units and emerging experiences in community environments are presented. Best practices in teaching, coaching, and facilitating learning in the clinical environment are discussed. Strategies for creating a positive clinical environment for learning are emphasized.

BACKGROUND

Clinical learning activities comprise a significant portion of nursing curricula. The primary purpose of clinical education is to provide learning opportunities for students to apply theory in practice. Consequently, most clinical experiences aim to provide opportunities for students to apply content encountered in the classroom and laboratory to the practice of caring for patients in authentic health care environments. Additionally, despite a demand for nurses in long-term care, community health, and primary care, undergraduate clinical practice experiences occur primarily in acute care facilities where learners are assigned to provide total care to one, two, or sometimes three patients, with a corollary written assignment of a nursing care plan (Leighton et al., 2021). This model of clinical education is no longer adequate or appropriate for preparing students in today's health care system. The increase in patient acuity requires students to have a higher level of knowledge, skills, and abilities to safely practice at even the novice level in complex acute care environments (Epp et al., 2022; Goers et al., 2022). The recent *Future of Nursing 2020–2030: Charting a Path to Achieve Health Equity* report (National Academy of Science, Engineering & Medicine [NASEM], 2021) calls for clinical experiences that prepare students with the competencies that address contemporary issues such as the Social Determinants of Health (SDOH) and health inequity (Sumpter et al., 2022). As health care in the United States transitions to value-based health care, new nurses must be prepared to apply foundational economic concepts and educated to contribute to innovations that support quality, safety, good patient outcomes, and lower the cost of care (Yakusheva et al., 2022).

New kinds of clinical education experiences informed by learning science are necessary because of a rapidly changing health care system, increasing complexity of nursing practice in acute care settings, expanding nursing roles focused on health promotion, chronic illness management in community-based settings and primary care (Giddens et al., 2022). Employers across the health care delivery spectrum need new graduate nurses who can: provide safe and quality patient centered-care, use evidence-based practice standards to deliver and evaluate care, make sound judgments, adapt knowledge and skills to novel situations, and function as a member of an interprofessional team.

OCNE CLINICAL EDUCATION MODEL

Challenges with clinical education have been identified over the past 10 to 15 years (Leighton et al., 2021; Ironside et al., 2014). Problems identified by the National League for Nursing (NLN) in 2009 continue to persist today (Goer et al., 2022; McNelis et al., 2014). The challenges are many and while nurse educators developed new approaches to clinical education in response to the global COVID-19 pandemic a lack of suitable clinical placements and a deficit of qualified clinical faculty persists as significant issues that plague nursing education programs.

The Oregon Consortium for Nursing Education (OCNE) launched a multiple-phase project in 2006 to enhance clinical education as a component of a shared competency-based curriculum developed by a statewide consortium of community colleges and Oregon's only public baccalaureate program provided by Oregon Health & Science University School of Nursing (Tanner & Gubrud-Howe, 2021). The first phase of the project involved a statewide assessment process that included workforce partners from a variety of settings (acute, long-term, community) and nursing faculty from all regions of the state. The assessment confirmed reliance on clinical placements focused primarily on total patient care was taxing faculty, health care organizations, and clinical staff (Gubrud-Howe et al., 2007). In response to these findings, OCNE organized a statewide group of educators and practice partners called the Clinical Education Redesign Group (CERG). The group met monthly for 6 months and identified a new model for clinical education.

The OCNE clinical model is used extensively in the consortium (Tanner & Gubrud-Howe, 2021) and has been adopted by other schools and programs (Epp et al., 2022; Niederhauser et al., 2012). Outcomes have been positive with students' successfully passing the NCLEX and employer satisfaction with new graduate proficiency (Tanner & Gubrud-Howe, 2021). With the transition to competency-based education (Giddens et al., 2022; NLN, 2023) the model has the potential to address current challenges resulting from dependency on clinical placements focused on students engaged in total patient care provided in acute care health care environments (Gubrud & Schoessler, 2009).

Central to the model is the notion there should be a clinical education curriculum with sequenced and progressive complexity of learning experiences as building blocks that intentionally provide students with the practice experience needed to apply theory to patient care across the health care continuum. This is in stark contrast to the more typical approach of students having clinical rotations through specialties in an acute care setting. In the OCNE model experiences are purposefully designed to comprise a

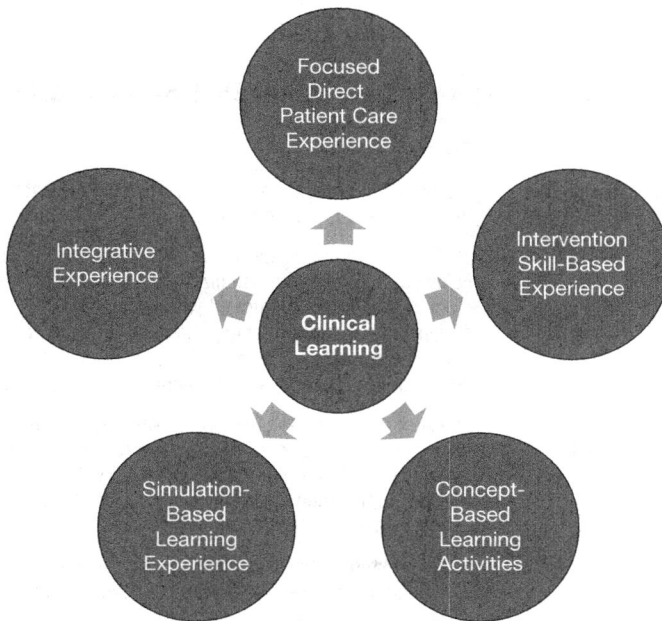

FIGURE 10.1 Elements of the OCNE Clinical Education Model.

variety of experiences including a new approach to total patient care named *focused direct patient care*. As the student develops more competency, the roles of students, faculty, and nursing staff change, and the learning experiences become more integrative. We have found the model reduces the burden clinical supervision places on faculty and staff nurses, focuses on learning clinical knowledge and skills, and uses a developmental approach to becoming clinically competent. Furthermore, the model makes more efficient use of clinical time for students.

The OCNE clinical education model plans and stages learning activities to accomplish course outcomes and is designed to address both the learning needs and developmental level of the student. The model also addresses the complexity and opportunities in the learning environment. The five types of learning experiences—or elements—of this model are illustrated in Figure 10.1.

Intervention Skill-Based Experience

The intervention skill-based experience element of the model builds proficiency in the "know-how" and "know-why" of nursing practice. These experiences include psychomotor skills, as well as techniques of assessment, interviewing, basic communication skills, and organizational skills such as prioritization, and delegation. Skill-based experiences include deliberate practice theory constructs where such repetition with active coaching will facilitate mastery and the development of embodied know-how (Gonzalez & Kardong-Edgren, 2017). Once students attain initial proficiency in a skill, it is

TABLE 10.1	
Progression of Learning in Interventional Skill-Based Learning	
Strategy	**Example**
Decontextualized learning in clinical lab setting	Students learn and demonstrate Foley catheterization using both male and female task trainers.
Contextualized learning on a low or mid-fidelity manikin	The circumstances regarding the order or decision to insert a Foley catheter are contextualized in a simple patient scenario and students are asked to interact with the manikin as they would a patient. The student must expand their performance beyond the psychomotor delivery of the skill and identify the purpose, risks, and evidence-based practice standards for follow-up care.
Contextualized learning in high-fidelity simulation scenarios	The scenarios are designed so the student may need to adapt the procedure to the particular patient (i.e., inserting a Foley in a patient with a fractured hip), interact with the patient and perhaps family members, and complete the task with time-based constraints.
Application in an authentic clinical environment	Once the student has demonstrated mastery of a skill in the simulated environment with minimal coaching, they have achieved a level of competency needed to safely perform the skill in the clinical environment under the supervision of faculty or designated staff nurse.

further developed by creating variable context. Mastery-learning theory and deliberate practice pedagogy (Gonzalez & Kardong-Edgren, 2017; McGaghie et al., 2020) informs this element of the model. Table 10.1 provides an illustration of these concepts.

Mastery Learning and Deliberate Practice

Mastery learning, an essential component of competency-based education, is designed so all learners demonstrate essential knowledge and skills to well-defined high standards (McGaghie, 2020). In mastery learning, the level of proficiency is fixed, but the time and process each learner engages in to reach competency vary (Gonzalez & Kardong-Edgren, 2017). Instructional design of mastery learning uses the pedagogy of deliberate practice and principles from behaviorism, constructivism, and self-efficacy learning theory (Gonzalez & Kardong-Edgren, 2017; McGaghie, 2020).

Expressions of behaviorism include integration of behavioral learning objectives, deliberate practice with coaching, immediate feedback, and most importantly reliable instruments and process used to measure observable behavior (McGaghie, 2020). Constructivism is evident as procedures such as Foley catheterization must be adapted to specific patient situations. The learner transfers and adapts a mastered skill or knowledge to a novel situation, constructing expanded expertise. Using the example of Foley catheter insertion, the use of sterile technique must be constant but, positioning the patient may need to be modified, interacting with the patient during the procedure will vary if the patient is confused or very anxious. Sometimes assistance is needed, and the student will need to include delegation and communication skills with the psychomotor skills already mastered. As the learner practices the skill in a variety of circumstances, they build a repertoire of approaches to completing the skill. Additionally, the student learns which patients are at risk for developing complications related to the procedure or skill and identifies strategies to mitigate risk. With experience, the student constructs deepening knowledge and skill. Self-efficacy is a learning theory developed by Albert Bandura that embodies the belief one has the capacity to execute the action needed to develop excellence (McGaghie, 2020). Actions to promote self-efficacy encourage the learner to assume responsibility for their performance and development toward achieving excellence through self-organization, proactive pursuit to improve, and self-reflection. A sense of accomplishment when a learner masters a skill based on objective and concise criteria contributes to developing self-efficacy.

Deliberate practices are intentional activities provided to optimize proficiency and improvement (McGaghie, 2020). Feedback by someone skilled in the task at hand is the cornerstone of deliberate practice. Feedback is given in the moment of performance, so the learner identifies when they have performed according to measurable expectations. Corrections in the moment are provided as the students learn a new skill. Feedback and coaching are also referred to as scaffolds and will vary depending on the baseline level of competency. As the learner develops proficiency, the expert coach minimizes the feedback provided, encouraging the student to self-reflect and self-regulate the amount of coaching needed. According to Reedy (2015), learners need to master simple tasks first and move to complex application of skills. When a skill is contextualized in a complex scenario the expert coach may need to provide more feedback. The assumption is students will master the skill according to expectations and need the opportunity to practice with coaching until they can perform independently, and scaffolds can be withdrawn. The time to mastery will vary among students.

Developing a mastery learning module includes several learning activities that involve independent study, group learning, and individual coaching with eventual demonstration of mastery. The general principles and resources presented in Chapter 7, *Backward Design: Aligning Outcomes, Assessments, and Activities,* can be applied to design mastery learning modules. See Table 10.2 for the elements of a mastery learning module.

Skill Decay

Due to pressures related to clinical placement scheduling, schools of nursing frequently front-load teaching and practicing skills at the beginning of a semester or quarter. Such practices do not support the science of learning principles discussed in Chapters 3 and 4. Additionally, studies have found there was a greater degree of skill decay when there is a longer interval between demonstrating mastery in a skills lab and using the skill in the clinical environment (Gonzalez & Kardong-Edgren, 2017). Consequently, programs should create opportunities for re-mastery, as when a skill is not used consistently the clinician's proficiency is likely to deteriorate (Gonzalez & Kardong-Edgren, 2017). Avoid referring to the re-mastery process as remediation due to the punitive interpretation associated with this word (Gonzalez & Kardong-Edgren, 2017). Skill decay is normal and expected when a skill has not been used for a period of time. Referring to the process of remastery as remediation may be seen as punitive and should be avoided. Resources should be available to assist and include procedural videos to review, practice using feedback and coaching. Learners

TABLE 10.2

Elements of a Mastery Learning Module

Element	Description
Assessment	➤ Clear measurable learning objectives—use SMART objective format; see Chapter 7, *Backward Design: Aligning Outcomes, Assessments, and Activities* ➤ Provide minimum passing standard (usually a checklist or scoring rubric)
Preparation	➤ Pre-reading assignment or screen-based content on the rationale and principles related to the skill ➤ Baseline diagnostic testing—this could be a written quiz or an initial attempt at performing the skill. Faculty should expect the results to be poor for many students. This is done because some students may have some baseline knowledge or experience and will need less practice time and provides formative feedback for learning.
Practice	➤ Demonstration of the skill by an expert—the expert describes each step in the skill as it is performed. The demonstration can be live, recorded, or both. ➤ Deliberate practice—practice with supervision and feedback from an expert. Practice sessions become more complex, increasing the real-world contextualization until mastery is demonstrated using the minimum passing standard.

should reflect on their experiences and identify when re-mastery is needed to grow self-efficacy as a professional.

Evaluation of Mastery Learning

A variety of methods used to determine if a learner has mastered a skill or intervention are delineated in Table 10.3. Using a checklist or rating scale, provide the learner with a clear description of the criteria used to assess mastery. Checklists typically use dichotomous assessments (i.e., competent/not competent) making establishing interrater reliability easier. However, most students perform in range of competency proficiency (i.e., not competent, partially competent, mostly competent, competent), especially when first learning. A checklist approach may not provide discrete feedback regarding strengths and areas for needed improvement. Instruments using rating scales provide more detailed feedback as each rating denotes a varying description of student performance. Monson et al., (2021) found using checklists to validate psychomotor skills was viewed favorably by students and helped them recall the sequence of steps, familiarity with equipment, and knowledge related to the purpose for performing the skill, assessment, and potential complications. They also concluded using formative assessment with immediate feedback improves student confidence and reduces student stress when performing the skill for the first time in the care setting (Monson et al., 2021). Student video recordings, if used, can be compared with an expert's performance recording, so the learner can self-evaluate and self-regulate their own practice.

Developing instruments using rating scales takes time and establishing interrater reliability is more challenging. Several nursing textbooks and skills manuals include instruments that can be used to assess mastery of skills. Faculty should work together to

TABLE 10.3

Evaluation of Mastery Learning

Assessment	Example
Cognitive skills interpretation and action needed after completing an assessment	➤ Accurate Subjective Objective Assessment Plan (SOAP) notes ➤ Verbal Situation Background Assessment Recommendation (SBAR) report
Knowledge needed to perform a particular skill	➤ Multiple-choice quizzes
Mastery of psychomotor skills	➤ Checklists and rubric-type instruments using rating scales can include supporting behavior such as patient communication and teaching. ➤ Video recording of student performance can be used for the learner to self-evaluate their performance using the checklist or rating scale. ➤ Self-evaluation should be considered as one lens to assess skill competency as this practice supports development of the self-efficacy required in the student's future as a professional.

establish a shared mental model about the criteria students need to demonstrate mastery of each skill. See Chapters 14, *Equitable Assessment Practices*, 15, *Item Writing and Analysis,* and 16, *Rubric Development* for related discussion on assessing competency.

In summary, the instructional design for the intervention-skill-based element of the OCNE Clinical Education Model integrates principles of backward design and mastery learning. The skills taught and mastered encompass psychomotor skills and other cognitive and team-based tasks such as communicating with patients and other colleagues and delegation. The instructional design used for the intervention-skill-based element of the OCNE model embraces formative assessment (assessment for learning) as the foundation for mastery learning with students having multiple opportunities to demonstrate clearly defined expectations of competency.

Concept-Based Learning Activities

Concept-based learning activities (CBLAs), based on early work by Heims and Boyd (1993) and expanded by Nielsen (2016), are designed to deepen and extend students' theoretical knowledge by studying how key concepts are exemplified in actual practice. CBLAs support the development of pattern recognition, and improve performance in clinical judgment (Nielsen, 2016; Nielsen et al., 2021). Through multiple encounters with clients who show variations on a particular problem, students learn patterns or clusters of cues associated with a specific concept, illness, disease, or health problem. The defining characteristic of this element of the model is that students study the concept or issue at hand through the study of the patient's record and patient assessment. See Chapter 11, *Concept-Based Learning in the Clinical Learning Environment* for an in-depth description.

Simulation-Based Learning Experience

Simulation-based Learning Experience (SLE) presents students with authentic clinical situations they will likely encounter in practice and provides opportunities for students to learn to think like a nurse through client case exemplars in simulated learning environments. This element of the model integrates research and The Health Care Simulation Standards of Best Practice™. Application of the SLE element presents clinical situations students will encounter in practice, with ambiguities and uncertainties, and as the situation unfolds over time. Simulation methods include using screen-based scenarios, high-fidelity manikins, or standardized patient simulation. SLE is designed to promote the development of clinical reasoning as situations unfold. Students learn to notice obvious and subtle clinical changes as they interpret findings, consider appropriate responses, communicate with physicians and other providers about their observations and interpretations, and reflect on practice. SLE also provides opportunities for developing team communication skills, and collaborating with physicians, pharmacists, and other health professionals as members of an interprofessional health care team. See Chapter 12, *Best Practices in Simulation Learning* for an in-depth discussion of developing and implementing SLE.

Focused Direct Patient Care Experience

Focused direct patient care experience is a derivative of the traditional model of the total patient care approach to clinical education. However, there are some distinct pedagogical and curricular assumptions of this element of the OCNE clinical education model. Focused direct patient care experiences enable students to gain progressive experience in the actual delivery of nursing care and to build and understand the role of developing relationships with patients. By having extensive time with individual patients and their families, students develop a deep understanding of the patient's experience, begin to identify the individual's typical pattern of responses, and know what is important to the client (Tanner, 2006; Tanner et al., 2022). Focused direct patient care differs from the tradition of total patient care with the focus on identifying the learning expectations appropriate for the student's developmental level and expected competencies. For example, beginning students are assigned to complete an assessment on healthy individuals in a community or home setting. Another example is focusing on managing medication administration and related assessments in a skilled care facility. These types of assignments focus on one or two aspects of care and allow the student to engage in repetitive practice that builds confidence and competence. Like the model of total patient care, faculty typically is present at the clinical site with a group of students in a care setting. The faculty assigns the focus of care and ideally aligns tasks performed with content from concurrent lab and theory courses. The assigned focus for a care experience allows the student to apply a growing knowledge and skill base to client care. Students learn to establish and nurture the nurse/client relationship and integrate the ethics of caring for individuals.

The focused direct patient care element of the model is informed by intentional learning pedagogy (Mollman & Candela, 2018) and constructivism. Epp and coauthors (2022) adapted the focused-direct patient care element of the model and applied findings from Mollman & Candela's concept analysis to implement a version of this element of the model. Application of intentional learning empowers the student to engage in clinical learning as they are equipped to use what knowledge, skills, and abilities they have already obtained in novel situations. Intentional learning is complementary to mastery learning as students are encouraged to use course outcomes and to focus their learning activities. As students gain experience they refine and expand their construction of knowledge through experience and reflection.

Faculty provide direct supervision and facilitation of learning in this element of the model. Because the patient care activity is focused, learning is at the forefront of faculty efforts as opposed to supervising random patient care tasks and procedures (Gubrud-Howe & Schoessler, 2008).

The focused direct patient care element of the model aims to facilitate the development of clinical judgment in a variety of settings (see Chapter 17, *Assessment of Clinical Judgment*). The student learns to notice the salient features of the situation by coming to know the patient's individual and unique responses to disease, illness, and treatment. Focusing on the patient's care needs also involves learning to interpret findings and craft responses tailored to the client. Because the learning occurs in an authentic clinical environment, students learn to incorporate the workflow of the agency into the care they are providing and continue developing tacit knowledge embedded in clinical practice. Students begin to learn to engage in the constant organization and prioritization activity that is required in dynamic care environments.

During the focused individual patient care experience, the student may or may not be responsible for all aspects of the client's care. For example, instead of providing all care the patient needs the student may focus on practicing delegation skills with certified nursing assistants (CNAs). In the OCNE baseline statewide assessment of the traditional total patient care model, students were providing all care for assigned patients yet employers noted new graduates were unskilled in delegation as novice nurses.

Communicating the focus of care the student will provide is key to successful implementation of this element of the OCNE model. The student is accountable for those aspects pertinent to the learning outcomes identified for the day, and for direct and clear communication with the patient's nurse regarding all patient care activities with an emphasis on sharing pertinent assessment findings. Students are expected to respond appropriately to any unexpected urgent situation that may arise. Students are also accountable for communicating with their faculty member regarding their learning related to care activities, client assessments, and findings.

The term "Patient" encompasses individual patients, families, communities, or populations as the focus of care, changing along with the course emphasis. In early clinical experiences of the curriculum, the focus is clearly on the individual patient. Students acknowledge the patient's interactions with family and community, but these aspects of the patient's situation are in the background as context. As student competency grows, the focus includes both the individual patient and family. Late in the curriculum, the focus is on communities, populations, and organizations, as students develop competencies in population-based care and leadership and outcomes management.

In summary, the focused direct patient care element of the model involves caring for patients in a variety of health care settings. One faculty supervises and facilitates the patient care learning activity for a small group of students. Development of clinical judgment is a key component of focus for teaching and learning activities. Focused direct patient care differs from traditional total patient care used in clinical education as the students focus on providing clearly delineated aspects of care with an emphasis on learning about the clinical reasoning nurses use to make clinical judgments.

Communicating with staff is a critical component of this element of the model to assure the staff nurse is aware of what aspects of care are provided by students.

Integrative Experience

Integrative experience provides an opportunity for the student to apply all elements of prior learning in an authentic clinical practice situation. Integrative experiences can be planned at various times throughout the curriculum and are of two main types: (1) the student undertakes a project that requires integration of their clinical knowledge and experience in the practice of leadership or community-based work; or (2) the student is engaged in a clinical practice setting, assigned to work with a professional nurse, and assumes increasing aspects of that nurse's work. The integrative practicum is a means to support the transition into practice. This is a common model used at the end of programs and is often referred to as a preceptorship or capstone clinical experience. Both project-focused and patient care experiences are integrative, and both require immersion in a setting to the extent necessary to do an adequate assessment of the organization, develop an understanding of the workflow, and become a participating member of the health care team.

Situated learning and cognitive apprenticeship are the pedagogies used to design and assess the efficacy of the *integrative experience* element of the OCNE model. Situated learning posits novices learn from experts by being situated in a community of authentic practice where learning is contextualized and the preceptor coaches the learner in the practical knowledge and skilled know-how and know-why embedded in the patient care environment (Benner et al., 2010; Woolley & Jarvis, 2007). The preceptor, under the guidance of the faculty, scaffolds the learning experience described in the six phases of a cognitive apprenticeship (Woolley & Jarvis). See Table 10.4.

In this element of the model, students are assigned to work with a nurse in a health care setting over a designated unit of time. The student works the same schedule as the nurse preceptor and engages in all activities, such as professional development sessions and committee meetings. The faculty is not always present in the setting and facilitates the preceptor placements, provides periodic teaching, and checks in with the preceptor and student to monitor student performance and progress in meeting defined course outcomes and competencies. The preceptor is responsible for assuring assigned patients receive safe, quality care and the nurse educator is responsible for facilitating learning and evaluating student performance. Much of the evidence the faculty uses to evaluate student performance is provided by the preceptor. The faculty makes periodic observations of a student's clinical behaviors in the setting, seeking feedback from the student and preceptor. Other stakeholders, such as the charge nurse and patients, may contribute to the evidence the faculty uses to determine if the student is progressing in developing competency according to expectations.

Preceptor role preparation—To prepare nurses for performing the role of a preceptor, OCNE developed a standard program that can be provided in a two-day workshop or accessed statewide through a web-based learning management system hosted by a hospital partner. The preceptor training emphasizes pedagogy that supports student-centered learning, communication skills, ways to facilitate a positive learning environment, coaching for clinical judgment, evidence-based practice, and strategies to use when providing students with performance evaluation and feedback. The training includes recorded scenarios

TABLE 10.4

Six Phases of Cognitive Apprenticeship

Phase	Description
Modeling	The expert models the skill and clinical competencies so the learner can observe and build a mental model of a mental model and process needed to accomplish expertise.
Coaching	The expert observes the learner, provides hints, guidance, feedback, and—if needed—further modeling with the aim of bringing the learner's performance closer to that of the expert.
Scaffolding	Learning is supported according to current skill level and activities are initiated to assist the learner to improve or stretch to a new level of competent behavior. Support is gradually removed (fading) until the student can perform the competency or skill independently.
Articulation/reflection (two phases)	The preceptor prompts the learner to articulate their knowledge, problem solving process and reasoning, and provides time for reflection of own performance and commitment for improvement (see Chapter 17, *Assessment of Clinical Judgment*).
Exploration	The preceptor pushes the student to problem solve independently actively beginning the process of transition into practice.

of difficult situations in which students and preceptors are to practice and debrief appropriate responses to common challenges periodically faced when precepting.

Multiple nurse education experts have identified characteristics that define a high-quality integrative practicum based on literature reviews, survey data, and evaluation of web-based training (Chicca & Shellenbarger, 2020a; Chicca & Shellenbarger, 2021; Ward & McComb, 2017; Wu et al., 2020). See Table 10.5 for a list of criteria synthesized from these four sources that promote optimum learning and achievement for integrative experiences.

In summary, the integrative experience is informed by situated learning and cognitive apprenticeship learning theory. This practicum is designed to achieve three major goals: (1) provide progressive experiences for the student to integrate prior learning; (2) provide opportunity for immersion in a clinical setting for a sufficient period of time that the student can be integrated as a member of the team, and begin to understand the impact of unit norms and values on care delivered; and (3) begin the transition to assuming full responsibilities of the registered nurse (RN).

Sequencing the Five Elements into the Curriculum

For early experiences, the concept-based, intervention skill-based, and simulation experiences that will facilitate the student's abilities required for increasing integration of focused-direct care experiences dominate (see Fig. 10.2). Students practice health assessment skills in the lab and apply those skills in simple simulation scenarios focused on identifying disease risk and promoting health. Through these building blocks, students are prepared to engage in *focused patient care activities*, often providing care

TABLE 10.5

Criteria for Successful Integrative Practicum

Criteria	Description
Preceptor selection and training	➤ Preceptor should be a match in terms of communication and work style ➤ Follow school and facility policy regarding requirements—i.e., years of experience and level of education ➤ Assure willingness of preceptor to assume role ➤ Review course outcomes and syllabi ➤ Review and practice best practices in coaching for clinical judgment (see Chapter 17, *Assessment of Clinical Judgment*) ➤ Review policies/procedures regarding task supervision emphasis on high-risk procedures such as IV medication administration ➤ Chain of command for addressing problems ➤ Faculty contact information
Preceptor roles	➤ Orient student to the unit and agency ➤ Plan care with student each shift ➤ Facilitate student integration as a member of the health care team on the unit ➤ Facilitate clinical learning through direct teaching and engaging in high-level discussions focused on clinical reasoning ➤ Provide constructive feedback ➤ Provide emotional support ➤ Communicate with designated faculty ➤ Provide faculty with assessment of student performance ➤ Support student's professional goals ➤ Model clinical care and expertise

Faculty roles	➤ Schedule and perform purposeful check-ins throughout the integrative practicum
	  ➤ Observe student engagement with patients during check-in visits
	  ➤ Seek preceptor feedback regarding student progress
	  ➤ Conduct high-level thinking conversations with student to facilitate clinical reasoning and judgment
	  ➤ Assist student to identify strengths and needed improvement with action plan
	  ➤ Provide formative feedback regarding student performance
	  ➤ Troubleshoot any emerging problems or challenges
	➤ Facilitate seminars and/or clinical conferences
	➤ Be available at all times and communicate contact information for student and preceptor. Identify backup communication plan if instructor can't be reached.
	➤ Evaluate Integrative Practicum experience—including preceptor performance, workload implications, and clinical environment as an optimum space for learning

TABLE 10.5

Criteria for Successful Integrative Practicum *(Continued)*

Criteria	Description
Student roles	➤ Demonstrate self-efficacy—coordinate with preceptor to meet personal professional goals and course outcomes ➤ Engage in self-reflection and self-evaluation with preceptor and faculty ➤ Demonstrate strong work ethic—be on time, engage as a team member, communicate changes in predetermined schedule
Clinical agency	➤ Provide a culture that supports students ➤ Establish and support a culture that embraces diversity, equity, and inclusion ➤ Express value for the student as a member of the health care team

Adapted from Chicca & Shellenbarger (2020a), Chica & Shellenbarger (2021), Ward & McComb (2017), & Wu et at. (2020).

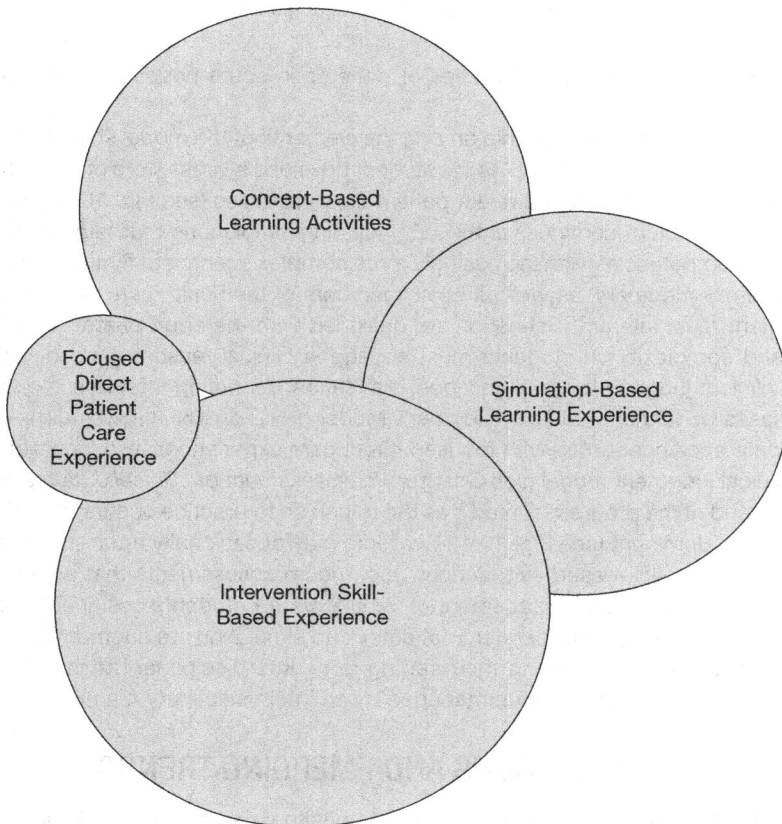

FIGURE 10.2 Early Clinical Learning Experiences.

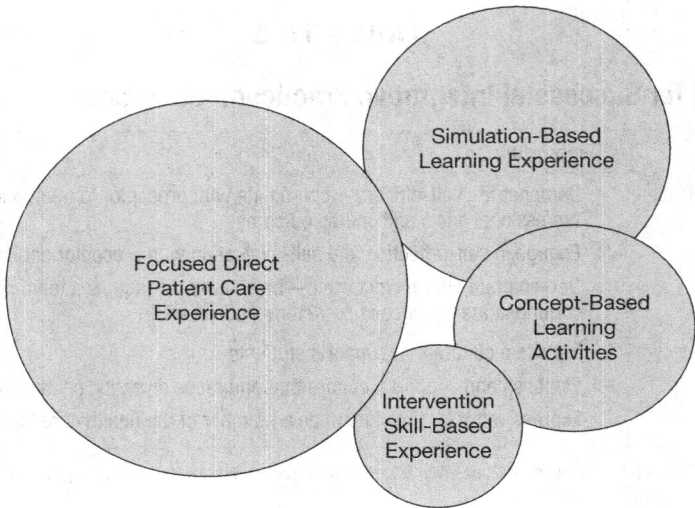

FIGURE 10.3 Mid-Program Clinical Learning Experience.

to residents in long-term care facilities or patients in acute hospitals experiencing an exacerbation of a chronic illness.

In later courses, the relationship among the elements of the model shifts to reflect the students' ongoing development. As the student develops a larger store of knowledge and skill, the emphasis on focused direct patient care increases (see Fig. 10.3). The clinical education curriculum continues with SLE, including simulations that require integration of several competencies with increasingly more complex scenarios. Simulations typically include family members, as well as other members of the health care team with whom the student must interact. Scenarios are designed with the appropriate level of uncertainty and complexity so students must engage in clinical reasoning needed to make sound clinical judgments. Pre- and post-simulation debriefing integrate the language and phases of Tanner's Clinical Judgment Model (Tanner & Gubrud-Howe, 2021). Pre- and post-conference conducted with focused direct care experiences also incorporate Tanner's clinical judgment model (see Chapter 17, *Assessment of Clinical Judgment*).

At the end of the program of study, as the transition to practice occurs, the integrative practicum is dominant (see Fig. 10.4). Students may occasionally return to the campus lab for specialty skill-based experiences (e.g., neuro assessments that are completed only on a particular unit; management of ventilators for students assigned to a facility with a focus on ventilator-dependent patients), and simulations to augment experiences students are able to acquire in their setting (e.g., interdisciplinary team conference; rapidly changing clinical situation managed by an interdisciplinary team).

ESTABLISHED INNOVATIONS AND EMERGING TRENDS

Changing demographics, improved access to health care through the Affordable Care Act, and exponential growth of health care science and technology have created a continuous and increasing demand for competent RNs. Over the last two decades, nursing

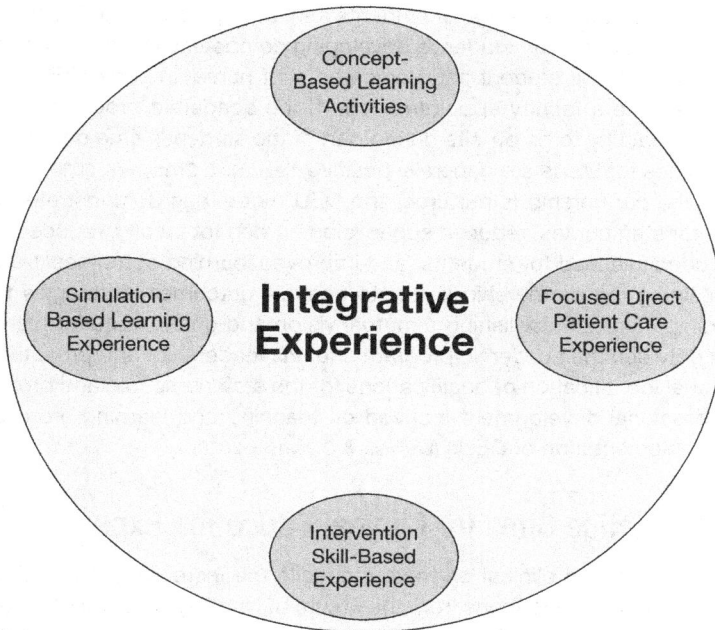

FIGURE 10.4 End of Program Clinical Learning Experience.

programs have expanded capacity creating a strain on clinical placements. All of this combined with recommendations from the Future of Nursing 2020–2030 report has prompted nurse educators, nursing workforce leaders, and clinical partners to rethink the utility of the traditional acute care clinical placement model (Jones-Schenk, 2021). The next section describes established innovations and emerging trends in clinical education.

Dedicated Education Units

A dedication education unit (DEU) is another model created to redesign clinical experiences. Originally created in Australia in the late 1990s, the DEU model has expanded across the United States (Musallam et al., 2021). The model employs collaboration between a health care organization and an academic nursing education program to create consistent and quality clinical experiences in a dedicated unit. The unit is developed to provide optimal teaching-learning environments within a larger hospital or other health care organizations such as long-term care and public health departments (Gubrud, in press). A key unique feature of DEUs focuses on the role of staff nurses and faculty. Much of the clinical teaching is done by competent staff nurses. The relationship between the staff nurse teacher and the student creates continuity of learning, supervision, and competency assessment. The student is paired with the same staff nurse every week during a clinical rotation. In traditional clinical rotations, students may work with a different staff nurse each week and learning activities are based on a particular patient assignment. In the DEU model, the staff nurse facilitates learning, provides oversight of each student's learning, and serves as a resource for students and faculty. Faculty maintain responsibility for assessing learning and student's developing competency which requires frequent communication with the student and dedicated staff nurse. In some DEU models, the staff nurses receive a faculty appointment with the academic program which allows the supervisory faculty to be off-site during part of the student's time on the unit.

The outcomes for DEUs are generally positive (Lapinski & Ciurzynski, 2020; Musallam et al., 2021). When the partnership is nurtured, the DEU model has demonstrated increased satisfaction for staff nurses, reduced supervision burden for faculty, reduced stress and decreased cognitive load for students, and improved learning outcomes (Musallam et al., 2021). Maintaining the partnership is key to positive outcomes. Strategies to support the partnership involve establishing a mutual vision and goals, frequent planned communication between the academic program and unit leadership, and proactive problem solving. Mutual identification of qualifications for the staff nurse role and providing continuous professional development focused on teaching and learning are essential for successful implementation of DEUs (Lapinski & Ciurynski, 2020).

Emerging Practice Sites for Clinical Education Experience

As nurse educators and clinical partners reconcile the increasing demand for clinical placements the recommendations from the Future of Nursing 2020–2030 report (NASEM, 2021) provide a vision for providing clinical education experiences aligned with the changing health care delivery system and emerging new roles for RNs. Community-based clinical learning placements have long been included in baccalaureate clinical education. The importance of including community and population-based clinical experiences is becoming a priority in clinical education for all levels of nursing education because of rapid changes in health care delivery and an emphasis on value-based models of care focuses on addressing health inequity (Buerhaus & Yakusheva, 2022; Rauch & Malloy 2020; Sumpter et al., 2022). Hassmiller and Wakefield (2022) published a call to action in response to the Future of Nursing 2020–2030 report purporting nurses must lead changes needed to close the gap in health care inequity through mitigating barriers to care. Clinical learning experiences in community-based settings need to expand so new graduates are prepared to practice at the top of their scope of practice, as well as to lead efforts to address health disparities for underserved populations by providing care in environments where individuals, families, and communities work, gather, live and play (Sumpter et al., 2022).

Application of the OCNE Model in Community

Nielsen and coauthors (2013) provide examples of how the OCNE Clinical Education model can be applied to designing clinical experiences in community and population-based settings. Learning in immunization clinics emphasizes the intervention-skilled base element of the model. After students demonstrate mastery of administering injectable medication in the skills lab on task trainers and manikins, they provide multiple immunizations in a clinic. The focus of the activity is to engage students in supervised repetitive practice to gain mastery of the skill. Concept-based experiences focus on activities designed to help students understand a community as client and other population-based concepts used in public health. Simulation-based learning involves a poverty simulation where students engage in a low-fidelity simulation and experience the daily challenges impoverished individual families face. The debriefing focuses on uncovering the barriers poverty creates to accessing needed health care. This simulation explores the nurse's role in mitigating challenges for individuals experiencing poverty and results in changing attitudes and values (Noone et al., 2012). Nielsen and co-authors address the integrative experience element of the model by describing a curricular learning plan and experiences for students that choose community or population health for their final integrative practicum with a nurse preceptor.

In summary, in preparation for a rapidly changing health care system preparing students to address health care inequity, clinical education needs ample experience in community environments focused on population-based care. Academic-Practice partnerships addressing population-based care, primary care, care coordination, telehealth, and other care experiences that prepare students for competencies needed across the health care continuum of care should be included in clinical education curriculums (Nahm et al., 2022; Rutledge et al., 2021). The OCNE model of clinical education provides a framework for developing meaningful clinical learning using a variety of experiences in traditional acute care and community environments. See Chapter 13, *Service-Learning* for further discussion of community-based and service-learning experiences.

CLINICAL FACULTY ROLES AND RESPONSIBILITIES

Creating learning experiences that also embrace safe quality care for patients and student-centered learning in complex patient care environments requires faculty expertise and unit staff who are committed to working together to achieve the best outcomes for all. The clinical faculty role is demanding, and the teacher must demonstrate knowledge and skill in applying teaching and learning theory and strategies, expertise in coaching and providing feedback, excellent communication with staff, and the ability to negotiate and problem solve as needed. The clinical faculty role involves assessing the clinical environment to assure students have ample opportunity to meet outcomes and develop competency, and the teacher must intervene when unnecessary barriers to learning arise. The clinical teaching role also involves continuous assessment of student competency, providing feedback, coaching, and instruction to assure students are developing as safe competent clinicians. In 2018, the NLN created core competencies relevant to the academic clinical nurse educator role. See Chapter 13, *Service-Learning* for discussion about the NLN Core Nurse Educator Competencies.

Teaching, Coaching, Facilitating

The expert clinical faculty must develop a toolbox of teaching-learning strategies to use according to desired learning outcomes, the context of the clinical situation, and the student's individual learning needs with consideration of the immediate clinical environment. Fey et al. (2022) provide a framework for simulation educators that can be modified and applied to all elements of the OCNE clinical model. The three broad categories of teaching/learning actions are: (1) Direct Teaching, (2) Coaching, and (3) Facilitating

TABLE 10.6

Categories of Clinical Teaching

Category	Description	Examples
Direct teaching	▸ In direct teaching, the teacher action is teaching-centered ▸ Use when sharing knowledge or modeling a skill when there is a gap in the students' understanding, there is a misunderstanding, or there is an urgent need to respond to a patient's situation or some other unit priorities related to workflow on the unit. ▸ Involves assuring the student has integrated the content provided and demonstrates they have included it in their plan and action.	▸ In intervention-skilled based element, demonstrates the skill live or using a recorded demonstration pointing out the salient and challenging aspects of a particular skill and provides rationale or further considerations. End the procedure by asking what was challenging and what, if any, follow-up learning or practice is needed. ▸ In the focused direct-care element, use when a student is going to administer an intravenous medication to a patient with the faculty supervising and the situation is time-sensitive. The faculty might say something like, "I want to review the safety considerations you must address when administering this medication." Because the situation is time-sensitive, the faculty lists the salient consideration to address when performing the procedure. ▸ Direct teaching may be used in post-conference such as reviewing a policy, or a common medication or procedure used in the clinical setting. For example, reviewing the blood administration policy and standards of practice on an oncology/hematology unit.
Coaching	▸ Coaching involves a student-centered stance ▸ Use to facilitate the learner to the next level of skill performance. ▸ May take more time and involves observation of performance, feedback, reflection, action, and correction with redemonstration. ▸ Conclude with a reflective conversation, identifying what went well and, if needed, strategies or thinking that should be considered to improve performance. ▸ Can be used for developing cognitive skills as well. See Chapter 17, *Assessment of Clinical Judgment* for an in-depth discussion on coaching for clinical judgment.	▸ Use coaching in skill-based intervention element while the student is practicing a skill. ▸ Use in focused-direct care and preceptors should coach when working with students in the integrative practicum experience. For example, in the patient care environment, the teacher might use coaching as a student prepares to insert a nasogastric tube for the first time and say something like "let's talk through the procedure before we go in the patient's room." The teacher can correct any omissions or missteps and assure the student has mentally rehearsed the steps of the procedure. The teacher will coach in the actual patient encounter, providing suggestions on when to advance the tube, adjusting the patient position, and how to troubleshoot any unforeseen challenges.

TABLE 10.6

Categories of Clinical Teaching *(Continued)*

Category	Description	Examples
Facilitating	➤ Facilitation uses a learning-centered focus with a back and forth sharing of knowledge, perceptions, and possible solutions. ➤ Much of the facilitated dialog focuses on building new knowledge is used in debriefing simulation scenarios (Fey et al., 2022).	➤ Use with individuals and in group sessions such as pre- and post-conference activities. ➤ Guide the learner to engage in reflection to analyze all phases of clinical judgments, with the aim of constructing new knowledge, enhancing a mental frame about a clinical situation, or reframing a mental model that did not result in the desired patient outcome. ➤ Ask probing questions that require the student to articulate their thinking and consider new or alternate strategies. ➤ Guide the exchange of ideas to assure the learners construct knowledge for practice based on evidence, empathy for the patient, and standards of best practice.

reflection and construction of new knowledge and skill. The key to expertise in clinical teaching is knowing when to employ which strategy. See Table 10.6 for a discussion of each category.

Direct teaching strategies, coaching, and facilitating are not mutually exclusive actions. The clinical teacher often uses all three strategies in one encounter with students and groups of learners. Being aware of these three categories prevents the clinical faculty from over-reliance on direct teaching by "telling" students what they need to know. Coaching provides guidance and promotes an eventual transition to independence. Facilitation leads to self-efficacy and a deeper understanding of knowledge the learner can adapt and transfer from one clinical situation to another.

Establishing a Learning-Centered Clinical Environment

Positive relationships are the foundation for establishing a positive clinical environment for learning. The clinical faculty is responsible for establishing relationships with students as individuals, with students as groups, and for facilitating relationships among students and with staff. Several studies have identified the attributes of clinical faculty that result in positive learning outcomes (Cant et al., 2021; Donavan et al., 2021; Hill et al., 2020; Reising et al., 2018; Subke et al., 2020). See Table 10.7 for a list of positive clinical teacher traits and actions based on the findings from these studies.

Regardless of the location or focus of learning for clinical learning, the clinical faculty is responsible for assuring the environment is a place where students feel welcome and

TABLE 10.7

Traits and Actions of Effective Clinical Teachers

Trait	Action

Interpersonal relationships	➤ Relationship with students
	  ➤ Establishes caring relationship with students
	  ➤ Learns about each student as individuals, learning preferences, strengths, needed areas for improvement
	  ➤ Demonstrates respect for learner's values and baseline levels of competency
	  ➤ Accepts differences among students
	➤ Relationship with staff and facility management
	  ➤ Is respectful of staff nurses
	  ➤ Does not gossip or complain about staff or management
	  ➤ Facilitates mutual respect with staff
	  ➤ Collaborates with staff to create a shared commitment to creating a positive learning environment

Creates an environment that supports learning	➤ Demonstrates knowledge of the practice area and uses available resources to facilitate learning ➤ Is friendly, approachable, and understanding toward students and staff ➤ Establishes a relationship with unit manager or leader ➤ Addresses bias or racism evident in the environment ➤ Shares enthusiasm for nursing and teaching ➤ Serves as a positive role model for students and staff ➤ Facilitates communication between staff and students
Professional competency and effective actions	➤ Demonstrates clinical competency ➤ Uses positive communication and questioning to help students think and reason ➤ Assists students to link theory from didactic courses with clinical learning ➤ Provides frequent feedback ➤ Demonstrates fairness in evaluation—does not show favoritism ➤ Encourages self-efficacy so students learn how to learn ➤ Encourages curiosity and exploration—does not penalize students for asking questions

Source: Cant et al., 2021; Donavan et al., 2021; Hill et al., 2020; Reising et al. 2018; Subke et al., 2020.

their contributions are embraced by all individuals with whom they interact to meet their learning goals (Cant et al., 2021; Chicca & Shellenbarger, 2020b; Noone, 2022). The Future of Nursing 2020–2030 report (NASEM, 2021) addresses the need to create an equitable learning opportunity for all students by challenging and eliminating practices that contribute to discrimination and racism and embracing practices that support inclusive learning environments. The clinical faculty must assess the environment for inclusivity and work with staff to assure all students are welcomed. Multiple studies have found under-represented minority groups (UMG) experience barriers to learning in clinical education environments (Graham et al., 2016; Englund, 2019; Metzger et al., 2020; Pusey-Reid & Blackman-Richards, 2022). In a scoping review, Metzger and co-authors (2020) found intervention by the clinical educator to be instrumental when a student is experiencing discriminatory behavior. Pusey-Reid & Blackman-Richards (2022) posit that discriminatory behavior often occurs in the form of microaggression and advocate for developing action plans for intervention that include the faculty, peers of the individual experiencing discrimination, the perpetrator, leaders, and bystanders. Pusey-Reid & Blackman-Richards acknowledge that resolving discriminatory situations is challenging and complex and that support for the student or students experiencing discrimination should be provided throughout the process. The clinical educator should seek guidance from supervising and course faculty and use program and college or university policy to guide their actions. See Chapter 5, *Creating Inclusive Learning Environments* for in-depth discussion of how to address microaggression in the clinical setting.

Clinical Competency Assessment

Assessing students' competency development is an essential component of the nurse educator role. Formative assessment occurs in every element of the OCNE clinical model. Assessing competency in the focused-direct care and integrative practicum element of the model must incorporate summative assessments. The NLN's visions for fair testing (2020) and for competency-based nursing education (2023) advocate for a systematic approach to summative assessments that include a variety of assessment methods. Typically, there is a clinical evaluation instrument the faculty uses to provide their assessment of developing competency of the student in clinical environments involving patient care. Providing constructive and timely feedback regarding the student's progress is an essential and complex responsibility and faculty should learn how to use the instrument as intended. Further discussion regarding best practices in assessing clinical competency is available in Chapter 17, *Assessment of Clinical Judgment* and Chapter 18, *Ethical and Legal Considerations in Assessment.*

CHAPTER SUMMARY

Clinical learning experience provides opportunities well beyond the application of theory to practice. Well-planned clinical activities can potentially help students develop and extend theoretical knowledge, learn how key concepts and skills are exemplified in practice, and develop competency needed to make sound clinical judgments and perform safe interventions.

The OCNE Clinical Education Model fundamentally changes how nurses are prepared for clinical practice. Elements of the model are deliberately planned to support attainment of curriculum competencies and provide the right amount of challenge and support for students' developmental levels. The five elements each address a different aspect of clinical judgment, relationship-centered care, evidence-based practice, and skillful intervention necessary for nursing practice. Learning activities are sequenced in a deliberate manner. More complex activities are planned as the student matures in skills and abilities. Redesigning clinical education is not an option; it is a requirement as described in the Future of Nursing 2020–2030 recommendations. The OCNE clinical education model moves clinical education from a random-access opportunity (Gubrud-Howe & Schoessler, 2008) to a structured learning experience in which students are prepared in real-world settings to think and act like practicing nurses. The model intentionally addresses the shortcomings of current clinical education, but more than that, it establishes a sound theoretical foundation for the development of the clinical knowledge and skills needed to practice nursing today and in the future.

References

Benner, P., Sutphen, M., Leonard, V., & Day, L. (2010). *Educating nurses: A call for radical transformation*. Jossey-Bass.

Buerhaus, P., & Yakusheva, O. (2022). Six part series on value-informed nursing practice. *Nursing Outlook, 70*, 89. https://doi.org/10.1016/j.outlook.2021.10005

Cant, R., Ryan, C., & Cooper, S. (2021). Nursing students' evaluation of clinical practice placements using the Clinical Learning Environment, Supervision and Nurse Teacher scale: A systematic review. *Nurse Education Today, 104*. https://doi.org/10.1016/jnedt.2019.104346

Chicca, J., & Shellenbarger, T. (2020a). Implementing successful clinical nursing preceptorships. *Nurse Educator, 45*(4), E41–E42. https://doi.org/10.1097/NNE0000000000000750

Chicca, J., & Shellenbarger, T. (2020b). Fostering inclusive clinical learning environments using a psychological safety lens. *Teaching & Learning in Nursing, 15*, 226–232.

Chicca, J., & Shellenbarger, T. (2021). Preparing, maintaining, and evaluating remote preceptorships: Considerations for nurse educators. *Teaching and Learning in Nursing, 16*, 396–400. https://doi.org/10.1016/jteln.2021.04.006

Donavan, L. M., Strunk, J. A., Lam, C., Argenbright, C., Robinson, J., Leisen, M., & Puuenburger, N. (2021). Enhancing the prelicensure clinical learning experience. *Nurse Educator, 47*(2), 108–113. https://doi.org/10.1097/NNE.0000000000001085

Englund, H. (2019). Nontraditional students' perceptions of marginalization in baccalaureate nursing education: Pushed to the periphery. *Nurse Educator, 44*(3), 164–169, https://doi.org/10.1097/NNE.0000000000000581

Epp, S., Reekie, M., Denison, J., deBosch Kemper, N., Wilson, M., & Marck, P. (2022). An innovative leap: Embracing new pedagogical approaches for clinical education. *Journal of Professional Nursing, 42*, 168–172. https://doi.org/10.1016/jprofnurs.2022.07.005

Fey, M. K., Roussin, C. J., Rudolph, J. W., Morse, K. J., Palaganas, J., & Szyld, D. (2022). Teaching, coaching, or debriefing with Good Judgment: a roadmap for implementing "with good judgment" across the SimZones. *Advances in Simulation, 7*(39). https://doi.org/10.1186/s41077-022-00235-y

Giddens, J., Douglas, J. P., & Conroy. (2022). The revised AACN Essentials: Implications for nursing regulation. *Journal of Nursing Regulation, 12*(4), 16–22.

Goers, J., Mulkey, D., & Oja, K. (2022). A call to reform undergraduate nursing clinical placements. *Nursing Outlook, 70*, 371–373. https://doi.org/10.1016/j.outlook.2022.01.006

Gonzalez, L., & Kardong-Edgren, S. (2017). Deliberate practice for mastery learning in nursing. *Clinical Simulation in Nursing, 13*(1), 10–14. https://doi.org/10.1016/j.ecns.2016.10.005.

Graham, C. L., Phillips, S. M., Newman, S. D., & Atz, T. (2016). Baccalaureate minority nursing students perceive barriers and facilitators to clinical education practices: An integrative review. *Nursing Education Perspectives*, *37*(3), 130–137. https://doi.org/10.1097/01.NEP.0000000000000003

Gubrud (in press). Teaching in the clinical setting. In D. M. Billings, & J. A. Halstead, *Teaching in Nursing: A Guide for Faculty. Seventh Edition*. Elsevier.

Gubrud-Howe, P., Driggers, B., Tanner, C. A., Shores, L., & Schoessler, M. (2007). White Paper-OCNE Clinical Education Redesign. Unpublished manuscript.

Gubrud-Howe, P., & Schoessler, M. (2008). From random access opportunity to a clinical education curriculum. *Journal of Nursing Education*, *47*, 3–4.

Hassmiller, S. B., & Wakefield, M. (2022). The future of nursing 2020–2030: Charting a path to achieve health equity. *Nursing Outlook*, *70*, S1–S9. https://doi/org/10.1066/j.outlook.2022.05.013

Heims, M. L., & Boyd, S. T. (1990). Concept-based learning activities in clinical nursing education. *Journal of Nursing Education, 29*, 249–254.

Hill, R., Woodward, M., & Arthur, A. (2020). Collaborative learning in practice (CLIP): Evaluation of a new approach to clinical learning. *Nurse Education Today*, *85*. https://doi.org/10.1016/jnedt.2019.104295

Ironside, P. M., McNelis, A. M., & Ebright, P. (2014). Clinical education in nursing: Rethinking learning in practice settings. *Nursing Outlook*, *62*(3), 185–191. https://doi.org/10.1016/j.outlook.2013.12.004.

Jones-Schenk, J. (2021). Redesigning clinical learning. *Journal of Continuing Education in Nursing*, *52*(9), 402–402. https://doi.org/10.3928/00220124-20210804-03

Lapinski, J., & Ciurzynski, S. (2020). Enhancing the sustainability of a Dedicated Education Unit: Overcoming obstacles and strengthening partnerships. *Journal of Professional Nursing*, *36*, 659–665. https://doi.org/10/1016/jprofnurs2020.09.007

Leighton, K., Kardong-Edgren, S., McNelis, A. M., Foisy-Doll, C., & Sullo, E. (2021). Traditional clinical outcomes in prelicensure nursing education: An empty systematic review. *Journal of Nursing Education*, *60*(3),136–142. https://doi.org/10.3928/01484834-20210222-03

McGaghie, W. C. (2020). Mastery learning: Origins, features and evidence from the health professions. In W. C. McGaghie, J. H. Barsuk, & D. B. Wayne (Eds.), *Comprehensive Health care Simulation: Mastery Learning in the Health Professions*. Springer.

McNelis, A. M., Ironside, P. M., Ebright, P. R., Dreifuerst, K. T., Avonar, S. E., & Conner, S. C. (2014). Learning nursing practice: A multisite, multimethod investigation of clinical education. *Journal of Nursing Regulation, 4*(4), 30–35.

Metzger, M., Dowling, T., Guinn, J., & Wilson, D. (2020). Inclusivity in baccalaureate nursing education: A scoping study. *Journal of Professional Nursing*, *35*, 5–14. https://doi.org/10.1016/j.profnurs.2019.06.002

Mollman, S., & Candela, L. (2018). Intentional learning: A concept analysis. *Nursing Forum*, *53*(1), 106–111. https://doi.org/10.1111/nuf.12222

Monson, N. L., Higbee, M., Brunger, C., Ensign, A., Gaul, R. A., & Taylor, N. (2021). Standardized skill pass-offs and nursing confidence: A qualitive study. *Teaching and Learning in Nursing*, *16*(2016), 194–198. https://doi.org/10.1016/j.teln.2021.04.003

Musallam, E., Alhaj, A., & Nicely, S. (2021). The impact of dedicated educational model on nursing students' outcomes. *Nurse Educator*, *46*(5), ED113–ED116. https://doi.org/10.1097/NNE.0000000000001022

Nahm, E. S., Mills, E. M., Raymond, G., Costa, L., Chen, L., Nair, P., Seidl, K., Day, J., Murray, L., Rowen, L., Kirschling, J., Daw, P., & Haas, S. (2022). Development of an academic-partnership model to anchor care coordination and population health. *Nursing Outlook*, *70*, 193–203. https://doi.org/10.1016/joutlook.2021.09.005

National Academies of Science, Engineering, and Medicine; National Academy of Medicine. (NASEM) (2021). Committee on the Future of Nursing 2020–2030. In J. L. Flaubert, S. Le Menestrel, D. R. Williams, & M. K. Wakefield (Eds.), *The Future of Nursing 2020–2030: Charting a Path to Achieve Health Equity*. National Academies Press.

Niederhauser, V., Schoessler, M., Gubrud-Howe, P., Magnussen, L., & Codier, E. (2012). Creating innovative model of clinical nursing education. *Journal of Nursing Education*, *51*(11), 603–608.

Nielsen, A. E., Noone, J., Voss, H., & Mathews, L. R. (2013). Preparing nursing students for the future: An innovative approach to clinical education. *Nursing Education in Practice*, *13*, 301–309. https://doi.org/10.1016/j.nepr.2013.03.015

Nielsen, A. (2016). Concept-based learning in clinical experiences: Bringing theory to clinical education for deep learning. *Journal of Nursing Education*, *55*(7), 365–371. https://doi.org/10.3928/01484834-20160615-02

Nielsen, A., Garner, A., Lanciotti, K., & Brown, L. (2021). Concept-based learning for capstone clinical experiences in hospital and community settings. *Nurse Educator*, *46*(6), 381–385. https://doi.org/10.1097/NNE.0000000000000964

NLN. (2020). *NLN Vision Series: The Fair Testing Imperative in Nursing Education. A Living Document from the National League for Nursing*. Accessed February 13, 2023. https://www.nln.org/docs/default-source/uploadedfiles/advocacy-public-policy/nln-fair-testing-vision-series.pdf

NLN. (2023). *NLN Publishes New Vision Statement: Integrating Competency-Based Education in the Nursing Curriculum*. Accessed February 13, 2023. https://www.nln.org/detail-pages/news/2023/02/09/nln-publishes-new-vision-statement-integrating-competency-based-education-in-the-nursing-curriculum.

Noone, J. (2022). Creating inclusive learning environments: Challenging and changing the paradigm. *Journal of Nursing Education*, *61*(3), 115–116. https://doi.org/10.3928/01484834-20220215-01

Noone, J., Sideras, S., Gubrud-Howe, P., & Mathews (2012). Influence of a poverty simulation on nursing student attitudes toward poverty. *Journal of Nursing Education*, *51*(11), 617–622.

Pusey-Reid, E., & Blackman-Richards, N. (2022). The importance of addressing racial microaggression in nursing education. *Nurse Education Today, 114*(105390). https://doi.org/10.1016/j.nedt.2022.105390

Rauch, L., & Malloy, S. (2020). Home hospitals: Maximizing nursing student clinical placements. *Journal of Nursing Education*, *59*(5), 269–273. https://doi.org/10.3928/01484834-201200422-06

Reedy, G. B. (2015). Using cognitive load theory to inform simulation design and practice. *Clinical Simulation in Nursing*, *22*(8), 355–360. https://doi.org/10.1016/j.ecns.2015.05.004–find it

Reising, D. L., James, B., & Morse, B. (2018). Student perceptions of clinical instructor characteristics affecting clinical experiences. *Nursing Education Perspectives*, *39*(1), 4–9. https://doi.org/10.1097/01.NEP.0000000000000241

Rutledge, C. M., O'Rourke, J., Mason, A. M., Chike-Harris, K., Behnke, L., Melhado, L., Downes, L., & Gustin, T. (2021). Telehealth competencies for nursing education and practice: The four P's of telehealth. *Nurse Educator, 46*(5), 300–305. https://doi.org/10.1097/NNE.0000000000000988

Subke, J., Downing, C., & Kearns, I. (2020). Pratice of caring for nursing students: A clinical learning environment. *International Journal of Nursing Sciences, 7*(2020), 214–219. https://doi.org/10.1016/j.ijnss.2020.03.005

Sumpter, D., Blodgett, N., Beard, K., & Howard, V. (2022). Transforming nursing education in response to the Future of Nursing 2020–2030 report. *Nursing Outlook*, *70*, S20–S31. https://doi.org/10.1016/j.outlook.2022.02.007

Tanner, C. A. (2006). Thinking like a nurse: A research-based model of clinical judgment in nursing. *Journal of Nursing Education*, *45*(6), 204–211.

Tanner, C. A., & Gubrud-Howe, P. (2021). The Oregon Consortium for Nursing Education: Delivering an innovative, competency based curriculum in the US. In I. Darmann-Finck, & K. Reiber (Eds.). *Development, Implementation and Evaluation of Curricula in Nursing and Midwifery Education*. Springer.

Tanner, C., Messecar, D., & Delawska-Elliott (2022). Chapter 13, Evidence Based Practice. In L. Joel (Ed.). *Advanced Practice Nursing: Essentials for Role Development*, 5th Edition. F.A. Davis.

Ward, A., & McComb, S. (2017). Precepting: A literature review. *Journal of Professional Nursing*, *33*(5), 314–325. https://doi.org/10.1016/j.profnurs.2017.07.007.

Woolley, N. N., & Jarvis, Y. (2007). Situated cognition and cognitive apprenticeship: A model for teaching and learning clinical skills in a technologically rich and authentic learning environment. *Nurse Education Today*, *27*, 73–79. https://doi.org/10.1016/j.nedt.2006.02.010

Wu, X. V., Chi, Y., Chan, Y., Wang, W., Ang, E. N. K., Zhao, S., Sehgal, V., Wee, F. C., Selvam, U. P., & Devi, M. K. (2020). A web-based clinical pedagogy program to enhance registered nurse preceptors' teaching competencies—An innovative process of development and pilot program evaluation. *Nurse Education Today*, *84*(104215). https://doi.org/10.1016/jnedt.2019.104215

Yakusheva, O., Rambur, B., & Buerhaus, P. I. (2022). Part 6. Education for value-informed practice. *Nursing Outlook*, *70*, 789–793. https://doi.org/10.1016/j.outlook.2022.08.002

11

Concept-Based Learning in the Clinical Learning Environment

Ann Nielsen, PhD, RN

CHAPTER OVERVIEW

To address the myriad of challenges in health care today, it is imperative that nurse educators maximize learning in the clinical environment, carefully selecting curricular content that addresses pressing needs, then focusing learning on the most important principles of care. This chapter describes concept-based learning activities (CBLAs), a clinical teaching strategy that supports the integration of theory and practice, as well as clinical judgment development that can be used to direct learners' attention to key aspects of nursing care and the associated decision-making. Current thought about CBLA use, efficacy, and best practices in implementation will be explained. The chapter focuses on how to create, implement, and debrief concept-based learning activities for use in the clinical setting. Tools, including design templates and ideas for the use of CBLAs in a variety of courses, are presented.

DEFINITION OF CONCEPT-BASED LEARNING ACTIVITIES

Conceptual approaches during nursing education have been associated with deep learning (Nielsen, 2016), as well as work readiness (Byrne & Connor, 2022). CBLAs, a strategy to enhance conceptual learning in the clinical environment, focus learners' attention on one aspect of care (a concept), in order to promote a better understanding of nursing practice. Learners prepare for the experience, then are assigned a patient or clinical situation to study. An educator-designed study guide directs them through a focused assessment and data gathering for the concept, then asks them to identify potential nursing problems or issues, propose interventions, and identify expected outcomes of those interventions. Debriefing with the nurse educator and other learners extends the learning by comparing and contrasting learners' clinical experiences, focusing on development of clinical judgment and decision-making. Reflection after the experience allows learners to process and solidify learning for use in future situations.

Nurse educators create CBLAs incorporating best practices in education. CBLAs are a way to chunk the complexity of learning in the clinical setting into smaller, more manageable, pieces to promote deeper understanding (Coffman et al., 2023). When CBLAs are framed by a clinical judgment model, they can be used to support understanding and integrate the elements of clinical judgment into patient care, underscoring the role of background understanding, toward effective decision-making in nursing practice. Use of principles of backward design (Chapter 7) facilitates development of CBLAs that are directed toward meeting learning goals, course outcomes, and program competencies.

CBLAs are an alternative or adjunct to the exclusive use of the traditional total patient care model of clinical education and have been shown to promote both clinical judgment and integration of theory and practice (Alfayoumi, 2019; Lasater & Nielsen, 2009; Nielsen, 2016). As noted in Chapter 10, CBLAs are particularly useful when students are early in the program but can support learning effectively when more experienced learners move to new clinical settings, including specialty settings. The sections below examine and describe in more depth the pedagogy, design, and use of CBLAs.

Concept-Based Learning Activities and Clinical Judgment

There is arguably no more important competency for nurses than clinical judgment, yet when total patient care is the only approach used in the clinical environment, learning often becomes task-focused, and opportunities to fully understand decision-making may be lost (Ironside et al., 2014). We know that thinking about nursing practice develops over time with experience (Benner, 2001). The process begins in nursing school and continues as new graduate nurses transition into practice. Making sound clinical judgments involves many factors and is informed by the nurse's background which includes theoretical knowledge, practical experience, nursing values, and ethics; the nurse's understanding of and collaboration with the patient; and the context of care (Tanner et al., 2022). Nurse educators influence this process in many ways, particularly by teaching theoretical knowledge (pathophysiology, pharmacology, nursing science, evidence-based practice, etc.) and providing practical experience. Integration of these two aspects of nursing practice is critical to the deep understanding needed to make clinical judgments (Benner et al., 2010). CBLAs support this integration. A recent integrative review suggests that teaching clinical reasoning is most effective when a model is used to frame learning (Tyo & McCurry, 2019). In the CBLAs presented in this chapter the Tanner Clinical Judgment Model, described in Chapter 17, is used as a framework for learning activity design (Tanner, 2006; Tanner et al., 2022).

Concept-Based Learning Activities and the Clinical Environment

In today's acute care settings, patients are often very sick and nursing care is fast paced. High patient acuity and the demands associated with caring for patients in this context can be daunting and drive task-focused rather than thinking-focused care (McNelis et al., 2014). This is particularly true for students earlier in nursing programs. In fact, research has shown that students taught using traditional total patient care models may not fully understand what is happening with their patient and yet do not reveal their questions of lack of understanding to their clinical teachers (Ironside et al., 2014).

Using a more deliberate approach by chunking related concepts and providing scaffolds such as cognitive aids, coaching, and feedback may support learners to better develop their thinking in practicum settings. Discussion during debriefing extends the learning. Reflection on the experience allows learners to process the learning, transfer knowledge, and transform it for use in future situations.

The complexity of acute care clinical settings impacts nurse educators as well. When supervising students who are doing total patient care, the clinical nurse educator's focus is often, appropriately, on assuring patient safety. Checking students' preparation and providing adequate supervision when giving medications and doing other nursing skills may preclude meaningful discussion of what is actually happening with the patient and what the student is thinking and understanding about patient care. Focusing on one concept of patient care (such as fluid and electrolyte balance, gas exchange, pain) in clinical, without responsibility for delivering patient care, frees up student and educator time for discussion of assessment findings, integrating findings with background science including pathophysiology, and development of thinking about care in the clinical environment. Robust discussion with nursing educators and other students is known to support understanding of care (National League for Nursing [NLN], 2015; Nielsen, 2016).

Although the situation is a bit different in the community, challenges to meaningful learning exist in this setting as well. Many believe the future of nursing is community practice with a focus on health promotion and managing chronic conditions so that acute care is avoided (Calma et al., 2019; Gorski et al., 2019; Institute of Medicine [IOM], 2010; Sumpter et al., 2022). While clinical study in the community is vital to learning concepts related to population health and gives students the opportunity to experience unique aspects of nursing care when patients are in their home and/or neighborhood environments, the unstructured nature of many community settings may preclude students' recognition of the embedded learning. Furthermore, the full scope of the nursing role has not been developed in many emerging practice settings in the community (IOM, 2010; Morton et al., 2019; Nielsen et al., in press). Development of specific learning activities that focus on key concepts (for example, chronic illness management in the community, population health, health equity, moral distress/moral courage, and school-based care) maximizes learning and assures that students make the clinical connections foundational to developing their nursing practice in the community (Nielsen et al., 2021).

While less has been published about the use of CBLAs in residency and internship programs, the underlying pedagogy is applicable to teaching in this situation, as well. New graduate nurses are often orienting to care of new patient populations. It is common for them to be overwhelmed with the demands of care and struggle with clinical decision-making (Kavanagh & Sharpnack, 2021). Well-designed CBLAs can support the transition of newly licensed RNs into nursing practice.

Health equity and social determinants of health remain persistent and serious challenges to health in the US (Hassmiller & Wakefield, 2022; Sumpter et al., 2022). CBLAs can be designed for learners to examine deeply the issues of health equity and/or social determinants of health. Furthermore, prompts can be woven into any CBLA that raise learners' awareness of underlying personal biases, perform key assessments in diverse populations, and develop interventions appropriate to the situation.

DESCRIPTION OF CBLAs

CBLA Design

Through intentional design of CBLAs, the nurse educator chooses and defines the concept being studied, identifies learning outcomes, assigns relevant preparation activities, then develops a study guide. In all aspects of design, the course or setting in which the CBLA will be used, the developmental level of the student, and intended outcomes should be considered. Use of a model to frame CBLAs helps students to develop thinking and decision-making about nursing care. In the approach presented, Tanner's Clinical Judgment Model is used to frame learning-focused learners' attention on salient elements of the concept, supporting interpretation of findings (including pattern recognition), and identifying appropriate nursing actions (Tanner, 2006; Tanner, 2022). A Backward Design approach, described in Chapter 7, facilitates development of well-targeted, effective CBLAs. (Table 11.1 and Box 11.1 can be used to guide CBLA design.)

TABLE 11.1	
CBLA Planning Guide	
CBLA Planning	**Nurse Educator Planning Notes**
Concept selection. Consider: ▸ Course outcomes/theory topics ▸ Clinical environment ▸ Nursing related to concept	**Concept:**

Design of study guide (see template below)
▸ Concept definition (and why the concept is important and how it is linked to nursing)
▸ Learning outcomes
▸ Student preparation—*Background*
▸ Guide to data collection/noticing, interpreting, responding, reflecting
  ▸ *Noticing*
  ▸ *Interpreting*
  ▸ *Responding*
  ▸ *Reflecting*
	Concept definition:
	Learning outcomes:
	Student preparation:
	Study guide prompts:

Student collaboration ▸ Alone ▸ Dyads ▸ Triads	

TABLE 11.1

CBLA Planning Guide *(Continued)*

CBLA Planning	Nurse Educator Planning Notes
Plan for student-faculty interaction ➤ Pre-conference (often used for clinical groups who are with faculty in the clinical setting) ➤ Plan for faculty-student interaction during clinical experience ➤ Patient "rounds" ➤ Post-conference debriefing	Interaction plan:
Plan for debriefing ➤ Structure ➤ Questions	Debriefing plan:
Plan for evaluation	
Plan for introducing CBLA to clinical site prn	

BOX 11.1

CBLA Study Guide Template

INTRODUCTION AND PREPARATION

Concept: (Example—*Nutrition*)

Definition: (Define the concept, *nutrition*, as it relates to nursing and the patient population.)

Learning Outcomes:

1. Notice and assess all pertinent data and physical findings to determine (*nutritional*) status of the patient.
2. Identify factors that influence (*nutrition*) of the patient.
3. Interpret patient findings and respond appropriately with interventions that promote adequate/appropriate patient (*nutrition*).
4. Evaluate the effectiveness of interventions, by nurses and other health care providers, to promote adequate/appropriate (*nutrition*).
5. Document findings accurately using appropriate descriptor of what is observed.

Student Evaluation:

1. Study guide completion—application of learning to course competencies.
2. Participation in discussion of patient(s) in rounds and in seminar.
3. Integration of knowledge about and experience with (*nutrition*) assessment and intervention into subsequent clinical practice.

(continued)

BOX 11.1

CBLA Study Guide Template *(Continued)*

Preparation:

1. Describe the plan for the day and any preparation that needs to happen in addition to the readings.
2. Do preparatory activities as assigned.
3. Consider your previous experiences with (patient nutrition) and how they might apply to this activity.

Readings and other preparatory activities:

(CBLA designer lists relevant required readings from text, journal articles, and internet sources.)

STUDY GUIDE DESIGN

Student:

Date of assessment:

Patient's/client's initials:

Medical diagnosis:

Admission date:

Briefly summarize the patient care situation:

Focused assessment prompts:

1. **Background**
   a. Based on the reading that you did in preparation for this activity and your previous experiences with patient problems related to *(nutritional)* issues, summarize your theoretical and practical knowledge about *(nutrition)* for your patient.
   b. What are the potential effects of your patient's medical condition on *(nutrition)*?
   c. What are the effects of prescribed therapies, medications, and other interventions on your patient *(nutrition)*? Please list ALL patient meds, whether or not you believe they have an impact on *(nutrition)*.

Therapy, medication, intervention
Describe potential effect on (*nutrition*)
   d. What developmental influences are there on *(nutrition)* in your patient?

Developmental characteristic
Influence on (*nutrition*)
   e. What data (including lab values) do you need about the patient before you begin your assessment? **List relevant lab tests done and the results here. Please note normal and abnormal values.**
   f. Considering what you know about *(nutrition)*, what will you make sure to notice when you go into the patient room?

2. **Noticing**
   a. Describe the general appearance of the patient from a *nutritional* perspective:
   b. *(CBLA designer develops the rest of the noticing section with prompts to guide the student through a complete focused assessment r/t the concept.)*

3. **Interpreting**
   a. Summarize your findings about the *(nutritional)* status of your patient. Use objective, clear health care terminology.
   b. Identify nursing problem(s)—actual or potential—in your patient regarding *(nutritional)* status. Include risk factors related to the concept in your statement.

BOX 11.1

CBLA Study Guide Template *(Continued)*

4. **Responding**
   a. What are the goals of your nursing care with regard to the *(nutritional)* status of your patient?
   b. What interventions will the nurse do to reach those goals?
5. **Reflection in action**
   a. Describe what happened with your patient. Did the patient meet the stated outcomes? Why or why not? What did or will you do next?
6. **Reflection on action**
   a. Describe three ways your nursing care skills expanded during this experience.
   b. Name three things you will do differently when you encounter a similar patient care situation in the future.
   c. What additional knowledge will you need when encountering this type of situation or similar situations in the future?
   d. Describe any changes in your values or feelings as a result of this experience.

Selecting Concepts

Nurse educators make important decisions about what will be taught in the curriculum. Distinguishing between essential learning, what is fundamental to nursing practice, and other less important content is imperative. When selecting concepts for CBLAs, consider course focus and outcomes, program competencies, and frequently encountered patient situations in the clinical setting in which the CBLA will be taught. For example, in an acute care clinical setting, fluid and electrolyte balance, oxygen-carbon dioxide exchange, pain, and nutrition might be particularly relevant to deepen learning about the physiology of acutely ill patients. In a clinic setting in the community, key concepts might be care coordination, telehealth, population-based care and management, health promotion and teaching, and team-based care (Nielsen et al., in press). In a leadership course, key concepts might be quality management, nursing leadership at the bedside, or interprofessional teamwork (Fletcher & Meyer, 2016). In a transition to a practice program, concepts may be more advanced, such as nursing management of patient care, advanced physiologic concepts, and dependent/independent scope of practice (Nielsen et al., 2017). In any setting, the use of a CBLA to focus learning on issues of health equity, diversity, and inclusion is appropriate and a way to examine those factors in context (Hassmiller & Wakefield, 2022; Sumpter et al., 2021). Examples of concepts for use in various clinical settings can be found in Table 11.2.

Concept Definition

CBLA design begins with concept definition. Learners need to have a clear understanding of the concept and why it is important to appreciate its relevance to nursing practice. The definition sets the stage for learning. For physiologic CBLAs, the

TABLE 11.2

Concept Exemplars for Various Clinical Environments

Physiologic	Patient Care Activities	Population Health	Leadership	Emerging Clinical Setting: Ambulatory Care	New Graduate Transition Programs
‣ Fluid & electrolyte balance ‣ O_2-CO_2 exchange ‣ Nutrition ‣ Pain management ‣ Skin integrity	‣ Wound care ‣ Bathing/skin care ‣ Medication administration ‣ Comprehensive physical assessment ‣ Care coordination and/or transitions management ‣ Supporting patient self-care management ‣ Patient teaching	‣ Health equity ‣ Management of patient populations	‣ Quality management ‣ Work environment ‣ Interprofessional collaboration ‣ Unit or agency leadership; formal and informal	‣ Team-based care ‣ Fiscal management and policy ‣ Informatics ‣ Patient safety in primary care ‣ Quality management ‣ RN support for chronic disease self-management ‣ Care coordination ‣ Telehealth simulation	‣ Self-management (responsibility and accountability for self-care and how it relates to care of patients/clients) ‣ Advanced respiratory ‣ Behavioral-cognitive assessment and care ‣ Therapeutic relationships ‣ Infection prevention, management, and care ‣ Independent and dependent scope of nursing practice

definition may be simple. For example, a definition of the concept of fluid and electrolyte balance:

> Fluid and electrolyte balance is defined as the maintenance of fluid and electrolyte homeostasis
> through physiological and therapeutic mechanisms.

For non-physiologic CBLAs, the definition may be more detailed to help the student
understand the link between the concept and nursing care. For example, a definition of
the concept of quality in a CBLA for use in primary care:

> Quality management is the use of data to monitor the outcomes of care processes and
> associated improvement methods to design and test changes to continuously improve the
> quality and safety of health care systems. Nurse-sensitive indicators of high-quality care
> include achievement of appropriate self-care, use of health-promoting behaviors, quality of
> life, perception of being well cared for, and effective symptom management. While these
> indicators are very pertinent to the primary care setting, the RN role in primary care settings
> is not well-defined, nor is the RN's role in quality management.

CBLA Outcomes

The next step is developing learning outcomes. Clear, specific outcomes capture the
intended learning and should be informed by course outcomes. Furthermore, learning
outcomes for CBLAs should be designed to align with course outcomes so students are
supported to meet broader course learning goals. Outcomes that describe thinking and
clinical judgment development underscore the importance of clinical decision-making.
Outcomes related to health equity, justice, diversity, and inclusion are appropriate to
build into many CBLAs. Framing outcomes around the elements of clinical judgment is
one effective approach to development. For example, for a fluid and electrolyte CBLA:

i. *Identify factors that influence the patient's fluid and electrolyte balance or
imbalance.*

ii. *Notice and assess all pertinent data and physical findings to determine fluid
and electrolyte status of the patient.*

iii. *Interpret patient findings and respond appropriately with interventions that
promote fluid and electrolyte balance.*

iv. *Evaluate the effectiveness of interventions, by nurses and other health care
providers, to promote fluid and electrolyte balance.*

v. *Document findings accurately using nursing language to describe what is
observed.*

Preparation Activities

The nurse educator identifies key preparation materials that will facilitate learner success in meeting intended outcomes. Readings about relevant theoretical background
(e.g., pathophysiology, pharmacology, current evidence, nursing theory, care models),
standards of care related to the concept, and videos demonstrating aspects of the
concept are only some examples of potential preparation activities. Asking students
to consider background elements including their personal values and biases and the
potential factors in the care environment (Tanner et al., 2022) helps students to understand
how factors beyond patient care itself might influence decisions.

Study Guide Prompts

The next step is to create prompts that support achieving stated outcomes. For developing consistency in thinking about patient care, prompts can be framed by a model. The Tanner Clinical Judgment Model is used in this chapter (Tanner, 2006; Tanner et al., 2022):

- The *Noticing* section guides learners through a focused assessment related to the concept so that they collect the needed data necessary to develop an appreciation of potentially salient findings. In some cases, it may be important to include prompts that direct students to aspects of interprofessional care that the patient is receiving. Depending on the situation and intended outcomes, consider including prompts that direct students to elements of diversity, health equity, and social justice.

- The *Interpreting* section asks learners to summarize key findings narratively, then identify potential problems or issues related to the concept. One of the goals here is for the learner to begin to identify most salient findings, recognize patterns, and understand what they see and why.

- The *Responding* section asks learners to propose appropriate interventions for the problems or issues they see. The patient may currently be receiving those interventions as a part of care, but the intent is for learners to make those specific connections between problems, the underlying factors (including pathophysiology), and interventions or nursing actions.

- The *Reflection-IN-Practice* section asks students to identify outcomes or anticipated outcomes of interventions, including how they would know that a patient's condition is improving or deteriorating.

- The *Reflection-ON-Practice* section invites students to consider the CBLA experience, identifying their learning and what they still wonder about.

Plan for Educator-Learner Interaction

The importance of educator-learner interaction, including group discussion, when using CBLAs cannot be overemphasized. A research study in which four academic nurse educator experts and their students were observed using physiologic CBLAs in acute and long-term care settings provided some insight into the effective implementation of CBLAs (Nielsen, 2016). All nurse educators built in robust time for discussion with students. Three of the four held a pre-conference to discuss the plan for the clinical day, the types of medical diagnoses the students might encounter, and to review relevant pathophysiology. During clinical, because the students were not responsible for direct patient care, the nurse educators were free to observe student assessments and ask or answer questions. In focus groups, students reported they greatly appreciated teacher questioning. It helped them both recognize what they knew and what they needed to find out more about. Some nurse educators did specific, direct clinical teaching. For example, one nurse educator on a cardiac unit made sure to review and interpret the EKG strips for each student's patient with them. Another did specific teaching about diabetes management and insulin administration. In post-conference, the focus was on debriefing each student's patient, connecting pathophysiology with what the students had seen in clinical, and comparing and contrasting among the students' patients. Nurse educators pointed out key assessment findings, patterns, and signs of patient trajectory of illness. In post-clinical focus groups, students in this study were emphatic that discussion and interaction with the nurse educator greatly impacted their learning (Nielsen, 2016; Nielsen, 2013).

Group Discussion

As in simulation, debriefing discussion structured by a specific model is recommended for CBLAs and the Tanner Clinical Judgment Model is one framework that can be used (Tanner, 2006; Tanner et al., 2022). In this model, understanding clinical judgment rests on situation-specific factors including the nurse's background (including theoretical and practical knowledge, values, biases, and ethical comportment), relationship with the patient, and the context of the situation. In CBLA discussion, these factors, particularly theoretical and practical knowledge, can be drawn upon to help students recognize what might influence clinical judgment. Once relevant background factors are discussed, the elements of clinical judgment described in the model—*noticing*, *interpreting*, *responding*, and *reflecting*—can guide the discussion, with a focus on noticing, interpreting, and to a lesser extent, responding (Nielsen et al., 2021).

Plan for Evaluation

CBLA participation and any associated written work can be used to understand learners' thinking about care. Because the focus of CBLAs is on learning, formative evaluation with feedback directed toward improvement is recommended. The Lasater Clinical Judgment Rubric (2007) operationalizes the Tanner Clinical Judgment Model and describes the development of thinking in the elements of noticing, interpreting, responding, and reflecting. This tool can be used to identify issues with learners' thinking, provide specific feedback, and guide the development of learners' thinking about practice. Stating clearly in the CBLA that application of learning going forward is expected, underscores the importance of integrating the learning into future nursing practice.

RECOMMENDATIONS
Use of CBLAs in Acute Care
Concept Selection

CBLAs in acute care are often designed for physiologic concepts, for example, fluid & electrolyte balance, oxygen-carbon dioxide exchange, nutrition, and pain. Other concepts closely linked to nursing care in a given setting, such as skin integrity, safety in the environment, and infection control, are also appropriate. When selecting CBLA concepts in acute care, it may be tempting to use a medical diagnosis as a concept. However, choosing nursing concepts rather than medical diagnoses can broaden the array of patients that can be assigned. For example, if the concept is congestive heart failure (CHF), learners need to have patients with this diagnosis to complete the activity. Whereas, if the concept of cardiac output is chosen, students can be assigned patients with CHF and any other condition that may impact cardiovascular function, such as dehydration, cardiomyopathy, myocardial infarction, shock, and hypertension.

Patient Assignment

For studies with CBLAs, learners do not need to be assigned patients ahead of time. They can do categorical preparation, per instructions on the CBLA document beforehand, then be assigned a patient on the day of study. Students report that it is easier to understand the concept when they are assigned to patients with actual manifestations of the problem, if possible. It is more difficult for students to see the connections between the clinical picture and the patient being "at risk for" the problem (Nielsen, 2016).

Learner Collaboration

Early in the program, learners—especially students—may benefit from working together in pairs (or triads) of students to one patient. They can support each other in assessment activities and share ideas about interpretation, not to mention simply provide a little mutual moral support to each other as they manage patient encounters. Assigning one patient to more than one student also limits the number of patients that the clinical instructor needs to access for students when using CBLAs in clinical groups.

Data Collection

Learners can collect data from a myriad of sources, including patient handoff/report, the electronic medical record, communication with the RN caring for the patient, and communication and physical assessment of the patient. Used early in the clinical experience, CBLAs can help orient learners to the variety of data sources available in the clinical environment, use of the electronic health record, and other resources.

Interaction in the Clinical Environment

As mentioned earlier, a key to implementation of CBLAs, especially when working with students early in the nursing program in the acute care environment, is nurse educator availability during the experience. Study using CBLAs in which the educator is freed from the responsibility of supervising higher-risk interventions shifts the role of the faculty from safety supervisor to teacher and guide (Heims & Boyd, 1990). The clinical educator can demonstrate assessment techniques, role model communication with patients, but more importantly, interact with students about their learning—asking and answering questions and helping learners to integrate theory and practice and develop their thinking about patient care.

Debriefing Acute Care CBLAs

Not unlike simulation, a large part of learning happens during debriefing CBLAs (Nielsen, 2016; Nielsen et al., 2021). One significant value of debriefing CBLAs is that learners gain experience with the patients of other students and therefore can learn how the concept presents in a variety of different patient situations, then compare and contrast them. This has the potential to increase the breadth of experience and thinking each learner brings to the next clinical situation. For example, in a student group on a pediatric acute care unit studying fluid and electrolyte balance, patients might include a 6-month-old with gastroenteritis, a 4-year-old with congenital heart disease, a 10-year-old with kidney disease, and a 14-year-old with an eating disorder. This variety of patients enriches the discussion and extends learning.

Using the Tanner Model to structure debriefing provides consistency between the study guide and the discussion and can underscore connections to thinking and decision-making in a variety of situations. Beginning the discussion with relevant background information theory (pathophysiology, pharmacology) or best practices related to the concept, then guiding the discussion through the elements of noticing, interpreting, responding, and reflecting supports the development of student thinking and decision-making in nursing practice. Emphasis on comparing and contrasting learners' clinical experiences, as well as best practices related to the concept, broadens understanding of nuances related to the concept (Nielsen et al., 2021).

While debriefing is an essential aspect of CBLA use, other approaches to learning about the patients of other students may be used to augment learning. For example, nursing rounds, visiting each other's patients, give students the opportunity to observe first-hand how a concept manifests in a variety of patients, as well as giving the student to whom the patient is assigned an opportunity to present their patient to others (Gonzalez, 2018; Heims & Boyd, 1990).

A Developmental Approach

While CBLAs are particularly useful in acute care when students are early in the program, they can support learning effectively when experienced learners move to new clinical settings, including during the transition to practice. For instance, students may do a pain CBLA at the beginning of their first acute care course, studying adult patients on a medical-surgical unit. Then, when beginning their capstone course, perhaps in the neonatal intensive care unit, they might use the very same CBLA to look at how pain presents and is managed in premature or sick neonates. Nurse educators' expectations of the quality of the student's work and understanding of the concept would of course be more advanced for the latter student. In fact, the faculty at one university uses a series of CBLAs (fluid and electrolyte, gas exchange, nutrition, pain, and growth and development) to orient students to specialty pediatric patient populations (pediatric medical and surgical acute care, pediatric oncology, pediatric and neonatal intensive care) at a children's hospital in an academic medical center. With a strong understanding of these concepts, faculty believe that students gain the foundational knowledge they need to orient to the patient population and provide safe care in these high-risk settings (Nielsen et al., 2021).

Innovations in Conceptual Learning in Acute Care

Gonzalez (2018) developed an entire clinical curriculum using principles of conceptual learning with a focus on the development of clinical reasoning. In this approach, students studied a different aspect of care each week (shift flow, documentation, focused assessment, data to diagnosis, priority diagnosis, communication, interventions, prioritization) in an adult medical-surgical nursing course, then during the last week of clinical focused on putting it all together (Gonzalez, 2018). Chunking and scaffolding in this way is another type of conceptual learning in clinical, supports the gradual development of students' understanding of the nurse's role in an acute care setting, and is an evidence-based approach to teaching (Gonzalez et al., 2021).

Orienting Staff

In clinical sites in which the traditional total patient care model has been used exclusively, introduction of CBLAs may represent a fairly large change in approach for unit staff. Staff understanding of the value of CBLAs, as well as knowing how they can support learners when using CBLAs, is important for successful implementation. To ensure patient safety, all staff need to know that learners will not be providing total patient care when CBLAs are being used. Discussion with the nurse manager ahead of time may help to understand and mitigate potential difficulties with implementation, as well as provide insight into potential approaches to staff orientation. When incorporating an innovative change in a clinical study, one group of faculty prepared staff by developing a newsletter about the change and preparing scripts to guide students' own explanation of the plan to RNs and other staff (Fletcher & Meyer, 2016).

Use of CBLAs in the Community

Studying nursing in the community can be an unstructured experience, and often happens without consistent clinical educator presence in the clinical environment. This situation also leaves students vulnerable to a lack of focus on key principles of nursing in the clinical setting, potentially missing critical learning. As in acute care, CBLAs can support deliberate learning of key principles of care in the community. Key learning in the community may include *population-based care,* in which students learn how to manage nursing care of specific groups of patients; *chronic condition management in the home,* in which students examine the complexity of self-management of chronic conditions in the client's home environment; *school-based care,* in which students examine roles of the school nurse from an evidence-based perspective. Similar to the curricular approach used by Gonzalez, described earlier, community clinical faculty in one bachelor's completion program for RNs designed an entire capstone practicum course around four key concepts in community nursing-health equity in nursing care of LGBTQ+ groups, care coordination, trauma-informed nursing, and emergency preparedness (Nielsen et al., 2021).

Working in the community with vulnerable patients, learners often come face-to-face with the realities of challenges that patients face in their everyday life. A well-designed health equity CBLA can help students analyze and understand this key principle of care across clinical settings. Encountering health disparities can also lead to considerable frustration related to social justice and client access to health care and other resources. Doing a CBLA focused on clinician moral distress/moral courage, allows learners to examine more deeply this aspect of being a nurse.

Use of CBLAs in Emerging Clinical Settings

In the current health care environment, emphasis has shifted to wellness, chronic condition management, and keeping people out of the hospital (Pitman, 2019). Significant roles for RNs working at the full scope of nursing practice in settings such as ambulatory care are emerging (Calma et al., 2019; Hassmiller & Wakefield, 2022; IOM, 2010; Kimble et al., 2020; Sumpter et al., 2022), yet RNs are often either not present in those settings or are not working at their full scope of nursing practice (Pitman, 2019). To learn the needed skills, nursing leadership organizations recommend inclusion of primary care content and clinical experiences in prelicensure nursing education (American Academy of Ambulatory Care Nursing [AAACN], 2021; American Association of Colleges of Nursing [AACN], 2021).

CBLAs are one way to manage these challenges and can be used to focus student attention on key learning in emerging settings, even in situations where students may not be able to directly observe best practices in nursing care. For example, in one school of nursing, CBLAs have been developed to support students' learning of key aspects of nursing care in primary ambulatory care settings. Concepts include *population health management*, *team-based care*, *fiscal management and policy*, *informatics*, *patient safety*, *quality management*, *nursing support for chronic disease management*, *triage*, and *care coordination*. All CBLAs examine how the concept presents specifically in primary care and emphasize best practices in order to account for the possibility that students may not actually see it or full aspects of it in the clinical setting (Nielsen et al., in press).

Debriefing CBLAs in the Community

Though it may look a little different, debriefing CBLAs used in community settings is as important as in acute care settings. Similar to acute care settings, when debriefing CBLAs used in the community, students learn from each other about how the concept presents in each other's clients or clinical situations (Nielsen et al., in press). Framing debriefing with a clinical judgment model is appropriate in this situation as well. The clinical educator can help guide students to *notice* the most salient aspects of situations in the context of the community, as well as identify patterns and reasons for the findings. Students can *interpret* and identify the problems or issues related to the concept in the community. Discussion of how we as nurses *respond* to address problems related to the concept develops thinking, decision-making, and understanding of the nursing role in the community. Students should identify commonalities and differences in patient or clinical situations and compare them with best evidence-based practices in community nursing.

Use of CBLAs to Teach Leadership Concepts

Traditionally in nursing leadership courses in nursing school, clinical study involves observational experiences with a nurse manager, if a clinical component is included at all. CBLAs can be used to broaden and deepen understanding of leadership and help learners, students, and practicing nurses, realize the distinctions between leadership and management, as well as the importance of early career nursing leadership. Studying key concepts in the clinical setting brings this learning to life. Potential concepts may be *staff nurse leadership* where learners observe a staff nurse and are guided to identify where the nurse needed to use leadership skills during the clinical day. Other concepts might include *interprofessional care*, in which learners identify the roles of other key professionals in the setting and perhaps spend a day interviewing, observing one or more of them and how they fit into the patient care team and collaborate with nurses. By studying the concept of *quality management,* students can learn about specific quality issues in their assigned clinical site, how they are identified, how trends are analyzed, and how interventions are evaluated. Learners can be guided to see the role of staff nurses in quality improvement. CBLAs can be used to support understanding *value-informed care*, a principle of care that is typically not emphasized in nursing school. This can help students understand what RNs bring to the care team and the interface with the realities of health care finance (Alley et al., 2021; Yakusheva et al., 2022). A related approach, referred to as Focus Learning Assignments was used to frame an educational model to teach QSEN concepts (Fletcher & Meyer, 2016).

Use of CBLAs in New Graduate Transition Programs

While not formally described in the literature, CBLAs can support newly licensed nurses as they transition into practice. In one academic medical center, CBLAs were created for an ICU internship program. Concepts included self-management (responsibility and accountability for self-care and how it relates to care of patients/clients); advanced respiratory care; behavioral-cognitive assessment and care; therapeutic relationships; infection prevention, management, and care; and independent and dependent scope of nursing practice. In evaluation of the internship, CBLAs were endorsed by new graduate nurses as effective learning experiences. Clinical nurse educators report that the result has enhanced professional nursing practice through the application of theory to practice and self-assessment to support the development of decision-making (Nielsen et al., 2017).

CHAPTER SUMMARY

CBLAs are an effective alternative or adjunct to total patient care or focused direct patient care learning in acute and community clinical settings. Used early in the nursing program or when learners are new to a clinical setting, CBLAs can focus assessment and data collection skills, facilitate analysis, integrate theory with practice, and help learners understand clinical decision-making. Effective implementation includes concept selection that allows learners to meet course outcomes, deliberate learning design, and implementation that includes robust opportunity for nurse educator interaction with learners. The learning gleaned can support development of clinical judgment and decision-making as learners engage in total patient care.

References

Alfayoumi, I. (2019). The impact of combining concept-based learning and concept-mapping pedagogies on nursing students' clinical reasoning abilities. *Nurse Education Today, 72*, 40. https://doi.org/10.1016/j.nedt.2018.10.009

Alley, R., Wilson, C., Carriera, E., & Pickard, K. (2021). Using nurse-sensitive indicators to assess the impact of primary care RNs on quality ambulatory patient care. *Nursing Economic$*, *39*(4), 200–207.

American Academy of Ambulatory Care Nursing (AAACN). (2021). The defining characteristics of ambulatory care nursing. https://www.aaacn.org/practice-resources/what-ambulatory-care-nursing/defining-characteristics

American Association of Colleges of Nursing (AACN). (2021). The essentials: Core competencies for professional nursing education. https://www.aacnnursing.org/Education-Resources/AACN-Essentials

Benner, P. (2001). *From Novice to Expert: Excellence and Power in Nursing Practice (Commemorative Ed.)*. Prentice Hall.

Benner, P., Sutphen, M., Leonard, V., & Day, L. (2010). *Educating Nurses: A Call for Radical Transformation*. Jossey-Bass.

Byrne, P., & Connor, S. (2022). Comparing work readiness for nursing students enrolled in a concept-based versus medical-based curriculum. *Nursing Education Perspectives*, *43*(6), E79–E81. https://doi.org/10.1097/01.NEP.0000000000000941

Calma, K., Halcomb, E., & Stephens, M. (2019). The impact of curriculum on nursing students' attitudes, perceptions, and preparedness to work in primary health care: An integrative review. *Nurse Education in Practice*, *39*, 1–10. https://doi.org/10.1016/j.nepr.2019.07.006

Coffman, S., Iommi, M., & Morrow, K. (2023). Scaffolding as active learning in nursing education. *Teaching and Learning in Nursing*, *18*, 232–237. https://doi.org/10.1016/j.teln.2022.09.012

Fletcher, K., & Meyer, M. (2016). Coaching model + clinical paybook = transformative learning. *Journal of Professional Nursing*, *32*(2), 121–129. https://doi.org/10.1016/j.profnurs.2015.09.001

Gonzalez, L. (2018). Teaching clinical reasoning piece by piece: A clinical reasoning concept-based learning method. *Journal of Nursing Education*, *57*(12), 727–735. https://doi.org/10.3928/01484834-20181119-05

Gonzalez, L., Cano, S., & Frost, L. (2021). Preparing the next generation nurse: Student experiences with a clinical reasoning clinical education curriculum. *The Maryland Nurse*, *22*(4), 16–17.

Gorski, M., Polanski, P., & Swider, S. (2019). *Nursing Education and the Path to Population Health Improvement*. Robert Wood Johnson, Future of Nursing Campaign for Action. https://campaignforaction.org/wp-content/uploads/2019/03/NursingEducationPathtoHealthImprovement.pdf

Hassmiller, S., & Wakefield, M. (2022). The future of nursing 2020–2030: Charting a path to achieve health equity. *Nursing Outlook*, *70*, S1–S9. https://doi.org/10.1016/j.outlook.2022.05.013

Heims, M., & Boyd, S. (1990). Concept-based learning activities in clinical nursing education. *Journal of Nursing Education*, *29*, 6, 249–254. https://doi.org/10.3928/0148-4834-19900601-05

Institute of Medicine (IOM). (2010). *The Future of Nursing: Leading Change, Advancing Health*. Washington, DC: The National Academies Press. https://www.ncbi.nlm.nih.gov/books/NBK209880/

Ironside, P., McNelis, A., & Ebright, P. (2014). Clinical education in nursing: Rethinking learning in practice settings. *Nursing Outlook*, *62*(3), 185–191. https://doi.org/10.1016/j.outlook.2013.12.004

Kavanagh, J., & Sharpnack, P. (2021). Crisis in competency: A defining moment in nursing education. *The Online Journal of Issues in Nurisng*, *26*, Manuscript 2. https://doi.org/10.3912/OJIN.Vol26No01Man02

Kimble, L., Phan, Q., Hillman, J., Blackman, J., Shore, C., Swainson, N., & Amobi, C. (2020). The CAPACITY professional development model for community-based primary care nurses: Needs assessment and curriculum planning. *Nursing Economic$*, *38*(3), 110–120, 148.

Lasater, K. (2007). Clinical judgment development: Using simulation to create an assessment rubric. *Journal of Nursing Education*, *46*, 496–503. https://doi.org/10.3928/01484834-20071101-04

Lasater, K., & Nielsen, A. (2009). The influence of concept-based learning activities on students' clinical judgment development. *Journal of Nursing Education, 48*(8), 441–446. https://doi.org/10.3928/01484834-20090518-04

McNelis, A., Ironside, P., Ebright, P., Dreifuerst, K., Zvonar, S., & Conner, S. (2014). Learning nursing practice: A multisite, multimethod investigation of clinical education. *Journal of Nursing Regulation, 4*(4), 30–35. https://doi.org/10.1016/S2155-8256(15)30115-0

Morton, J., Weierback, F., Sutter, R., Livsey, K., Goehner, E., Lieseveld, J., & Goldschidt, M. (2019). New education models for preparing pre-licensure students for community-based practice. *Journal of Professional Nursing, 35*, 491–498. https://doi.org/10.1016/j.profnurs.2019.05.004

National League for Nursing (NLN). (2015). Debriefing across the curriculum: A living document from the National League for Nursing. Retrieved from: https://www.nln.org/docs/default-source/uploadedfiles/professional-development-programs/nln-vision-debriefing-across-the-curriculum.pdf

Nielsen, A. (2013). *Concept-based learning in the clinical environment* (Doctoral Dissertation). Retrieved from CINAHL Plus with Full Text. (Accession Order No. AAT 109864436)

Nielsen, A. (2016). Concept-based learning in clinical experiences: Bringing theory to clinical education for deep learning. *Journal of Nursing Education, 55*(7), 365–371. https://doi.org/10.3928/01484834-20160615-02

Nielsen, A., Tutsch, A., & Lasater, K. (2017, May 24). Concept-based learning in academia and practice: Supporting new nurses as they transition into practice. 7th International Skills Conference, Prato Italy. https://internationalclinicalskillsconference.com/uploads/2017-PRATO-Abstract-book.pdf

Nielsen, A., Garner, A., Lanciotti, K., & Brown, L. (2021). Concept-based learning for capstone clinical experiences in hospital and community settings. *Nurse Educator, 46*(6), 381–385. https://doi.org/10.1097/NNE.0000000000000964

Nielsen, A., Taylor, C., Claudson, R., Keller, G., & Barfield, P. (in press). Creating a Clinical Curriculum for Prelicensure Students in Primary Care Clinical Experiences. *Nurse Educator*, accepted for publication February 2023.

Pittman, P. (2019). Activating nursing to address unmet needs in the 21st Century. *Robert Wood Johnson Foundation*. Princeton, NJ. March 12, 2019. https://publichealth.gwu.edu/sites/default/files/downloads/HPM/Activating%20Nursing%20To%20Address%20Unmet%20Needs%20In%20The%202021st%20Century.pdf.

Sumpter, D., Blodgett N., Beard, K., & Howard, V. (2022). Transforming nursing education in response to the Future of Nursing 2020–2030. *Nursing Outlook, 70*, S20–S31. https://doi.org/10.1016/j.outlook.2022.02.007

Tanner, C. A. (2006). Thinking like a nurse: A research-based model of clinical judgment in Nursing. *Journal of Nursing Education, 45*, 204–211. https://doi.org/10.3928/01484834-20060601-04

Tanner, C. A., Messecar, D. C., & Delawska-Elliott, B. (2022). Chapter 13, Evidence based practice. In L. Joel (Ed.), *Advanced practice nursing: Essentials for role development* (5th ed.). F.A. Davis.

Tyo, M. B., & McCurry, M. K. (2019). An integrative review of clinical reasoning teaching strategies and outcome evaluation in nursing education. *Nursing Education Perspectives, 40*(1), 11–17. https://doi.org/10.1097/01.NEP.0000000000000375

Yakusheva, O., Rambur, B., & Buerhaus, P. I. (2022). Value based care series part 6: Education for value-informed nursing practice. *Nursing Outlook, 70*, 789–793. https://doi.org/10.1016/j.outlook.2022.08.002

12

Best Practices in Simulation Learning

Ashley E. Franklin, PhD, RN, CNE, CHSE-A
Jeremy Hutson, MSN, RN

CHAPTER OVERVIEW

This chapter presents current research and simulation best practices for nursing and health professions. Topics include learner preparation, scenario design, pre-briefing, and debriefing simulation experiences. Current simulation standards are introduced, and various simulation modalities are presented, with a focus on aligning scenarios with course and curricular goals. The chapter concludes with an overview of assessment in simulation.

SIMULATION DEFINED

Simulation is an experiential teaching strategy allowing learners to practice psychomotor and clinical judgment skills in a safe environment without risk of patient harm. Educators and academic programs recognize the many strengths simulation pedagogy offers, especially its safe, timely, and prescriptive approach to meeting specific learning objectives for individual courses, larger curricula, and academic programs (Franklin & Blodgett, 2021). Simulation has gained traction, especially in pre-licensure education, because it enhances learning while avoiding obstacles from traditional clinical settings such as downtime, workarounds, or low patient census (Waxman et al., 2019). Simulation is a safe and intentional teaching strategy focused on developing practice-ready nurses (Bryant et al., 2020). This chapter provides exemplars for effective simulation using a scenario involving a transgender male post-operative patient experiencing pneumonia following a mastectomy, with the intent of highlighting opportunities to weave health equity, social determinants of health, and population health throughout a simulation curriculum.

Simulation has a long history of application across multiple disciplines, and definitions of the term vary from generalized to specific. Gaba (2004) described simulation as "a technique...to replace or amplify real experiences with guided experiences that evoke or replicate substantial aspects of the real world in a fully interactive manner" (i2). This definition captures the essence of simulation; however, a more comprehensive description brings clarity to its use within the context of nursing education. In this chapter, the term "simulation" refers to "a technique that creates a situation or environment to allow persons to experience a representation of a real event for the purpose of practice, learning, evaluation, testing, or to gain understanding of systems or human actions" (Lioce et al., 2020).

HISTORICAL OVERVIEW

Educators have included simulation learning experiences in nursing education for decades; however, focused efforts to shape effective simulation teaching strategies began in the early 2000s. Since 2003, the National League for Nursing (NLN) has transformed the way nurse educators develop, test, and integrate simulation to promote learning. The NLN sponsored the first national study (Jeffries & Rizzolo, 2007) that launched a movement toward using simulation as an essential teaching strategy and measuring learners' outcomes (Forneris et al., 2017). In 2007, the NLN launched a Simulation Innovation Resource Center which provides scaffolded educational programs and professional development resources. The NLN has since conducted research to study high-stakes simulation, spearheaded facilitator professional development, provided access to unfolding scenarios through the Advancing Care Excellence series, and sustained a simulation leadership development program.

Three seminal papers support simulation integration across curricula. First, the landmark National Council of State Boards of Nursing (NCSBN) National Simulation Study, compared outcomes from learners across the United States (U.S.) who completed either 10, 25, or 50 percent of traditional clinical hours in standardized, high-quality simulation implemented by trained facilitators; results provided substantive evidence that high doses of simulation learning did not detract from knowledge, clinical competency, critical thinking, or readiness for practice (Hayden et al., 2014). The National Simulation Study prompted many state boards of nursing to allow simulation to replace traditional clinical hours. Subsequently, the NLN published two vision statements encouraging a paradigm shift from nursing faculty as teachers to facilitators of knowledge co-creation (Forneris et al., 2017). The *Vision for Teaching with Simulation* (NLN Board of Governors, 2015a) provides recommendations for nursing deans and directors, faculty, and communities of interest particularly focused on collaboration between simulation facilitators and faculty peers as well as academic and clinical partners. The NLN forged the path to emphasize simulation facilitator professional development and curriculum integration (Franklin & Blodgett, 2021). Finally, the vision statement for *Debriefing Across the Curriculum* (NLN Board of Governors, 2015b) was co-created with the International Nursing Association for Clinical Simulation in Learning (INACSL) and extends beyond simulation into traditional and classroom teaching. The debriefing vision statement emphasizes the importance of reflection to help learners question their practice and reorder how they think, act, and understand (Forneris et al., 2017).

There are several significant milestones to consider as nurse educators unpack the strengths of simulation pedagogy (see Table 12.1). Starting in 2011, INACSL published the Standards of Best Practice: Simulation[SM] as living documents with guidelines to anchor simulation teaching and learner evaluation. Over time, interprofessional and international colleagues contributed to Standards updates and added topics relevant to our maturing simulation discipline. In 2015 as a response to the National Simulation Study, NCSBN published Simulation Program Guidelines (Alexander et al., 2015) to

TABLE 12.1

Significant Milestones in Health Care Simulation

Date	Artifact	Citation	Website
2005	Nursing Education Simulation Framework	Jeffries, P. R. (2005). A framework for designing, implementing, and evaluating simulations used as teaching strategies in nursing. *Nursing Education Perspectives, 26*(2), 96–103.	—
2007	NLN Simulation Innovation Research Center	—	https://sirc.nln.org
2011	First INACSL Standards of Best Practice	INACSL Board of Directors. (2011). Standards of best practice: Simulation. *Clinical Simulation in Nursing, 7*, S1–S20.	https://inacsl.memberclicks.net/healthcare-simulation-standards-history
2013	Revision, INACSL Standards of Best Practice	INACSL Board of Directors. (2013). Standards of best practice: Simulation. *Clinical Simulation in Nursing, 9*, S1–S32.	—
2014	NCSBN National Simulation Study	Hayden, J. K., Smiley, R. A., Alexander, M., Kardong-Edgren, S., & Jeffries, P. R. (2014). The NCSBN National Simulation Study: a longitudinal, randomized, controlled study replacing clinical hours with simulation in prelicensure nursing education. *Journal of Nursing Regulation, 5*, S1–S64.	—
2015	NCSBN Simulation Program Guidelines	Alexander, M., Durham, C. F., Hooper, J. I., Jeffries, P. R., Goldman, N., Kardong-Edgren, S., Kesten, K. S., Spector, N., Tagliareni, E., Radtke, B., & Tillman, C. (2015). NCSBN simulation guidelines for prelicensure nursing programs. *Journal of Nursing Regulation, 6*, 39–42.	—
2016	Revision, INACSL Standards of Best Practice with new Standards for Simulation Design, Interprofessional Education, and Operations	INACSL Standards Committee. (2016). INACSL standards of best practice: Simulation^SM. *Clinical Simulation in Nursing, 12*, S1–S50.	—
2016	Jeffries Simulation Framework Elevated to Mid-Range NLN Jeffries Simulation Theory	Jeffries, P. R. (2016). *The NLN Jeffries simulation theory.* Wolters Kluwer.	—

(continued)

TABLE 12.1

Significant Milestones in Health Care Simulation *(Continued)*

Date	Artifact	Citation	Website
2019	2:1 model for sim:clinical time	Sullivan, N., Swoboda, S. M., Breymier, T., Lucas, L., Sarasnick, J., Rutherford-Hemming, T. Budhathoki, C., & Kardong-Edgren, S. (2019). Emerging evidence toward a 2:1 clinical to simulation ratio: A study comparing traditional clinical and simulation settings. *Clinical Simulation in Nursing, 30,* 34–41. https://doi.org/10.1016/j.ecns.2019.03.003	—
2021	Name change from INACSL Standards to Healthcare Simulation Standards of Best Practice with new Standards added for Pre-Briefing and Professional Development	Watts, P., Rossler, K., Bowler, F., Miller, C., Charnetski, M., Decker, S., Molloy, M., Persico, L., McMahon, E., McDermott, D., Hallmark, B. (2021). *Preamble. Clinical Simulation in Nursing,* https://doi.org/10.1016/j.ecns.2021.08.006	https://www.inacsl.org/healthcare-simulation-standards
2022	INACSL Endorsement Program Pilot	—	https://www.inacsl.org/endorsement-program

highlight the need to establish policies and allocate resources—such as dedicated simulation staff, faculty development, evaluation of learner and faculty competency, as well as a commitment to pre-briefing and debriefing—to ensure continuity between facilitators and within simulation programs.

In 2016, the NLN Jeffries Simulation Framework was elevated to a middle-range theory (see Figure 12.1). Supported by a robust body of literature, the NLN Jeffries Simulation Theory illustrates the influence of context, background, and facilitator-learner interactions on effective simulation experiences. It builds on Chickering and Gamson's (1987) principles to improve undergraduate education, including active learning, prompt feedback, learner/faculty interaction, collaborative learning, high expectations, allowing for diverse styles of learning, and time on task. The NLN Jeffries Simulation Theory broadened our understanding of simulation outcomes from exclusively learner outcomes to include patient and system-level outcomes as well.

As educators seek to define simulation versus traditional clinical hours, a 2019 study provides evidence for awarding 2:1 clock hours for time spent in simulation versus clinical (Sullivan et al., 2019). Sullivan and colleagues compared nursing tasks, thinking, and time spent in simulation versus traditional clinical settings. Because learners function independently in simulation with specific objectives for each 20-minute scenario, they have more opportunities to practice assessment, skills, and patient teaching in simulation

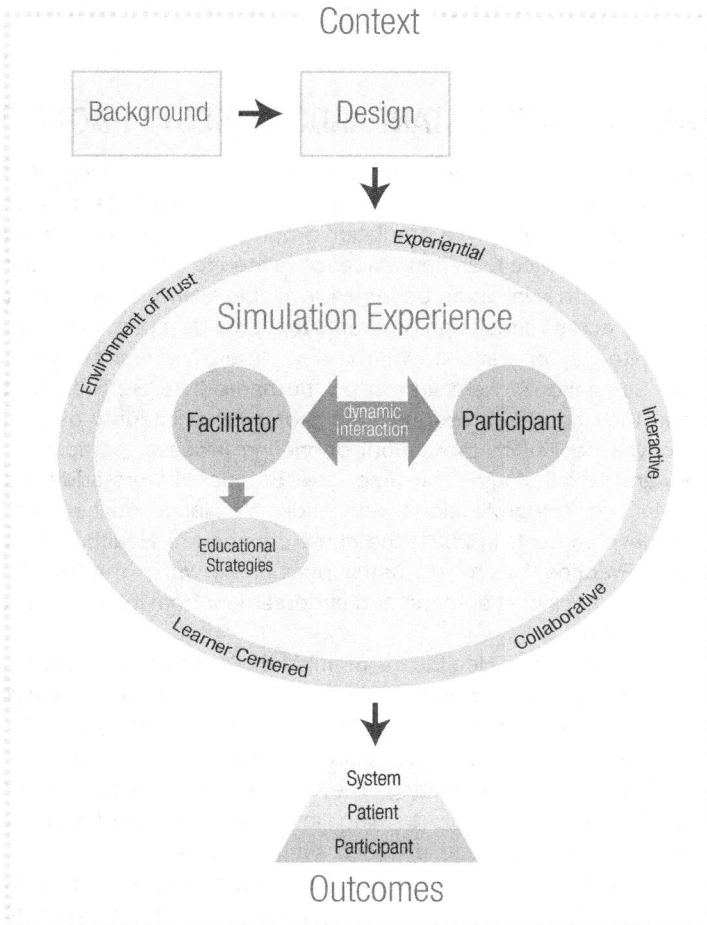

FIGURE 12.1 Diagram of the NLN Jeffries Simulation Theory. (Reprinted with permission from Jeffries, P. R. [2016]. The NLN Jeffries Simulation Theory [Fig. 3.1]. Wolters Kluwer.)

than in traditional clinical and accomplish those tasks more efficiently. Sullivan and colleagues provide evidence supporting simulation as a concentrated, efficient teaching methodology with a greater focus on the application of knowledge compared to recalling diagnoses or medicine names in traditional clinical settings. In the study, simulation learners spent 51 percent of time articulating steps in nursing decision-making at the "Knows How" level of Miller's Pyramid compared to 12 percent in a traditional clinical setting (Miller, 1990). Similarly, learners performed 66 percent of activities at the highest "Does" level of Miller's Pyramid in simulation, compared to 46 percent in traditional clinical settings. As a result, many academic programs adopted a 2:1 ratio counting simulation experiences as double time spent in traditional clinical settings; for example, a 4.5-hour simulation experience could count as 9 hours spent in traditional clinical settings when calculating hours required to meet course or program requirements.

HEALTHCARE SIMULATION STANDARDS OF BEST PRACTICE™

The Healthcare Simulation Standards of Best Practice™ advance the science of simulation, share best practices, and provide evidence-based guidelines for the practice and development of a comprehensive simulation program. They are peer-reviewed, living documents updated cyclically as new evidence related to simulation design, implementation, debriefing, and evaluation becomes available (Sittner, 2016). The Standards increase consistency across simulation programs and provide a process for evaluating and improving day-to-day operations (Waxman et al., 2019). The first seven Standards of Best Practice: Simulation™ were known by the name INACSL Standards beginning in 2011, and their content areas included professional integrity of participants, participant objectives, facilitator, facilitation, debriefing process, participant assessment evaluation, and terminology. Over time, new Standards were added pertaining to simulation-enhanced interprofessional education, simulation design, pre-briefing, and professional development. In 2021, the name changed to Healthcare Simulation Standards of Best Practice™ to reflect better positioning within the field of simulation, input from interprofessional authors, and endorsement from interprofessional and international associations.

To further the impact of the Healthcare Simulation Standards of Best Practice™, INACSL launched an endorsement program in 2021 to recognize simulation programs in academic and practice settings that demonstrate sustained application of the "Core Four" Standards, which include: pre-briefing—preparation and briefing; facilitation; professional integrity; and debriefing. The endorsement program recognizes all simulation modalities, including skills training, low-fidelity to high-fidelity manikins, augmented reality, virtual reality, and distance simulation. Endorsement encourages ongoing evaluation and performance improvement with a long-term goal of improving health care education and patient safety through promotion and practice of high-quality simulation. A summary of the "Core Four" Standards with exemplars for application will follow.

Pre-Briefing: Preparation and Briefing

Through simulation preparation and pre-briefing, educators work to ensure learners are ready for educational content and aware of ground rules for simulation experiences (INACSL Standards Committee et al., 2021a). Preparation activities prior to the simulation day and just-in-time pre-briefing orientation decrease learners' cognitive load and increase the effectiveness of simulation experiences. Both elements of simulation design help learners and facilitators share a common mental model, so they are able to accomplish *a priori* objectives.

In a simulation focused on the care of a transgender male patient experiencing postoperative pneumonia following mastectomy surgery, preparation materials might include evidence-based recommendations from the American Psychological Association, websites about local gender-affirming health services, patient education materials about antibiotics and incentive spirometry, or a review of abnormal breath sounds. Briefing should include orientation to simulation roles and objectives, a tour of the simulation environment and equipment, and a discussion on patient-centered communication, use of preferred pronouns, and strategies to identify the patient before giving medications. Learners can lead a conversation about their plan of care using the Situation, Background, Assessment, and Recommendations format. Most prelicensure learners will benefit from a discussion of the patient's background and problem list tied to individualized, priority-focused assessments and interventions. Educators can implement well-planned briefing activities in as little as 20 minutes.

Facilitation

Simulation facilitation helps learners develop psychomotor skills, critical thinking, clinical judgment, and apply theoretical knowledge. Effective facilitation requires educators to tailor teaching methods (e.g., pre-simulation activities/briefing, delivery of cues during simulation, debriefing) to meet expected outcomes (INACSL Standards Committee et al., 2021b). Facilitation will vary based on learners' needs and expected outcomes. A key component of effective facilitation is facilitator competency, especially ongoing peer evaluation and personal reflection on facilitators' skills, knowledge, and performance.

An example of applying facilitation techniques and principles of sociocultural learning theory during pre-briefing and debriefing is open-ended prompts to promote peer learning rather than "sage on the stage" lectures. An open-ended prompt could be "What did you think about ...?" in pre-briefing or "How did you decide what to do first when ...?" during debriefing. To continue with the scenario focused on care of a transgender male patient experiencing post-operative pneumonia, it would be important to facilitate a discussion around learners' values and beliefs about transgender individuals and how personal assumptions intersect with nursing care. Delivering a cue during simulation from the patient such as "Thank you for being kind. The Emergency Room was stressful. There was a staff member who was so disrespectful and called me 'It.' She was really nasty ..." provides learners an opportunity to think on their feet and respond in action, while the facilitated debriefing discussion allows learners time to reflect on action and consider their culture, past interactions, and aspirations for providing patient-centered care. A broad debriefing prompt could be "He told you about a difficult situation in the Emergency Room. How did you respond in that situation?" A follow-up prompt aimed to engage simulation observers could be "How did you see the team of nurses show our patient they cared for him?" The subsequent teaching point could focus on service recovery strategies and chain of command such as nurse to charge nurse and charge nurse to patient advocate and/or educator.

Debriefing

The debriefing process includes feedback, debriefing, and guided reflection, which educators may blend according to the level of the learner, objectives, and evaluation goals (INACSL Standards Committee et al., 2021c). Debriefing should be guided by a theoretical framework to encourage self-analysis, exploration of knowledge, and mitigation of performance gaps while maintaining psychological safety and confidentiality. The Clinical

Judgment Model (Tanner, 2006) is an example of a nursing-specific theoretical framework that can be used to structure debriefing and promote reflection. Debriefing can be accomplished on-demand at a stopping point in a scenario and/or as a post-scenario activity. Debriefing incorporates individual, team, and system-level analysis. Although debriefing should not be a "sage on the stage" lecture, much learning occurs during the debriefing process (INACSL Standards Committee et al., 2021c).

Debriefing commonly starts with a reactions phase to allow learners to decompress after the scenario and identify salient discussion points, followed by an analysis phase wherein participants explore their experiences and connect theoretical knowledge to the scenario. In the summary phase, participants recap the experience, identify insights, and explore how to transfer learning from simulation to actual patient care settings. A trained debriefer helps identify knowledge and performance gaps and provides feedback to close gaps, often using the advocacy/inquiry method. Advocacy/inquiry is appropriate to help a facilitator and group of learners understand a peer's rationale for behavior or decisions made (Eppich & Cheng, 2015). Using both advocacy and inquiry, a trained facilitator shares an observation, an assertion, and a question to engage conversation (Rudolph et al., 2006). For example, "Sarah, I noticed you used female pronouns in reference to our transgender male patient, and I'm concerned he might consider them as insensitive. I'm curious about what you were thinking when talking to Mr. Vaughn and about his care to your preceptor in simulation."

The ultimate goal of debriefing is to promote reflective thinking centered on scenario objectives. Reflection can lead learners to new interpretations and cognitive reframing wherein learners look at a situation from a different perspective, which is a skill essential to maintaining professional competencies (INACSL Standards Committee et al., 2021c). In our exemplar focused on the care of a transgender male patient, debriefing provides opportunities for cognitive reframing related to culturally competent care and hormone replacement therapy. For example, delivering a cue during simulation from the patient such as "I'm supposed to get my T today, and I really don't want to miss my dose. It's in my backpack" provides learners an opportunity to respond in action. A debriefing prompt like "He said he needed his T. What was he talking about?" and then "What interprofessional resources can we use to promote care coordination?" allows for a debriefing conversation about local access to gender-affirming health services, social discrimination, gatekeepers, and insurance-related barriers to hormone therapy.

Professional Integrity

Professional integrity requires that participants (i.e., learners, faculty, staff, and standardized patients) adhere to ethical and practice standards, demonstrate respect and inclusivity, and maintain confidentiality to create a physically and psychologically safe learning environment (INACSL Standards Committee et al., 2021d). The Society for Simulation in Healthcare's Simulationist Code of Ethics (Park et al., 2018) addresses professional integrity and its role in positive simulation experiences. Simulation requires all participants to be vulnerable during simulation as well as in pre-briefing and debriefing conversations because they are charged to consider another's perspective. The core of professional integrity relies on simulation environments built upon psychological safety and environmental safety that removes the risk of patient harm.

In our simulation exemplar, learning objectives around cultural competence and patient-centered communication exemplify the aspirational value of mutual respect from the Healthcare Simulationist Code of Ethics. Facilitators model ethical behavior, especially in pre-briefing conversations about use of preferred pronouns and strategies to identify the patient before giving medicine. Interprofessional simulationists have adopted The Basic Assumption™ from the Center for Medical Simulation, which states "We believe that everyone who comes to simulation is intelligent, well trained, cares about doing their best, and wants to improve the way they care for patients." The Basic Assumption™ exemplifies professional attitudes when modeled by facilitators, simulation staff, and shared publicly with simulation communities of interest. Simulationists honor The Basic Assumption by respecting confidentiality and dignity when following policies to share learner performance details and avoiding disclosure of simulation errors unless dictated by legal or ethical regulations. Learners should know what errors are disclosed and the rationale for disclosure as part of orientation to simulation and pre-brief in order to preserve the integrity of the simulation environment and promote transparency.

SIMULATION PEDAGOGY

Simulation is integral to nursing education because it fills curricular gaps with active learning scenarios, guided by specific learning objectives, which reflect practice, include teamwork, and improve patient safety (Bryant et al., 2020). Simulation experiences allow learners to develop and enhance knowledge, skills, and attitudes, as well as analyze and respond independently to realistic patient care situations (Morse et al., 2019). We know from a recent meta-analysis that simulation has the greatest outcomes on psychomotor and cognitive skills (Kim et al., 2016), and in order to maintain these, simulation must continue to evolve from teaching stand-alone skills to focusing on higher-order thinking, which underpins quality nursing care (Bryant et al., 2020).

While simulation literature commonly describes nursing simulation as a teaching strategy employing manikins to represent simulated patients, modern simulation is expanding beyond manikins. In fact, educators use multiple simulation modalities to meet learner needs and curriculum objectives. Manikins, standardized patients, and various forms of virtual technology provide realism to engage and challenge learners.

SIMULATION MODALITIES
Manikin-Based

Manikin-based simulation is a flexible strategy to address learner needs and *a priori* objectives across levels of nursing education. A manikin is a full or partial-body simulator with varying levels of physiologic function, which determines its designation as low- or high-fidelity (Lioce et al., 2020). Low-fidelity manikins, or task trainers, are designed to train learners on key elements of procedural skills, such as intravenous catheter insertion, and they may use mechanical or electronic interfaces to teach and give feedback on skills, such as injection technique or auscultation technique (Lioce et al., 2020). High-fidelity manikins mimic human body functions like chest rise, palpable pulses, breath sounds, and interactive pupils, at a very realistic level (Lioce et al., 2020). Given the realism of high-fidelity manikins, learners often apply knowledge and higher-order thinking skills more readily (Kim et al., 2016). Regardless of the level of fidelity, manikins offer flexibility in simulation as their appearance can be easily altered with various clothing items and moulage allowing for multiple patients with varying conditions to be represented through one single manikin.

Educators should choose a manikin and level of fidelity during simulation design to align with learning objectives. It is important to remember that learning outcomes do not correlate with fidelity level and that, although simulation research with high-fidelity manikins has larger cognitive and affective effect sizes compared to those with low-fidelity manikins, low-fidelity manikins produce more learning for psychomotor skills (Kim et al., 2016). Therefore, simulation educators should prioritize learning objectives, choose the simulation modality to match objectives, and design simulations according to Healthcare Simulation Standards of Best Practice™ (Kim et al., 2016).

Standardized Patients

Standardized patients are collaborators in simulation education who bring patient experiences and voices to life (Bradley et al., 2023). Standardized patients foster both cognitive and affective learning outcomes (Kim et al., 2016) when they serve as simulation patients, family members, or embedded health care team members to guide learners to meet desired objectives (Lewis et al., 2017). The terms standardized patient, simulated participant, and embedded patient are often used interchangeably and refer to a person trained to portray a patient in realistic and replicable simulation experiences (Lewis et al., 2017). Standardized patients require training to portray roles, give feedback, and complete assessment tools, and they deserve the same preparation, training, feedback, and guided reflection as learners (Lewis et al., 2017). Depending on the setting and resources available, volunteers, educators, students, retired faculty, or actors may serve as standardized patients (Rutherford-Hemming et al., 2019); educators should choose the individual standardized patients and provide training with tenets of professional integrity (e.g., it may be important learners are not familiar with the standardized patient). An example of individualized training, standardized patients may follow a full script, partial script representing the gestalt of a patient or scenario. To enhance authenticity the standardized patient will need some ability to deviate from the planned script and respond with flexibility to students' communication and behavior with the patient during the scenario.

To continue our example of focused care of a transgender male patient, a standardized patient could portray a spouse and add depth to the consideration of patient-centered care and challenge assumptions about family structure in transgender communities. Standardized patients add opportunities for providing physical cues in simulation environments. For example, a standardized patient could pick up a backpack or retrieve supplies to deliver a testosterone injection from a home medication supply and lead the way into a debriefing conversation about the nursing scope of practice with medicine reconciliation and responsibility to check medicines, document, and refine technique for families who administer medicines long term.

Virtual, Augmented, and Extended Reality

Virtual reality (VR) and augmented reality (AR) simulations have gained popularity in recent years, and simulationists are working to apply the Standards to these new modalities as they develop, facilitate, debrief, and evaluate simulation experiences (Aebersold et al., 2023). The term VR commonly refers to computer technology to create an interactive three-dimensional world in which objects have a sense of spatial presence (Lioce et al., 2020); VR may involve screen-based simulation or a head-mounted display (HMD). VR increases learner engagement, allows active learning, and provides authentic experiences because learners experience essential clinical activities and interact with a virtual environment without the risk of patient harm or the cost of in-person simulation (Choi et al., 2021). AR adds the element of interacting with a physical environment as AR overlays digital content through a tablet, HMD, or smartphone; AR became popular through Snapchat and Instagram applications using AR filters (Aebersold et al., 2023). The term extended reality (XR) is an umbrella term to capture VR, AR, and other alternate realities (Aebersold et al., 2023).

There is a growing body of evidence that XR supports efficient and reliable cognitive learning as well as psychomotor practice for intravenous and urinary catheter insertion, basic life support, and needlestick prevention (Choi et al., 2021). XR is effective to support critical thinking and clinical reasoning by providing opportunities for pattern recognition across clinical scenarios (Sim et al., 2022). XR provides uniform content delivery, allows practice with high-acuity but low-frequency situations, and meets learner and program needs flexibly (Roye et al., 2021). It is important to emphasize learners need debriefing after XR simulation, whether through review of feedback provided by virtual software, self-debriefing with reflection, or facilitator-guided synchronous debriefing (Roye et al., 2021).

Nursing is in a good position to use XR simulation because manikin and standardized patient simulations are well-established (Aebersold et al., 2023). Other health care disciplines have used XR to scale learning experiences to accommodate large learner cohorts. For example, educators used AR with the HoloLens 2 to deliver live-streamed, remote access, interactive teaching rounds with medical students (Bala et al., 2021). XR brings new physical and emotional safety concerns to simulation experiences, particularly when learners wear an HMD and are susceptible to injuring themselves or damaging the physical environment; XR simulations may trigger or induce trauma and cybersickness related to the intense reality (Aebersold et al., 2023) and concurrent stimulus of multiple senses. XR also introduces new concerns related to data protection and privacy in education settings, such as internet protocol (IP) addresses and biometric data, which warrants consultation with information technology and legal departments during contract negotiations with vendors. At the time of this publication, research surrounding XR simulation has focused mostly on usability (Aebersold et al., 2023) and learner satisfaction; more research is needed to define the dose of XR simulation required to impact learners and transfer knowledge and skills from XR to actual patient care settings.

CURRICULUM INTEGRATION

As schools continue to replace clinical hours with simulation, the need to develop integrated, sustainable, simulation-based curricula for competency-based education increases (Bryant et al., 2020). Curriculum integration represents a coordinated and purposeful use of simulation to meet predetermined learning goals (Franklin & Blodgett, 2021). Integrating simulation throughout the curriculum allows facilitators to build on previous learning to promote higher-order thinking (Leighton, 2017) and gives learners an opportunity to apply and synthesize didactic and clinical knowledge over time (Aul et al., 2021)

TABLE 12.2

Miller's Pyramid of Clinical Competence

	Stage of Professional Practice	Professional Competencies	Evidence
Novice	Level 1	Knows	Recognizes facts in traditional multiple-choice questions or true/false items
	Level 2	Knows How	Applies knowledge to case studies, essays, or extended matching type test items
	Level 3	Shows	Demonstrates skill and application of knowledge in simulation or objective structured clinical exam
Expert (includes mastery of levels 1–3)	Level 4	Does	Independently integrates knowledge into practice with actual patients

Adapted from Miller, G. E. (1990). The assessment of clinical skills/competence/performance. *Academic Medicine, 65*(9), s63–s67.

in a scaffolding format of increasing complexity. Since the inception of high-fidelity simulation in health professions education, the evidence has been strongly supportive of curriculum integration as a simulation feature leading to the most effective learning (Issenberg et al., 2005).

Factors shaping curriculum integration include learner demographics, local needs identified by a community of interest, trends, and accreditation requirements (Franklin & Blodgett, 2021). A framework for curriculum design includes a needs assessment, curricular mapping, scaffolding, resource utilization, planning, and evaluation (Franklin & Blodgett, 2021). A needs assessment should include faculty perspectives and willingness to adjust the type, scope, and amount of simulation. Curriculum mapping links simulation content, objectives, and competencies to didactic, clinical, and lab courses. We recommend comprehensive initial and ongoing faculty development and a systematic approach to selecting simulation scenarios, facilitating them, and evaluating simulation experiences for how they fit into a larger curriculum (Aul et al., 2021). When educators design, test, and evaluate scenarios, careful attention should be given to how learners accomplish the "shows" and "does" competencies from Miller's Pyramid (see Table 12.2; Miller, 1990). In such an evaluation process, it is also wise to link scenarios to course objectives, competencies, and program outcomes. For example, educators should critically examine each scenario to determine how the *content* (i.e., knowledge of oxygenation) can be intentionally linked to *context* (i.e., care of patients with respiratory distress) across care environments (Franklin & Blodgett, 2021; Waxman et al., 2019).

Sequential "Unfolding" Simulations

Sequential or "unfolding" simulation allows for both flexibility in curriculum integration and a deeper focus on patient and disease trajectories. Sequential simulation situates learners in scenarios that depict the progression of one patient over time (Leighton, 2017). Scenarios can take place during one simulation day or may be spread across multiple simulation experiences. Sequential simulation allows learners to address a patient holistically by "seeing" elements of multiple comorbid conditions, and gives context for understanding the impact of an illness or illnesses on the patient and family members. Sequential simulations also provide opportunity for repetative practice with key concepts.

Utilizing our exemplar with a transgender male patient in a sequential simulation, the case could be presented as three separate scenarios. The first scenario could require learners to care for this patient pre-operatively to accomplish learning objectives related to patient teaching, informed consent, and care coordination between outpatient and inpatient care environments. In the second scenario, learners could provide pain relief during the immediate post-operative period as well as care for surgical drains. In the third scenario, learners could encounter the patient weeks to months later with post-operative pneumonia. There are two main strengths to sequential simulation. First, sequential simulation maps to curriculum integration when content and skills practice occur at the same point in the semester for didactic and simulation experiences. Second, sequential simulation decreases stress on the learner to get to know a new patient so they instead focus on salient concepts and curricular threads that may otherwise be overlooked, such as psychosocial concerns and gender-affirming care in our exemplar case.

Utilizing Simulation Observers

Educators often overlook the amount of time learners spend in a simulation observer role and downplay observer outcomes (Johnson et al., 2023); however, there is growing evidence about observers' positive learning experiences. Early simulation leaders suggested simulation learning includes observation (Gaba, 2004). Many simulation programs accommodate growing numbers in academic cohorts and nurse residency programs by assigning learners to observer roles (Rogers et al., 2020). Observers may watch the simulation from an external debriefing room, within the simulation room in a non-participant role, or by actively participating in the scenario as a family member (O'Regan et al., 2021). We now know observers construct knowledge similarly to active simulation participants when a theoretically derived and evidence-based debriefing follows observation (Johnson, 2019). Positive observer outcomes include clinical skills, teamwork and collaboration, confidence, critical thinking, clinical judgment, insight, and conceptual thinking (Rogers et al., 2020).

Positive observer outcomes depend in part on simulation design. For example, simulation observers should participate in pre-briefing and complete the same preparation assignments as active simulation participants. Additionally, educators may use written guides to direct observers' noticing of salient behaviors mapped to learning objectives; notes observers make in turn allow them to give peers specific feedback during debriefing (Johnson et al., 2023). Observation guides increase some learners' motivation, attention, and retention and make the observer role more active (Johnson, 2019), particularly when items on the observation guide change over time and are novel from learners' perspectives. Finally, the Tag-Team simulation model engages active simulation participants and observers, especially in large groups, when participants "tag" in or out so everyone shares responsibility for nursing interventions and outcomes (Johnson et al., 2023).

ASSESSING LEARNERS' SIMULATION PERFORMANCE

Simulation allows educators to evaluate learners' knowledge, skills, attitudes, and behaviors firsthand (INACSL Standards Committee et al., 2021e). Most educators align standardized simulation assessments with the "shows" or "does" levels of Miller's Pyramid of Clinical Competence (see Table 12.2), wherein we objectively evaluate learners' behaviors and how they apply knowledge. Not only do simulation performance assessments represent higher levels of clinical competence, but they also reflect the maturity of our simulation discipline because we have moved beyond using subjective, self-report measures alone to show simulation effectiveness. Miller's seminal model introduced performance-based assessments in medical education, and it informs the competency-based education movement across nursing and health professions today. A major focus in measurement is the use of a valid and reliable assessment tool with trained raters using an *a priori* criteria to determine passing scores. To follow evaluation best practices, facilitators should measure interrater reliability in at least ten percent of the cohort. The assessment tool should have been used with a similar group of learners previously and the simulation scenario pilot tested before assessing learner performance. Both the Evaluating Healthcare Simulation website (www.sim-eval.org) and INACSL's Repository of Instruments (search on https://www.inacsl.org) provide references and resources for an assortment of assessment tools. Regardless of the assessment tool used, it is important implications or consequences of assessment are explained to learners in advance (INACSL Standards Committee, 2021e).

Formative Assessment

Assessment happens along a continuum from informal or formative assessment to high-stakes assessment. Formative assessment focuses on providing specific feedback and repetitive practice to maximize simulation learning (Issenberg et al., 2005). An example of formative assessment is feedback structured around the categories and behavioral descriptors from a valid and reliable assessment tool. Formative assessment fosters development and assists learners to progress toward desired outcomes (INACSL Standards Committee, 2021e). Constructive feedback influences learners' perceptions and motivation (Sultan & Victor, 2021). Feedback is a cornerstone of the teaching and learning process, especially in formative assessment, because it bridges gaps in learning and performance. Formative and immediate feedback on specific knowledge and performance elements addresses gaps and provides suggestions for improvement (Sultan & Victor, 2021).

Feedback should be given either immediately or well before the next simulation activity (Sultan & Victor, 2021). Written feedback that is clearly constructed can be a powerful tool to improve performance, as learners can refer to it often; written feedback may be delivered in the learning management system in response to a post-simulation reflection assignment. Facilitators deliver some feedback during debriefing to provide immediate evaluation and foster reflection (Bryant et al., 2020). The advocacy/inquiry method structures debriefing around uncovering learners' cognitive frames that underpin behavior performance and allows educators to provide mini-teaching to close performance gaps; though group presence sometimes creates tension between feedback, psychological safety, and professional integrity thereby necessitating more specific, written feedback directed at individual learners. Verbal feedback can be difficult to use when learners struggle with retention, comprehension, and implementation. Nursing learners report they receive more verbal feedback but have difficulty remembering or implementing behavior change over time (Sultan & Victor, 2021).

Repetitive practice is a key to formative assessment allowing educators to monitor the trajectory of behavior performance. Learners need opportunities to repeat psychomotor skills in simulation more than once to ensure competency (Bryant et al., 2020). Educators can build repetitive practice experiences and formative assessments across a curriculum with scaffolding scenarios of increasing complexity that move from stand-alone skill performance to holistic patient care. We can also use repetitive practice for cognitive and communication skills. For example, the NLN provides examples of reflection assignments called Finish the Story in the Advancing Care Excellence series; Finish the Story assignments use the sequential simulation format where learners visit the patient or a family member at a future point in time and respond in writing by describing their unfolding clinical judgment or communicating with the patient in first person.

Summative Assessment

Summative assessment focuses on measuring outcomes at a discrete point in time, such as at the end of a course (INACSL Standards Committee et al., 2021e). Ideally, learners have previous exposure to the simulation environment, similar patient experiences, and an opportunity to become familiar with the assessment tool in formative experiences before a summative assessment (INACSL Standards Committee et al., 2021e), and simulation assessments are just one method to assess whether or not learners pass a course. We need to use caution with summative assessment until facilitators have adequate training and establish interrater reliability (Bryant et al., 2020) and intrarater reliability. Summative assessment prioritizes scoring learners' behavior at a discrete point in time over providing feedback to supplement learning and skill acquisition.

There are many barriers to summative assessment. Although many educators are skilled at giving feedback to improve learning and behavior performance, few are prepared to use simulation for summative assessment owing to the complexity of scenario design, testing for validity and reliability of the scenario and assessment tools, and rater training (Oermann et al., 2016). Summative assessment involves inherent time pressure that may increase learners' anxiety because it takes place at a discrete point in time compared to the ongoing nature of learning promoted by formative assessment (Arrogante et al., 2021).

High-Stakes Assessment

High-stakes assessment measures outcomes and has significant implications or consequences, such as merit pay, academic or job progression, or course grades (INACSL Standards Committee et al., 2021e). Our colleagues in medicine have used high-stakes simulation assessments in the form of computer-based objective structured clinical examinations (OSCEs) as part of the Step 3 examination for U.S. Medical Licensure (Boulet, 2008), but there are fewer descriptions in the nursing literature.

To follow evaluation best practices, high-stakes assessment involves multiple scenarios representing a variety of situations in which to apply knowledge and demonstrate skill. OSCEs require students to rotate through scenarios designed to assess competency. Assessment involves a combination of direct observation, checklists, learners' verbal presentation, and follow-up activities (Lewis et al., 2017). Typically, there are eight to ten stations lasting three to ten minutes each, and stations focus on developing discrete competencies (Oermann et al., 2016). In nursing, high-stakes simulation assessment could focus on end-of-program competencies. Rizzolo et al. (2015) investigated the feasibility of using simulation for end-of-program assessment by pilot testing and revising scenarios targeting physical assessment and interventions, clinical judgment, quality and safe care, and teamwork skills.

SIMULATION IN PRACTICE SETTINGS FOR PROFESSIONAL DEVELOPMENT

Simulation continues to add value at the later stages of learning and training, such as post-licensure residencies (Bryant et al., 2020). Yet, the evidence surrounding simulation effectiveness with post-licensure clinicians is not as strong as the body of literature for pre-licensure nurses. Systems issues, including supplies, time, and cost, may prohibit simulation research in practice settings and contribute to the gap in the literature (Cantrell et al., 2017). There is evidence around the effectiveness of simulation to help new nurses practice medication administration (Myroniak & Elder, 2021) as well as team training in resuscitation scenarios (Abildgren et al., 2022). Virtual simulations are a promising modality, especially because they are flexible enough for learners to choose the time and place without detracting from direct patient care (Rouleau et al., 2022).

CHAPTER SUMMARY

The Healthcare Simulation Standards of Best Practice™ guide simulation design, implementation, evaluation, and facilitator training. A robust body of evidence supports simulation and formative assessment across care environments. Maturity in our simulation disciplines allows for performance assessment at the levels of learner, patient, and system across modalities. A focus on curriculum integration allows for competency-based education and communication of simulation outcomes across simulation programs.

References

Abildgren, L., Lebahn-Hadidi, M., Mogensen, C. B., Toft, P., Nielsen, A. B., Frandsen, T. F., Steffensen, S. V., & Hounsgaard, L. (2022). The effectiveness of improving healthcare teams' human factor skills using simulation-based training: a systematic review. *Advances in Simulation, 7*, Article 12. https://doi.org/10.1186/s41077-022-00207-2

Aebersold, M., Lee, D., & Nelson, J. (2023). In P. R. Jeffries (Ed.), *Clinical Simulations in nursing education: Advanced concepts, trends, and opportunities* (2nd ed., pp. 177–194). Wolters Kluwer.

Alexander, M., Durham, C. F., Hooper, J. I., Jeffries, P. R., Goldman, N., Kardong-Edgren, S., Kesten, K. S., Spector, N., Tagliareni, E., Radtke, B., & Tillman, C. (2015). NCSBN simulation guidelines for prelicensure nursing programs. *Journal of Nursing Regulation, 6*, 39–42.

Arrogante, O., González-Romero, G. M., López-Torre, E. M., Carrión-García, L., & Polo, A. (2021). Comparing formative and summative simulation-based assessment in undergraduate nursing students: nursing competency acquisition and clinical simulation satisfaction. *BMC Nursing, 20*, Article 92. https://doi.org/10.1186/s12912-021-00614-2

Aul, K., Bagnall, L., Bumbach, M. D., Gannon, J., Shipman, S., McDaniel, A., & Keenan, G. (2021). A key to transforming nursing curriculum: integrating a continuous improvement simulation expansion strategy. *SAGE Open Nursing, 7*, 1–7. https://doi.org. 10.1177/2377960821998524

Bala, L., Kinross, J., Martin, G., Koizia, L. J., Kooner, A. S., Shimshon, G. J., Hurkxkens, T. J., Pratt, P. J., & Sam, A. H. (2021). A remote access mixed reality teaching ward round. *The Clinical Teacher, 18*(4), 386–390. https://doi.org/10.1111/tct.13338

Boulet, J. R. (2008). Summative assessment in medicine: the promise of simulation for high-stakes evaluation. *Academic Emergency Medicine, 15*, 1017–1024. https://doi.org/ 10.1111/j.15532712.2008.00228.x

Bradley, C. S., Flaten, C. B., Muehlbauer, M. K., Woll, A., & Clark, L. (2023). Engaging standardized patients in nursing education. In P. R. Jeffries (Ed.), *Clinical Simulations in Nursing Education: Advanced Concepts, Trends, and Opportunities* (2nd ed., pp. 210–225). Wolters Kluwer.

Bryant, K., Aebersold, M. L., Jeffries, P. R., & Kardong-Edgren, S. (2020). Innovations in simulation: Nursing leaders' exchange of best practices. *Clinical Simulation in Nursing, 41*(C), 33–40. https://doi.org/10.1016/j. ecns.2019.09.002

Cantrell, M. A., Franklin, A. E., Leighton, K., & Carlson, A. (2017). The evidence in simulation-based learning experiences in nursing education and practice: An umbrella review. *Clinical Simulation in Nursing, 13*, 634–677. https://doi.org/10.1017/j.ecns.2017.08.004

Chickering, A. W., & Gamson, Z. F. (1987). Seven principles for good practice in undergraduate education. *AAHE Bulletin*, 3–7. Accessed December 16, 2022. https://files. eric.ed.gov/fulltext/ED282491.pdf

Choi, J., Thompson, C. E., Choi, J., Waddill, C. B., & Choi, S. (2021). Effectiveness of immersive virtual reality in nursing education: systematic review. *Nurse Educator, 47*, E57–E61. https://doi.org/10.1097. NNE.000000000001117

Eppich, W., & Cheng, A. (2015). Promoting excellence and reflective learning in simulation (PEARLS): Development and rationale for a blended approach to health care simulation debriefing. *Simulation in Healthcare, 10*, 106–115. https://doi.org/ 10.1097/SIH.0000000000000072

Forneris, S. G., Tagliareni, M. E., Jeffries, P. R., & Rizzolo, M. A. (2017). National League for Nursing and Simulation Innovation Resource Center. In C. Foisy-Doll, & K. Leighton (Eds.), *Simulation champions: Fostering courage, caring, and connection* (pp. 61–69). Wolters Kluwer.

Franklin, A. E., & Blodgett, N. P. (2021). Simulation in undergraduate education. In T. Schneidereith (Ed.), *Annual Review of Nursing Research: Healthcare Simulation, Volume 39*, (pp. 3–31). Springer. https://doi.org. 10.1981/0198-8794.39.3

Gaba, D. A. (2004). The future vision of simulation in healthcare. *Quality and Safety in Health Care, 13*(supp1), i2–i10.

Hayden, J. K., Smiley, R. A., Alexander, M., Kardong-Edgren, S., & Jeffries, P. R. (2014). The NCSBN National Simulation Study: A longitudinal, randomized, controlled study replacing clinical hours with simulation in prelicensure nursing education. *Journal of Nursing Regulation, 5*, S1–S64.

INACSL Board of Directors. (2011). Standards of best practice: Simulation. *Clinical Simulation in Nursing, 7*, S1–S20.

INACSL Board of Directors. (2013). Standards of best practice: Simulation. *Clinical Simulation in Nursing, 9*, S1–S32.

INACSL Standards Committee. (2016). INACSL standards of best practice: Simulation[SM]. *Clinical Simulation in Nursing, 12*, S1–S50.

INACSL Standards Committee, McDermott, D. S., Ludlow, J., Horsley, E., & Meakim, C. (2021a). Healthcare simulation standards of best practice prebriefing: Preparation and briefing. *Clinical Simulation in*

Nursing, *58*, 9–13. https://doi.org/10.1016/j.ecns.2021.08.008

INACSL Standards Committee, Persico, L., Belle, A., DiGregorio, H., Wilson Keates, B., & Shelton, C. (2021b). Healthcare simulation standards of best practice facilitation. *Clinical Simulation in Nursing*, *58*, 22–26. https://doi.org/10.1016/j.ecns.2021.08.010

INACSL Standards Committee, Decker, S., Alinier, G., Crawford, S. B., Gordon, R. M., & Wilson, C. (2021c). Healthcare simulation standards of best practice the debriefing process. *Clinical Simulation in Nursing*, *58*, 27–32. https://doi.org/10.1016/j.ecns.2021.08.011

INACSL Standards Committee, Bowler, F., Klein, M., & Wilford, A. (2021d). Healthcare simulation standards of best practice professional integrity. *Clinical Simulation in Nursing*, *58*, 45–48. https://doi.org/10.1016/j.ecns.2021.08.014

INACSL Standards Committee, McMahon, E., Jimenez, F. A., Lawrence, K., & Victor, J. (2021e). Healthcare simulation standards of best practice evaluation of learning and performance. *Clinical Simulation in Nursing*, *58*, 54–56. https://doi.org/10.1016/j.ecns.2021.08.016

Issenberg, S. B., McGahie, W. C., Petrusa, E. R., Gordon, D. L., & Scalese, R. J. (2005). Features and uses of high-fidelity medical simulations that lead to effective learning: A BEME systematic review. *Medical Teachers*, *27*(1), 10–28.

Jeffries, P. R. (2005). A framework for designing, implementing, and evaluating simulation used as teaching strategies in nursing. *Nurse Education Perspectives*, *26*(2), 96–103.

Jeffries, P. R., & Rizzolo, M. A. (2007). Designing and implementing models for the innovative use of simulation to teach nursing care of ill adults and children: A national, multi-site, multi-method study. In P. R. Jeffries (Ed.). *Simulation in Nursing Education, From Conceptualization to Evaluation* (pp. 147–159). Wolters Kluwer.

Jeffries, P. R. (2016). *The NLN Jeffries Simulation Theory*. Wolters Kluwer.

Johnson, B. K. (2019). Simulation observers learn the same as participants: The evidence. *Clinical Simulation in Nursing*, *33*, 26–34. https://doi.org/10.1016/j.ecns.2019.04.006

Johnson, B. K., Zulkosky, K., & O'Regan, S. (2023). Observer roles: their purpose, power and value to health care simulation. In P. R. Jeffries (Ed.), *Clinical Simulations in Nursing Education: Advanced Concepts, Trends, and Opportunities* (2nd ed., pp. 146–162). Wolters Kluwer.

Kim, J., Park, J., & Shin, S. (2016). Effectiveness of simulation-based nursing education depending on fidelity: A meta-analysis. *BMC Medical Education*, *16*, 152. https://doi.org/10.1186/s12909-016-0672-7

Leighton, K. (2017). Curriculum development in nursing simulation programs. In C. Foisy-Doll & K. Leighton (Eds.), *Simulation Champions: Fostering Courage, Caring, and Connection* (pp. 397–428). Wolters Kluwer.

Lewis, K., Bohnert, C. A., Gammon, W. L., Hölzer, H., Lyman, L., Smith, C., Thompson, T. M., Wallace, A., & Gilva-McConvey, G. (2017). The Association of Standardized Patient Educators (ASPE) Standards of Best Practice (SOBP). *Advances in Simulation*, *2*, 10. https://doi.org/10.1186/s41077-017-0043-4

Lioce, L. (Ed.), Downing, D., Chang, T. P., Robertson, J. M., Anderson, M., Diaz, D. A., Spain, A. E. (Assoc. Eds.), & the Terminology and Concepts Working Group (2020). Healthcare Simulation Dictionary—Second Edition. Rockville, MD: Agency for Healthcare Research and Quality; September 2020. AHRQ Publication No. 20-0019. https://doi.org/10.23970.simulationv2

Miller, G. E. (1990). The assessment of clinical skills/competence/performance. *Academic Medicine*, *65*(9), s63–s67.

Morse, C., Fey, M., Kardong-Edgren, S., Mullen, A., Barlow, M., & Barwick, S. (2019). The changing landscape of simulation-based education. *American Journal of Nursing*, *119*(8), 42–48. https://doi.org/10.1097/01.naj.0000577436.23986.81

Myroniak, K., & Elder, S. (2021). Improving safe medication in new RNs using simulation. *Journal of Continuing Education in*

Nursing, 52(1), 30–33. https://doi.org/ 10.3928/00220124-20201215-08

National League for Nursing Board of Governors. (2015a). Vision for teaching with simulation. NLN Vision Series. http:// www.nln.org/docs/default-source/about/ nln-vision-series-(position-statements)/ vision-statement-a-vision-for-teaching-with-simulation.pdf?sfvrsn=2

National League for Nursing Board of Governors. (2015b). Debriefing across the curriculum. NLN Vision Series. http:// www.nln.org/docs/default-source/about/ nln-vision-series-(position-statements)/ nln-vision-debriefing-across-the-curriculum. pdf?sfvrsn=0

Oermann, M., Kardong-Edgren, S., & Rizzolo, M. A. (2016). Summative simulation-based assessment in nursing programs. *Journal of Nursing Education, 55*, 323–328. https://doi. org/10.3928/0148434-20160516-04

O'Regan, S., Molloy, E., Watterson, L., & Nestel, D. (2021). 'It's a different type of learning.' A survey-based study on how simulation educators see and construct observer roles. *BMJ Simulation & Technology Enhanced Learning, 7*, 230–238. https:// doi.org/10.1136/bmjstel.-2020-000634

Park, C. S., Murphy, T. F., & the Code of Ethics Working Group. (2018). Healthcare Simulationist Code of Ethics. http://www.ssih.org/ Code-of-Ethics

Rizzolo, M. A., Kardong-Edgren, S., Oermann, M. H., & Jeffries, P. R. (2015). The National League for Nursing project to explore the use of simulation for high-stakes assessment: process, outcomes, and recommendations. *Nursing Education Perspectives, 36*, 299–303. https://doi.org/10.5480/ 15-1639

Rogers, B., Baker, K., & Franklin, A. E. (2020). Learning outcomes of the observer role in nursing simulation: a scoping review. *Clinical Simulation in Nursing, 49*, 81–89. https://doi.org/10.1016/j.ecns.2020.06.003

Rouleau, G., Gagnon, M., Cote, J., Richard, L., Chicoine, G., & Pelletier, J. (2022). Virtual patient simulation to improve nurses' relational skills in a continuing education context: a mixed-methods study. *BMC Nursing,*

21, Article 1. https://doi.org/10.1186/ s12912-021-00740-x

Roye, J., Anderson, M., Diaz, D. A., & Rogers, M. (2021). Considerations for the effective integration of virtual simulation in the undergraduate curriculum. *Nursing Education Perspectives, 42*(6), e173–e175. https://doi.org/10.1097/01. NEP.0000000000000740

Rudolph, J., Simon, R., Dufresne, R., & Raemer, D. (2006). There's no such thing as "Nonjudgmental Debriefing": A theory and method for debriefing with good judgment. *Simulation in Healthcare, 1*(1), 49–55.

Rutherford-Hemming, T., Alfes, C. M., & Breymier, T. L. (2019). A systematic review of the use of standardized patients as a simulation modality in nursing education. *Nursing Education Perspectives, 40*(2), 84–90.

Sim, J. J. M., Rusli, K. D. B., Seah, B., Levett-Jones, T., & Liaw, S. Y. (2022). Virtual simulation to enhance clinical reasoning in nursing: A systematic review and meta-analysis. *Clinical Simulation in Nursing, 69*, 26–39. https://doi.org/10.1016/j.ecns. 2022.05.006

Sittner, B. S. (2016). Extra! Extra! Read all about it! The INACSL Standards of Best Practice[SM] have been revised! *Clinical Simulation in Nursing, 12*, s1–s2. https://doi. org.10.1016/j.ecns.2016.10.002

Sullivan, N., Swoboda, S. M., Breymier, T., Lucas, L., Sarasnick, J., Rutherford-Hemming, T., Budha-thoki, C., & Kardong-Edgren, S. (2019). Emerging evidence toward a 2:1 clinical to simulation ratio: A study comparing the traditional clinical and simulation settings. *Clinical Simulation in Nursing, 30*, 34–41. https://doi.org/ 10.1016/j.ecns.2019.03.003

Sultan, B., & Victor, G. (2021). Bachelor of science in nursing students' perceptions regarding educator feedback. *Journal of Nursing Education, 60*(10), 577–581. https:// doi.org/10.3928/01484834-20210729-07

Tanner, C. A. (2006). Thinking like a nurse: A research-based model of clinical judgment in nursing. *Journal of Nursing Education, 45*, 204–211. https://doi.org/ 10.3928/01484834029960601-04

Watts, P., Rossler, K., Bowler, F., Miller, C., Charnetski, M., Decker, S., Molloy, M., Persico, L., McMahon, E., McDermott, D., & Hallmark, B. (2021). Preamble. *Clinical Simulation in Nursing*. https://doi.org/10.1016/j.ecns.2021.08.006

Waxman, K. T., Bowler, F., Forneris, S. G., Kardong-Edgren, S., & Rizzolo, M. A. (2019). Simulation as a nursing education disrupter. *Nursing Administration Quarterly*, *43*(4), 300–305. https://doi.org/10.1097/NAQ.00000000000000369

13

Service-Learning

Heather C. Voss, PhD, RN

CHAPTER OVERVIEW

This chapter provides an overview of service-learning as a critical pedagogy and clinical teaching-learning strategy to prepare nurses to be leaders in diverse health care environments now and in the future. Topics include alignment with nursing education initiatives, values, and best practices on design and implementation of service-learning in collaboration with clinical partners. Service-learning exemplars are discussed.

INTRODUCTION

Service-learning is a structured and experiential teaching strategy used in many disciplines to integrate theory and practice through service and community engagement (Murray, 2013; Yancey, 2016). It requires careful planning and preparation, community-academic partnering, and clear linkages to curricular goals and activities. Students engaged in service-learning collaborate with clinical partners to address an identified need. Service-learning is most commonly defined as a teaching and learning strategy that integrates meaningful experiential community service with instruction and reflection to enrich the learning experience, teach civic responsibility, and strengthen communities (Voss, 2016).

Service-Learning in Nursing Education

Specific to nursing education, service-learning is a credit bearing clinical learning experience whereby nursing students participate in an organized service activity that addresses an identified community/organizational need and uses reflection to gain further understanding of course content, broader appreciation of the discipline, and an enhanced sense of personal values and civic responsibility (Murray, 2013; Deal et al., 2020).

Service-learning is not a course or discipline in itself but rather a method that engages students through active learning in authentic clinical environments. This active learning helps to develop professional competencies including social awareness and responsibility related to social justice and cultural competence with diverse populations (Alpin-Snider et al., 2023). Reflection facilitates the connection between theory and practice, fosters critical thinking, and leads to deeper understanding of professional values (Curtin et al., 2015).

Nursing faculty have adopted service-learning as a pedagogical strategy for authentic learning by exposing students to real life health challenges in community and hospital-based settings; including experiences in interprofessional collaboration, problem solving, ethical decision-making, change management, and cultural competence (O'Shea et al., 2013). Service-learning has been documented to increase civic responsibility, communication skills, awareness of health care disparities, social injustices, cultural proficiency, and personal growth (Murray, 2013; Deal et al., 2020; Alpin-Snider et al., 2023).

EVIDENCE SUPPORTING SERVICE-LEARNING IN NURSING CLINICAL EDUCATION

Studies have shown positive correlation between service-learning and the development of the professional nurse role and values (Alpin-Snider et al., 2023). A few seminal studies are offered here. Loewenson and Hunt (2011) observed stronger beliefs related to the contribution of structural causes of homelessness, and an understanding that personal causes are not responsible for homelessness in a pre-post service-learning experience. Their study provided evidence that nursing students were more comfortable affiliating with homeless individuals and had stronger beliefs in finding solutions to address homelessness after their service-learning experience. They were among the first to report an increase in positive attitudes and non-stigmatizing attitudes toward homeless individuals when students had opportunities to confront stigmatizing attitudes and better understand the experiences of a marginalized population to foster more compassionate and culturally competent nursing care.

In a more recent study, students participating in a four-hour service-learning foot soak clinic for people experiencing homelessness (PEH) demonstrated improved attitudes toward homelessness after the service-learning experience (Richmond & Noone, 2020). A pre-posttest using the Attitudes Toward Homelessness Inventory and thematic analysis of student reflections substantiated findings from similar service-learning programs with PEH that included a decreased belief that homelessness is the result of an individual's behaviors, and increased empathy and comfort with affiliating with people who are unhoused.

Jarrell et al. (2014) measured empathy toward individuals living with poverty among students who participated in a service-learning experience. In the post intervention assessments, students reported that they believed society had a responsibility to help poor people and there was a decrease in blaming of poor individuals for their status. Multiple students in this study noted that clients' inability to comply with their treatment was due to lack of resources (i.e., structural barriers), not knowledge as they had originally believed. The findings in the Jarrell et al. study demonstrated that student awareness of the influence of societal pressures on health and health care resulting in greater empathy for people who are economically disadvantaged. Subsequent studies substantiated the findings in the Jarrell study (Alpin-Snider et al., 2023).

In their seminal study, Groh, Stallwood & Daniels (2011) measured impact of service-learning on leadership and social justice in 306 undergraduate nursing students. In their analysis of findings, they found an overall increase in self-reported leadership skills and social justice interest.

In a systematic review of qualitative studies on service-learning, Taylor and Leffers (2016) identified the following themes of service-learning outcomes: professional competency development, integration of knowledge for professional nursing role, greater understanding of community strengths and needs, collaboration and teamwork, civic engagement, emotions and adjustment, transformation and personal growth, and cultural awareness and competency.

Alignment with Nursing Education Initiatives

Service-learning is a valuable pedagogy for preparing nursing students for professional nursing practice with an emphasis on the socio-political and structural influences on health. Service-learning aligns with current and emerging nursing education initiatives in the United States and can aid in meeting educational competencies for students (O'Shea et al., 2013; Murray, 2013).

National League for Nursing Competencies

The National League for Nursing (NLN) developed competencies to facilitate clinical education excellence (NLN, 2019). The Academic Clinical Nurse Educator competencies are specific to the facilitation of learning that occurs primarily in the clinical setting within an academic program of nursing education (NLN, 2018). The NLN Academic Clinical Educator Competencies are:

▸ Function within the Education and Health Care Environments

▸ Function in the Clinical Educator Role

▸ Operationalize the Curriculum

▸ Abide by Legal Requirements, Ethical Guidelines, Agency Policies, and Guiding Framework

▸ Facilitate Learning in the Health Care Environment

▸ Demonstrate Effective Interpersonal Communication and Collaborative Interprofessional Relationships

▸ Apply Clinical Expertise in the Health Care Environment

▸ Facilitate Learner Development and Socialization

▸ Implement Effective Clinical and Assessment Evaluation Strategies

Service-learning aligns with the NLN competencies and creates a unique opportunity for clinical faculty to integrate clinical teaching that best meet course outcomes in both traditional and non-traditional health care environments, and develop and sustain reciprocal relationships with clinical partners and students through authentic learning.

Faculty tend to choose service-learning pedagogy due to prior service-learning experience and/or work with the nonprofit sector, a personal commitment to civic duties through student engagement with communities and real-world issues, and impact on students and contributions that students made in the community. Service-learning is a transformative experience that is meaningful to faculty as well as students. Service-learning as a critical pedagogy creates an opportunity for clinical faculty to apply their expertise, participate in and contribute to community and clinical partner initiatives, and strengthen academic presence in their community (Cooper, 2014).

The NLN competencies for graduates (2022) guide nurse educators to design curricula that best prepares nurses for contemporary and emerging health care environments, and that is informed through context, relevance, and best evidence. The NLN competencies for graduates are *Human Flourishing; Nursing Judgment; Professional Identity, and Spirit of Inquiry*. Students who participate in service-learning during their nursing education program are exposed to and articulate with the human condition in diverse and often compromised circumstances that leads to problem identification, critical appraisal and reflection, assessment of personal and professional values, impacts of policy, ethical questions, and moral comportment. Whether service-learning projects take place in hospitals or in community-based settings, students and their clinical faculty are members of a team to improve health and contexts of care through inquiry, critical appraisal, and collaborative decision-making.

Future of Nursing Competencies

The 2020–2030 Future of Nursing Report (National Academies of Science, Engineering and Medicine, 2021) moves nursing education toward prioritizing health equity in curriculum to address the health disparities and improve health for all members of society. In order to best prepare nurses to address systemic inequities in health care, nurse educators will need to ensure that students are exposed to and articulate with social influences on health and have longitudinal community-based learning experiences where they interact with diverse groups of people with varied cultural beliefs and backgrounds across the life span, collaborate with other professions, and participate in thinking and action to remove barriers associated with structural racism in health care and associated educational institutions (NAS, 2021).

The NLN (2019) provided the following recommendations for ensuring clinical faculty are integrating social influences (determinants) of health recommended by the report into Nursing Education Curricula (NLN, 2019, p. 6):

> Utilize the NLN toolkit to provide evidence-based approaches to teaching/learning strategies related to the SDH [social determinants of health].

> Raise students' consciousness about SDH, how to develop an inclusive understanding of the SDH, and how recognizing the shared impact of the SDH on health and wellness leads to new perspectives related to differences and mitigates bias and racism.

> Create partnerships with community agencies to provide experiences that intentionally expose students to address the impact of SDH on patients, families, and communities.

> Thread SDH education throughout the program of learning in varied educational settings (e.g., classroom, clinical settings, and simulation-learning environments).

> Be intentional about providing opportunities for students to assess and implement actions to address SDH in a variety of health care settings.

> Develop curricula that strengthen the links between SDH, health equity, and nursing's social mission.

The emphasis of service-learning is on collaborating with communities to address community concerns and SDH. Service-learning's reciprocal and principle centered partnering between community and academia uses critical reflection and mutual problem solving to address systematic inequalities that lead to poor health (Gillis & MacLellan, 2010; Voss, 2016). The NLN competencies for nurse educators, graduates, their recommendations for ensuring students are exposed to the broader context of health and wellness, and the 2020–2030 Future of Nursing Report provide an unequivocal imperative that service-learning be a standard teaching-learning strategy in nursing education and the preparation of nurses in alignment with nursing's vision, values, and mission.

SERVICE-LEARNING AND NURSING EDUCATION THEORY, VALUES, AND MISSION

Service-learning has been described as a philosophy, a program, and a high impact approach to meet educational goals (Richmond & Noone, 2020; Deal et al., 2020; Yancey, 2016; Cooper, 2014). In service-learning, nursing students apply professional values, behaviors and skills necessary for competent and safe practice in complex health care delivery models. Students who participate in service-learning gain important insights into nursing's professional scope of practice in broad societal contexts whereby the provision of direct health services may not be the most important factor in becoming or staying healthy (Wros et al., 2015).

Service-learning provides opportunities for transformational experiences consistent with nursing's values early in professional formation. Transformational learning occurs when assumptions are challenged, stigmatizing beliefs and inequities are acknowledged, and worldviews are redefined to reflect socio-political truths (Mezirow, 2003). Experiential Education, Emancipatory Knowing, Transformational Learning, and Critical Pedagogy provide foundational theoretical frameworks for service-learning.

Experiential Education

Experiential learning occurs through the construction of knowledge and meanings from real life experiences and is rooted in constructivist epistemology. Characteristics of constructivist learning include the active participation of learners in their learning, ackowledgment of prior learning as foundational to current learning, interaction with others leading to greater understanding and shared meanings, and a focus on real world or authentic activities (Hedin, 2010). Experiential education places the student at the center of the learning process so that learning itself becomes a process of interacting with the environment resulting in an outcome as a consequence of the interaction (Carver, 1997).

Central to experiential education is the importance of reflection, and the notion of reciprocity in the learning process. Service-learning is situated within authentic experiential contexts relevant to the development of professional nursing competencies and values through the provision of a service or need. Nursing students are provided opportunities to actively engage with their environment in order to link new experiences and meanings with prior experiences and meanings. Assimilation and accommodation of new meanings occur first through recognition of commonalities between new and previous experiences, and then through identification and exploration of what is different and why. It is the exploration of commonalities and differences which lead to refinement and extension of existing knowledge (Yardley et al., 2012).

Emancipatory Knowing

In 2008 Chinn and Kramer introduced the Pattern of Emancipatory Knowing: the praxis of nursing (Chinn & Kramer, 2011; Peart & MacKinnon, 2018). They chose the term emancipatory because of its link to underlying critical social perspectives and its inference as an outcome of nursing practice. Emancipatory knowing is defined as "the ability to recognize social and political problems of injustice or inequity, to realize that things could be different, and to identify or participate in social and political change to improve people's lives" (Chinn & Kramer, 2011, p. 64). The awareness of and reflection on the social, cultural, and political status quo that results in institutional inequities provides a beginning dialog in the identification of cultural and social norms needed to create fair and just conditions; such dialog cultivates understandings of how problematic social conditions converge, reproduce, and remain in place to sustain inequities within society (Chinn & Kramer, 2011).

Emancipatory knowing, as the fifth pattern of knowing, is integrated into nursing's four fundamental patterns developed by Carper (1978): Personal, Empiric, Aesthetic, Ethics. While it focuses on developing an awareness of social problems and action to create social change, it does not exist independently of ethical, personal, aesthetic, or empirical knowing. Acting comes in the form of praxis, and praxis in nursing occurs when all the knowing patterns are integrated in a way that supports social justice (Kagan et al., 2014). Emancipatory knowing provides a critical framework for nursing students to learn how to advocate for social justice and to question structural barriers that result in health disparities and health care inequity. The emancipatory knowing framework challenges nursing educators to push students beyond theorizing and toward praxis in preparation for professional nursing in today's complex health care environment. Service-learning is a valuable pedagogical approach for developing emancipatory praxis in nursing students.

Critical Pedagogy

The term critical service-learning was introduced into the service-learning literature in 2008 (Mitchell, 2015; Latta et al., 2018) and helps distinguish between traditional and critical approaches to service-learning pedagogy. Critical Service-Learning is focused on activities that are focused on social justice, social change, power and privilege, and authentic relationships with community members (Latta et al., 2018; Harkins et al., 2020). Critical service-learning focuses on analysis of power structures and social changes that works to redistribute power through authentic relationships, reciprocity and an emancipatory nursing lens (Gillis & MacLellan, 2010). In their early description of Critical Service-Learning, Gillis & MacLellan suggested that in traditional service-learning student outcomes are emphasized over community change; that students were viewed as service providers; that community partners were presented as in need of something; and that relationships were based on a power orientation. Gillis and MacLellan proposed that in order to prepare competent and caring nurses for professional practice, educators need to incorporate a critical perspective into nursing education through critical service-learning.

DESIGN AND IMPLEMENTATION OF NURSING SERVICE-LEARNING

Service-learning experiences require dedicated faculty who are committed to experiential learning and who embody a teaching philosophy that is consistent with the critical and transformative nature of service-learning. Community-academic partnership, reciprocity, deep learning, and a critical philosophic orientation are central to service-learning in today's socio-political health care context. Community-academic partnerships are the cornerstone for service-learning in nursing clinical education. An infrastructure that creates reciprocity between community partners (inpatient and outpatient) provides essential resources for faculty to develop longstanding relationships with clinical partners for service-learning projects (Voss, 2016).

A Community-Academic Partnership focused on addressing population and system level gaps through the establishment of mutual goals is essential for successful service-learning implementation (Voss, 2016; Harkins et al., 2020). Clinical partners need to be involved in the development and evaluation of service-learning projects and projects must align with the everyday life of the agency in order to be sustainable. As partnership also benefits the students. In a recent study by Harkins et al. (2020), positive relationships between students, their community partner, and their professors resulted social justice attitudes, reciprocity, and reflective processes among the learners.

The Community-Campus Partnership for Health (CCPH) published principles for greater collaboration between academic institutions and community partners. The Guiding Principles of Partnerships are:

- The Partnership forms to serve a specific purpose and may take on new goals over time.
- The Partnership agrees upon mission, values, goals, measurable outcomes, and processes for accountability.
- The relationship between partners in the Partnership is characterized by mutual trust, respect, genuineness, and commitment.
- The Partnership builds upon identified strengths and assets, but also works to address needs and increase capacity of all partners.
- The Partnership balances power among partners and enables resources among partners to be shared.
- Partners make clear and open communication an ongoing priority in the Partnership by striving to understand each other's needs and self-interests, and developing a common language.
- Principles and processes for the Partnership are established with the input and agreement of all partners, especially for decision-making and conflict resolution.
- There is feedback among all stakeholders in the Partnership, with the goal of continuously improving the partnership and its outcomes.
- Partners share the benefits of the Partnership's accomplishments.

> ▸ Partnerships can dissolve, and when they do, need to plan a process for closure.
> ▸ Partnerships consider the nature of the environment within which they exist as a principle of their design, evaluation, and sustainability.
> ▸ The Partnership values multiple kinds of knowledge and life experiences.

The CCPH principles (2013) serve as standards of reciprocity for service-learning within community academic partnerships and provide a foundation for service-learning that includes shared decision-making and joint responsibility for the successes, failures communications, and modifications to service-learning projects. Reciprocity between preceptor, clinical faculty and student, intentional planning and project clarity, meaning-ful and authentic experience, and valued and beneficial contributions which address a need are cornerstones to successful service-learning experiences (Voss, 2016). The Community-Campus Partnership for Health website https://ccphealth.org/ provides tools and information on best practices partnership development within a social justice and health equity framework for community action. The American Association of Colleges of Nursing also provides a valuable resource on developing practice partnerships: https://www.aacnnursing.org/Academic-Practice-Partnerships/Implementation-Tool-Kit.

Faculty Preparation for Service-Learning

Faculty who use a service-learning model apply the principles of good partnership to guide the planning and implementation of the service-learning project. In addition, fac-ulty need to assess the appropriateness of the project for the level of student learning relevance to student learning goals, and alignment with the clinical partner and organi-zational project goals.

Clearly articulated roles and responsibilities of students, faculty, and preceptors are critical to planning and implementation and create the foundation necessary in relation-ship building between student, faculty and preceptor (Voss, 2016; CCPH, 2013). Use of a project outline to co-create the service-learning project provides a guide for mutual understanding, planning, and goal alignment (Voss, 2016). Table 13.1 provides a template for a project outline and a sample.

The clinical faculty and the preceptor develop the project outline together before the students begin their term. The co-created project outline is shared with the students at the beginning of the term and during initial meetings with the preceptor and the faculty. The project outline serves as the roadmap for service-learning projects and becomes a working document for students, preceptor, and faculty to refer to during the term. An agreement that outlines student contribution to the project can also be helpful (Box 13.1).

Preceptors report better experiences when they and the clinical faculty identified service-learning projects which aligned both with coursework and organizational priori-ties, and when realistic goals and student expectations were identified (Voss, 2016).

Clinical Partner Preparation for Service-Learning

Clinical partners benefit when provided with the course information and student learning outcomes. As partners in the service-learning project, they should be consulted about opportunities to facilitate student learning needs as well as the project or initiative the

TABLE 13.1

Project Outline Template and Sample

Project Outline Template	Project Outline Sample
Partnering Agency	CBO.US
Project Name	Navigating resources for low income families with high needs children
Preceptor Name/Contact	
Student(s) Name/Contact	
Faculty Name/Contact	
Desired Project Outcome	Improved navigation of resources and services as demonstrated through increased self-sufficiency among I-CAN clients and providers Reduced barriers to self-sufficiency and health literacy among I-CAN clients as demonstrated through I-CAN Self-Sufficiency Matrix.
Project Goals for the Term	Identify high risk population Identify barriers to resource navigation/health literacy Analyze causes of poor resource navigation among at-risk population Enroll and engage up to four at-risk individuals in the I-CAN program Use client-centered, trauma-informed nursing approach Use evidence to guide nursing actions
Project Activities (to meet goals) for the Term	Literature review Key informant interviews: clients, staff, service providers Develop service navigation algorithm/concept map for clients and providers Attend coalition meetings Home/client visits Agency huddles
Project Time Line for the Term	Wk 1: Meet with preceptor/faculty, review outline, discuss roles and responsibilities, begin population assessment Wk 2 etc.:
Meeting Times	Every Wed at 2:00 PM at agency
Project Team, Roles, and Responsibilities	Preceptor: Faculty: Student:

students are collaborating on. This approach provides a reciprocal relationship between student and the preceptor/organization. The clinical preceptor collaborates with nursing faculty, and at times students, to identify service-learning projects that address a gap in health-related services, surveillance and program evaluation, or a specific community or organizational need, and that aligns with the student's academic coursework. Common service-learning projects include population-specific needs assessments to

---

BOX 13.1

Service-Learning Project Agreement

Student name: Date:

Agency: Project contact person:

Contact information (phone and email):

Describe in detail planned student contribution to project (Use project outline information)
Specific deliverable student will produce:
Due date for presentation of project work to key stakeholders _____
Due date for submission of deliverable to contact person _____
Amendments (include dates):

---

identify gaps in community resources, programs, structural barriers, and inequities of resource distribution; program development and evaluation related to health impact assessments; community outreach efforts; programmatic adjustments; public policy and purpose; and direct services. Hospital-based service-learning projects often correlate with quality and process improvement initiatives.

Clinical partners collaborate with faculty on learning opportunities, serve as a resource, and provide guidance for students, and contribute to and oversee student learning. Service-learning preceptors may come from diverse professional backgrounds such as mental health/psychology, social work, medicine, public health, education, and administration as well as nursing.

Faculty presence is critical to the community academic partnership (Voss, 2016). Routine check-ins with the preceptor and the students provide opportunities for clarifying questions, linking coursework to project activities, and role clarity. Preceptors report greater satisfaction when faculty meet regularly with them, but also allow autonomy in directing the project and the students (Voss, 2016). Preceptors should anticipate that students present their project to all stakeholders, and receive a hand-off summarizing the student's work (Table 13.2).

Service-learning projects are rarely completed in a single academic term. The hand-off ensures continuity over multiple terms and demonstrates a longitudinal commitment to the partnership. For example, students may conduct a community needs assessment for a population/community health course in collaboration with a community-based partner and then develop an implementation plan for a leadership course later in their program. The handoff is an opportunity to demonstrate accountability to the project and those involved. Students who are part of an ongoing project benefit from reading the project hand-offs from their peers establishing context, history, and continuity.

Student Preparation for Service-Learning

Students should be oriented to the concept of service-learning (Shea et al., 2022), the principles of partnership (CCPH, 2013), the project details, the stakeholders/population, and the desired outcomes. In service-learning, students are active members of a project or health care team. Accountability to the project/stakeholders and active learning to

TABLE 13.2

Sample Handoff

Criterion	Description
Situation	➤ Summary of project ➤ Potential or actual impact of project on individuals, population, and/or organization
Background	➤ Brief history of project
Assessment	➤ Data collected during the term ➤ Tools used ➤ Interventions or implementation plan
Recommendation	➤ Recommendations for next steps ➤ Resources and contacts used during the term ➤ Pearls of wisdom or advice for next student(s)

address course outcomes are important elements to review. Expectations, role clarity, linkages to course outcomes and professional nursing development are integral to the student's experience and deep learning. Engagement of students in the project planning, providing opportunity for input, and shared decision-making enhances meaningfulness of the experience. Students should be prepared for active learning in authentic and at times, unpredictable environments, and difficult conversations on systemic and structural racism, inequity, social change, and analysis of societal power structures.

Students may feel uncomfortable with the population they are working with, may experience moral distress due to circumstances of people's lives, and may need to confront their own experience with trauma, inequity, stigma, and bias. In today's trauma-informed culture, students need to be aware of their own points of sensitivity, pain, and triggers, and have a plan for addressing them should they arise.

Pre-brief/debrief provide opportunity for faculty, students, and the preceptor to dialog about difficult circumstances; collaborate on mutual goals and actions to address concerns, moral discomfort and distress; offer alternative perspectives; and deepen the relationship. Table 13.3 provides examples of pre-brief, debrief, and reflection prompts that can be tailored to any service-learning project.

Reflection is a fundamental component of service-learning (Curtin et al., 2015). Critical Reflective Inquiry (CRI) is one framework to guide reflection that leads students toward action-oriented development. Three phases comprise CRI: descriptive, reflective, and critical/emancipatory (Curtin et al., 2014).

ASSESSMENT OF SERVICE-LEARNING: STUDENT AND COMMUNITY BENEFIT

A framework for measuring impact of service-learning projects provides an opportunity for reciprocity between student learning, the community being served, and the partnering agencies; ensures that students are exposed to outcomes-driven practice;

TABLE 13.3

Example of Discussion Prompts

Pre-Brief	Debrief	Critical Reflective Inquiry
What do I/we know about the situation/population?	What additional information did we learn from ____?	Descriptive: the situation or circumstance
What are the causes of causes?	How am I feeling about ____?	What went well/didn't go well?
How am I feeling about the situation/working with the population/project?		
What is the purpose/goal of ____?		
What don't I/we know?	What questions remain unanswered about ____?	Reflective:
Why is this happening to ____ (a group, as situation, an individual)?	What resources are available to help address the questions raised?	Re-examination of a situation, in relationship to standards, theories, and knowledge, the student's intentions, attitudes, values, and emotions, and influences on the outcome.
	How am I feeling about the situation?	How am I feeling about what happened?
		What was learned/challenged?
What do I/we need to know before moving forward?	What are the barriers preventing ____?	Critical/emancipatory:
How will the ____ (population/community) be impacted by____?	What steps need to be taken in order to move forward?	What needs correcting?
What are the barriers preventing ____?		What will I change for next time?
What steps need to be taken in order to move forward?		What is my role in making a change?
		How will I apply what I learned to future situations?

and captures the positive impact of nursing students on community health and organizational goals. Clinical evaluation metrics that measure student learning should reflect course outcomes. Service-learning specific measures should be assessed relative to the goals identified on the project outline, reviewed regularly through the term, and especially at the end of the term with the students, preceptor, and faculty. The student hand-off mentioned above provides documentation of student contribution, data collected and recommendations/next steps, and service-learning goal attainment and evaluation. For projects that are ongoing (i.e., over multiple academic terms), the handoff serves as a longitudinal measure of impact on community and organizations, support the community academic partnership, and facilitate opportunities for faculty scholarship.

The literature is rich with the positive impacts service-learning has on nursing student professional role development, but less has been published on the impact of service-learning projects on community, organization, and individuals (Yancey, 2016; Mitchell, 2015). Metrics for measuring service-learning require collaborative community partnerships; access to clients/community, data collection methods focused on outcomes, and consistent engagement of faculty and students over time (Voss et al., 2012). Outcome metrics using the critical service-learning approach focus on community, population, organizational, and system-policy level outcomes in addition to those associated with student learning and competencies.

EXEMPLARS OF SERVICE-LEARNING IN NURSING EDUCATION

Exemplars of service-learning can be found in the literature. Four are highlighted here with discussion of community academic partnership, preparation, course linkages, and assessment. Street Nursing and Home Visiting are Service-Learning Programs that were initiated through grant funding. The High School Completion and Hospital Based Quality Improvement are service-learning projects that were developed between faculty and clinical partners. All four serve as clinical placements for population/community health and/or leadership courses in a baccalaureate nursing program. Students participate in clinical experiences that address course outcomes and clinical course competencies while engaging in projects/initiatives that address an identified gap or need in the community or organization. The projects described below are the result of strong community-academic partnerships and ongoing community engagement.

Street Nursing

Consistent with nursing's values and mission, and in alignment with the Future of Nursing Report recommendations, the Street Nursing Program is a service-learning experience whereby students and faculty partner with community-based organizations and health care providers to develop relationships, coordinate care, and provide vital nursing care to people who are experiencing homelessness (PEH). In their study, Richmond and Noone (2020) describe a foot soak clinic and the impact the service-learning experience had on nursing student's attitudes toward homeless people. The students participated by washing, massaging, and applying essential oils and lotions to feet of unhoused individuals: guests of the clinic. Students sat on stools below the level of the guest and followed the guest's lead as to how much or how little conversation occurred, creating space for relationship and trust building.

The foot soak clinic was situated inside a church. In addition to the foot soak clinic there was a mobile health van operated by a local federally qualified health center and a free meal provided by the church. Students received orientation and preparation materials prior to the four-hour foot soak experience that included readings and videos on empathy, power structures, common health problems among people who are unhoused, and a guided reflection (Richmond & Noone, 2020).

The foot soak clinic provided an opportunity for students to meet people "where they are," use their developing nursing knowledge and the art of nursing to gain trust, develop empathy, and in some cases provide direct service. For the majority of students, it was an opportunity to meet and talk with PEH for the first time. The foot soak clinic provided episodic and longitudinal clinical experiences for all junior-level students for seven years. During that time community partnerships solidified, and trust among the unhoused community strengthened.

A critical element to service-learning programs and projects is the continuous presence and long-standing relationship with the community partner(s) and the people served. Faculty continued to operate the foot soak clinics when students weren't in session. Foot soak clinics continued during the Covid-19 pandemic and were faculty led until students returned to in-person clinical learning. In 2022, the foot soak clinic received local and federal funding for the development of a Street Nursing program.

Street Nursing provides opportunity for critical service-learning for both undergraduate and graduate students. Students in collaboration with their faculty and community partners address health and social consequences related to the Covid-19 pandemic, reproductive (sexual) health, mental/behavioral health, and substance use disorder, specifically related to opioids. The street nursing faculty supervise and guide students in culturally-aligned care, management of social influences on health, and barriers to health equity. Students build trusting relationships, assist people with immediate needs, help with navigation of health and social services, implement harm reduction strategies, and facilitate telehealth visits with federally qualified health centers (FQHC) from the field. In addition to the foot soak clinics and street rounds, students participate in population level projects that focus on structural, societal, cultural, and political contexts, and health care response and action. The project outline and handoff provide longitudinal documentation of project progression and outcomes.

Graduate students in the Masters in Nursing Education program design and develop curriculum to prepare and support students during their service-learning rotation on the street team. Psychiatric Mental Health Nurse Practitioner Students gain valuable insights into innovative mental/behavioral health care that meets people where they are and guides them toward safer environments.

All students are introduced to the Street Nursing program. Radical Humility, Trauma and Violence Informed Care, Social Determinants of Health, Structural Racism, and Harm Reduction concepts and practices are integrated in the curriculum and practiced during the clinical experiences on the Street Nursing Team. Pre-brief, debrief, and reflection are key to the student's learning, and occurs regularly. Students along with their faculty and preceptors unpack their thoughts, feelings, and frustrations about the systemic barriers that often prevent PEH from moving out of homelessness and potential and real actions that are needed to improve health outcomes.

Addressing Social Influences of Health with Interprofessional in Home Visiting

Home visiting has historical significance in community health nursing, but has not been as common in the United States due to institutionalization of health care. The Interprofessional Care Access Network (I-CAN) is an interprofessional education (IPE) home visiting program whereby health professional students and nursing faculty partner with community-based organizations and health care providers to assess and address challenges to accessing care associated with social influences and structural barriers (Wros et al., 2015). The I-CAN program is a service-learning model that provides services to improve health and health outcomes of people who are negatively impacted by social influences such housing and income instability, health literacy, stigma/bias, language barriers, and generational poverty. The I-CAN community partners refer clients to the program based on co-created criterion. Student teams along with the nursing instructor meet clients where they are: at home or in the community. Students learn about the complexity of people's lives and gain perspectives of the challenges when navigating health and social services. Students participate and contribute to care coordination, resource finding, and health education. Students use and develop active listening, culturally appropriate communication and teaching, patient centered approaches, and interprofessional collaboration to address the client's needs and self-identified goals (Bradley et al., 2018). Consistent with the critical element of reciprocity, I-CAN has demonstrated positive impact on the clients who participate in the program including improved housing, medication management, primary care access, and reduced utilization of emergency services (Bradley et al., 2018).

The I-CAN program has been replicated and is a model for long-standing community academic partnerships, community networking and service, and interprofessional education through service-learning. As with the street team exemplar, faculty continue to meet with clients and community during the time students are off session. Consistent faculty engagement provides an opportunity for faculty to practice nursing in their community, develop their critical pedagogy, and collaborate with clinical partners in service to their community.

High School Completion Service-Learning Project

An eight-year service-learning project called the "Big Idea" was developed in partnership with a United Way Chapter and School of Nursing faculty to address poor academic success among high school students. Students collaborated with elementary school, middle school, and high school leaders with a commitment that the community's class of 2020 would have a 100% high school completion.

Starting in 2011, nursing students developed tools to assess academic success and related barriers. Each year students surveyed the class of 2020 (starting when they were in fourth grade). Based on responses, schools created programs to address identified needs. For example, one of the middle schools added a graduation coach to their staff. Students participated in programs and initiatives to address identified needs including support for bullying, substance use, unstable housing, food insecurity, and mental health support. The nursing students reported the anonymous survey results to the United Way Board of Directors each year which resulted in strategic funding and community support programs.

The Big Idea service-learning project provided nursing students with an intimate experience of how social influences impact child and teenage health and health trajectory, well-being, and academic success. Students used age and culturally appropriate communication, collaborated across sectors and professions to address student identified concerns, and contributed to resource allocation and program development. The Big Idea Class of 2020 was a success and saw an increase in graduates who completed high school on time (https://unitedwayofjacksoncounty.org/big-idea-time/). The United Way and the School of Nursing continue their partnership through a second longitudinal service-learning project called the Big Idea Next. The Big Idea Next focuses on students who do not complete high school within four years. This ongoing collaboration and partnership are hallmarks of service-learning and a School of Nursing's commitment to community.

Hospital-Based Service-Learning: Quality Improvement Projects

Service-learning for hospital-based clinical learning may be less common, but is ideal for leadership courses. Quality improvement, change management, and organizational policy change provide rich opportunities for nursing students to learn about health care systems, patient safety, and quality initiatives. Leadership concepts such as shared decision-making, interprofessional collaborative practice, accreditation and regulation scope of nursing practice, the work environment and unit culture, and workplace violence are integrated in service-learning projects and create unique opportunities for the development of professional nursing competencies.

Hospital-based service-learning, like community-based service-learning, is developed through building and sustaining mutual goals that meet both the student's academic needs (i.e., course outcomes and clinical learning) and the organization/project goals. Students who are paired with a nurse leader on a quality or process improvement initiative benefit from role modeling and contributions to a practice/process change. Service-learning projects may be self-limiting such policy revision, or ongoing. A root cause analysis of falls in one term, and then implementation of safety measures and evaluation in subsequent terms, is an example of an ongoing project. The project outline, agreement for student contribution, presentations to stakeholders, and the project hand-off provide opportunities for students to learn about role clarification, accountability, shared decision making, and professional commitment.

CHAPTER SUMMARY

Service-learning pedagogy is an evidenced-based teaching-learning strategy for clinical nursing education that aligns with nursing values and priorities. Faculty who develop and engage in service-learning are central to ensuring deep student learning and community partnership through mutual goals, meaning that both student learning needs and the community/organizational project goals are met. Successful service-learning requires strong, longitudinal community partnerships that address a need or gap in the community or organization and identified by the members of the community; clear linkages to course outcomes and learning; student, clinical partner, and faculty preparation; shared decision-making for achievement of mutual goals; and, faculty presence.

Critical service-learning provides an opportunity for students and their faculty in collaboration with the community they are partnering with to articulate with health inequity and disparity related to social-political constructs, professional nursing values, and ethical-moral comportment. Service-learning's impact is dependent on facilitating student engagement from knowledge attainment to action. Faculty who engage in service-learning have the opportunity to practice nursing and critical pedagogy while contributing to the development of nurses as leaders committed to social change and advocates for improved health and health outcomes for all.

References

Alpin-Snider, C., Behnke, L., & Fulks, E. (2023). A school of nursing and a community service agency close the gap for rural families with health disparities during covid-19: A novel approach to clinical education and service-learning. *The Journal of Service-Learning in Higher Education, 16,* 93–108. Retrieved from https://files.eric.ed.gov/fulltext/EJ1382268.pdf

Bradley, K. J., Wros, P., Bookman, N., Mathews, L. R., Voss, H., Ostrogorsky, T. L., & LaForge, K. (2018). The interprofessional care access network (I-CAN): Achieving client health outcomes by addressing social determinants in the community. *Journal of Interprofessional Care.* https://doi.org/10.1080/13561820.2018.1560246

Carper, B. (1978). Fundamental patterns of knowing in nursing. *Advances in Nursing Science, 1*(1), 13–23.

Carver, R. L. (1997). Theoretical underpinnings of service learning. *Theory into Practice, 36*(3), 143–149.

Community-Campus Partnership for Health. (2013). *Community Campus Partners for Health Board of Directors. Position statement on authentic partnerships.* Community-Campus Partnerships for Health. https://ccphealth.org/

Cooper, J. R. (2014). Ten Years in the Trenches: Faculty Perspectives on Sustaining Service-Learning. *Journal of Experiential Education, 37*(4), 415–428. https://doi.org/10.1177/1053825913513721

Chinn, P., & Kramer, M. (2011). *Integrated theory and knowledge development in nursing* (8th ed.). Elsevier Mosby.

Curtin, A. J., Martins, D. C., Schwartz-Barcott, D., DiMaria, L. A., & Ogando, B. M. S. (2015). Exploring the use of critical reflective inquiry with nursing students participating in an international service-learning experience. *Journal of Nursing Education, 54*(9), 95–98. https://doi.org/10.3928/01484834-20150814-17

Deal, B., Hermanns, M., Marzilli, C., Fountain, R., Mokhtari, K., & McWhorter, R. R. (2020). A faculty-friendly framework for improving teaching and learning through service-learning. *Journal of Service Learning in Higher Education, 10*(2020). Retrieved from https://files.eric.ed.gov/fulltext/EJ1242880.pdf

Gillis, A., & MacLellan, M. (2010). Service learning with vulnerable populations: Review of the literature. *International Journal of Nursing Education Scholarship, 7*(1), 1–27.

Groh, C. J., Stallwood, L. G., & Daniels, J. J. (2011). Service-learning in nursing education: Its impact on leadership and social justice. *Nursing Education Perspectives, 32*(6), 400–405.

Harkins, D. A., Grenier, L. I., Irizarry, C., Robinson, E., Ray, S., & Shea, L.-M. (2020). Building relationships for critical service learning. *U.S. Department of Education.* Retrieved from https://files.eric.ed.gov/fulltext/EJ1272313.pdf

Hedin, N. (2010). Experiential learning: Theory and challenges. *Christian Education Journal, 7*(1), 108–117.

Jarrell, K., Ozymy, J., Gallagher, J., Hagler, D., Corral, C., & Hagler, A. (2014). Constructing the foundations for compassionate care: How service-learning affects nursing students' attitudes towards the poor. *Nurse Education in Practice, 14*(3), 299–303.

Kagan, P. N., Smith, M.C., & Chinn, P. L. (Eds.). (2014). *Philosophies and practices of emancipatory nursing: Social justice as praxis.* Rutledge.

Latta, M., Kruger, T. M., Payne, L., Weaver, L., & VanSickle, J. L. (2018). Approaching critical service-learning: A model for reflection on positionality and possibility. *Journal of Higher Education Outreach and Engagement, 22*(2), 31–55.

Loewenson, K. M., & Hunt, R. J. (2011). Transforming attitudes of nursing students: Evaluating a service-learning experience. *Journal of Nursing Education, 50*(6), 345–349.

Mezirow, J. (2003). Transformative learning as discourse. *Journal of Transformative*

Education, 1(1), 58–63. https://doi.org/10.1177/1541344603252172

Mitchell, T. D. (2015). Using a critical service-learning approach to facilitate civic identity development. *Theory into Practice, 54*(1), 20–28.

Murray, B. (2013). Service-learning in baccalaureate nursing education: A literature review. *Journal of Nursing Education, 52*(11), 621–626.

National Academies of Sciences, Engineering, and Medicine. (2021). *The future of nursing 2020–2030: Charting a path to achieve health equity.* The National Academies Press. https://doi.org/10.17226/25982.

National League for Nursing. (2019). NLN core competencies for nurse educators. A vision for integration of the social determinants of health into nursing education curricula a living document from the national league for nursing. Retrieved from https://www.nln.org/education/nursing-education-competencies/core-competencies-for-academic-nurse-educators

National League for Nursing. (2022). Competencies for graduates of nursing programs. Retrieved from https://www.nln.org/education/nursing-education-competencies/competencies-for-graduates-of-nursing-programs

O'Shea, E., Planas, J., Quan, M., Greiner, L., Kazer, M., Babington, L. (2013). Service-learning initiatives in nursing education. *Journal of Catholic Higher Education, 32*(2), 265–281.

Peart, J., & MacKinnon, K. (2018). Cultivating Praxis Through Chinn and Kramer's Emancipatory Knowing. ANS. *Advances in Nursing Science, 41*(4), 351–358. https://doi.org/10.1097/ANS.0000000000000232

Richmond, R., & Noone, J. (2020). The impact of a service-learning foot soak experience on nursing students' attitudes towards the homeless. *Nursing Forum, 55*(2), 236–243. https://doi.org/10.1111/nuf.12421

Shea, L. M., Harkins, D., Ray, S., & Grenier, L. I. (2022). How critical is service-learning implementation? *Journal of Experiential Education, 1*(46), 1–18. https://doi.org/10.1177/10538259221122738

Taylor, S. L., & Leffers, J. M. (2016). Integrative review of service-learning assessment in nursing education. *Nursing Education Perspectives, 37*(4), 194–200.

Voss, H. (2016). Preceptors' experience of nursing service-learning projects. *Journal of Nursing Education, 55*(3), 150–154.

Wros, P., Mathews, L. R., Voss, H., & Bookman, N. (2015). An academic-practice model to improve the health of underserved neighborhoods. *Family Community Health, 38*(2), 195–203.

Yancey, N. R. (2016). Community-centered service-learning. *Nursing Science Quarterly, 29*(2), 116–119.

Yardley, S., Teunissen, P. W., & Dornan, T. (2012). Experiential learning: AMEE guide no. 36. *Medical Teacher, 34*, 102–115.

3

Assessment of Learning

14

Equitable Assessment Practices

Rana Halabi Najjar, PhD, RN, CPNP

CHAPTER OVERVIEW

This chapter reviews best practices in the equitable assessment of students. Topics include avoidance of high-stakes testing and other grading practices that do not contribute to the assessment of learning. Multiple strategies for equitable assessment and grading are discussed.

HISTORY OF GRADING

I begin this chapter by presenting a brief overview of the history of grading practices and how we arrived at the current grading system. This historical grounding between assessment, grading, and equity is a starting point rather than a comprehensive review of assessment and grading in the United States (US) education system. Examining our history is a way to understand how racism and discrimination are embedded in our systems and structures and extend to our assessment practices.

The earliest documented form of grading in the US was developed at Harvard University in 1646 using exit exams before awarding degrees; Yale University was the first to create a grading scale in 1785 (Espinola, 2017). Around the same time, at Cambridge University in England, a professor of chemistry, William Farish, employed a grading system that attempted to quantify learning (Hartmann, 2000). Before Farish, pedagogical approaches utilized an apprenticeship model with students receiving individualized training and feedback. Lecture halls were reserved for occasional speeches by famous philosophers and authors. Farish transformed educational spaces into lectures and numerical grades, eliminating the mentor model, which included individualized student learning and evaluation; thus promoting a learning approach of rote memorization and preoccupation with grades (Hartmann, 2000). In 1832, Yale extended their 4-point system from exit exams to individual classes, and the grade point average (GPA) was born. By 1837, Harvard began utilizing numerical grading, with educators shifting to the 100-point system. This grading method, spread across the US and the world, with many universities adopting some form of the numerical scheme. Educators recognized the harmful impact of grading, such as fostering competition, and chose to keep grades secretive to discourage student discord and conflict (Espinola, 2017).

Feldman (2019), in his book *Grading for Equity,* provides an overview of the history of grading, detailing five reasons for the impact of the political, social, economic, and scientific events that shaped schools in the US. He discusses the rise of manufacturing, migration and immigration, the development of intelligence testing, belief in universal education, and scientific discoveries of behaviorism (Feldman, 2019). I will discuss intelligence and standardized testing below. Behaviorism will be further discussed within the concepts of intrinsic and extrinsic motivation.

Standardized Testing

Alfred Binet, a psychologist, and his colleague, Theodore Simon, were the first to develop a standardized test to quantify intelligence by assessing memory, attention, and the use of logic (problem-solving skills). Binet aimed to improve the education system for children with learning challenges. Although he believed these skills could not be quantified into a single innate intelligence score since a number of factors, including background and experiences, could impact the results of this test, his work triggered the development of other forms of intelligence testing (McFadden, 2017). These tests reinforced the misguided and immoral belief that intelligence is innate and race-based. Soon the use of these tests to exclude, criminalize, and discriminate against Black and Brown people became widespread (Rosales & Walker, 2021). Binet criticized the fixed mindset ideology and stated, "A few modern philosophers assert that an individual's intelligence is a fixed quantity, a quantity which cannot be increased. We must protest and react against this brutal pessimism . . . with practice, training . . . we manage to increase our attention, our memory, our judgment and literally to become more intelligent than we were before" (Dweck, 2006, p. 5). One hundred years later, Binet's assertion continues to be supported by the research on the neuroscience of learning and growth mindset (discussed in Chapter 3, *The Science of Learning*).

Horace Mann is known as the father of American education and was influential in establishing a unified school system. He saw education as the 'great equalizer' and felt all children, regardless of income, class, or ethnicity, should have access to education (Carleton, 2009). In 1845, Mann recommended implementing tests to replace oral examinations to ensure proper documentation and evaluation of the educational environment. The results of this process were similar to the use of standardized testing today, including the narrowing of the curriculum to teach to the test, cheating scandals, public shaming of teachers, and poor performance of students from various ethnic and racial backgrounds (Lehigh University, 2013). Mann's purpose may have been to monitor the quality of education at that time, but what emerged was an administrative mechanism with oppressive political and philosophical ramifications (Garrison, 2020).

Tests have cultural underpinnings with social reproduction of what is deemed as valuable knowledge or behavior and are usually used to sort individuals (Garrison, 2020). Recently, universities began eliminating standardized testing as part of the admission requirement because it creates a barrier to increasing student diversity (Tugend, 2019). The elimination of these tests should be done not only to increase diversity but rather to achieve justice by righting a wrong that has been perpetuated for over a century.

ASSESSMENT AND GRADING

The etymology of the word assessment comes from the Latin root *assidere* which means "to sit beside." As educators, how much of our grading is "assessment" where we 'sit beside' our students, and how much of it is to keep them accountable, or worse, punish them? How much of our feedback is based on our judgment which comes from our ways of knowing and doing? Assessment is considered an important aspect of education, providing feedback for educators and students on learning outcomes. It may be graded or ungraded and can heavily impact pedagogical approaches. We should reflect on whether our thoughts, approaches to grading, and the discipline paradigm in nursing education align with best practices in equitable grading.

PROBLEMS WITH CURRENT GRADING AND ASSESSMENT PRACTICES
Lack of Knowledge of Students

Often, we begin teaching without pre-assessing gaps in student learning. Pre-assessments, individual or collective, can provide a road map of how we should approach a concept or topic and may activate prior knowledge for students. The discussion on the science of pre-assessments and ways to incorporate them in a learning plan is discussed extensively in Chapter 3, *The Science of Learning* and Chapter 7, *Backward Design: Aligning Outcomes, Assessments, and Activities*, respectively.

Instructor-Centered

Although faculty have implemented varied ways of assessing students, grades continue to be the method by which students' knowledge and abilities are assessed and recognized. We also use grades to control behaviors focusing on nonacademic factors such as punctuality, attendance, and participation. Conversely, we may reward other behaviors by awarding bonus points or extra credit that may not reflect learning (Feldman, 2019; Wormeli, 2018). In nursing, behaviors tend to be referred to as 'professionalism'. We must ask ourselves where the criterion for professionalism comes from and the relation to assessing learning outcomes. Are we grading on learning or compliance? Could the non-compliance be because of diversity or divergent ways of processing and learning and as a result of innovative thinking? If we want to build a more equitable assessment model, we should consider positioning all assessments from a student-centered approach. Henry Giroux, an educational theorist, says, "The first question is: Can learning take place if in fact, it silences the voice of the people it is supposed to teach? And the answer is Yes. People learn that they don't count" (Giroux, 2005, p. 15).

Motivation

Daniel Pink's book *Drive* discusses the research on motivation and the evolution of what 'drives' humans. He states that foundationally, human motivation was to survive, to seek food, water, and shelter. (Motivation 1.0) In the era of industrializa-tion, motivation shifted to focus on reward and punishment. Pink (2012) calls this 'operating system' Motivation 2.0, or what we commonly refer to as extrinsic motiva-tion. According to research, Motivation 2.0 still works sometimes for *routine* tasks but is deeply unreliable, outdated, encourages competition, and impedes lifelong learning (Baygi et al., 2017). Eminent scholars in learning and the alignment of teaching and assessment outcomes state that extrinsic motivation stifles curiosity, increases fear of failure and anxiety, and encourages surface learning (Biggs & Tang, 2011; Biggs e al., 2022). Extrinsic motivation negatively impacts mental well-being and encourages shortcuts and academic dishonesty because the focus is the end goal (the grade) and not the journey (learning) (Biggs & Tang, 2011). Academic dishonesty includes accept-ing help from external resources, plagiarism, lying, and cheating on assignments or exams. Although reasons for academic dishonesty are numerous and complex, evi-dence indicates a higher incidence of cheating among students that are grade- and not learning-oriented (Baran & Jonason, 2020; Yu et al., 2017).

There is an incongruence between what science has uncovered about motivation and what the educational system currently utilizes in assessment and grading prac-tices. Our goal as educators should be to facilitate intrinsic motivation for multiple reasons. Intrinsic motivation promotes creativity and life-long learning, increases self-esteem and resilience, buffers anxiety, and is more enduring for behavior change (Bayg et al., 2017; Gajda et al., 2017). In a meta-analysis of 120 studies spanning six decades of evidence on motivation and academic achievement, researchers concluded that creativity and academic achievement are closely linked (Gajda et al., 2017). We can limit extrinsic motivation and increase intrinsic motivation using the trauma-informed prac-tices outlined in Chapter 5, *Creating Inclusive Learning Environments*. Establish positive relationships with students to build safety and trust, and develop pedagogical activities to promote peer support and collaboration between faculty and students. Empower students by using a student-centered approach and providing voice and choice in their demonstration of learning and assessment practices (discussed below under building equitable practices). There is a misconception that trauma-informed practices would decrease rigor; however, the science on motivation indicates the opposite. The lack of progress and change in assessment and grading practices, a focus on grades rather than learning is what holds us back from creating rigor and academic robustness in our classrooms.

Unreliable and Unfair

From a quantitative perspective, the utilization of a 100-point scale is deeply flawed. Consider the 9- to 10-point interval between A (90–100), B (80–89), C (70–79), D (60–69), and the 60-point interval of an F (0-59). When students receive a 0 or a missed or even a 40 on a failed assignment, it presents challenges for educators and students. First, the 0 does not provide any information on the student's learn-ing which defeats the purpose of an assessment. Second, if the grade was used to motivate a student, again, it did not meet that purpose. Rather, a 0 may create the opposite situation with future assignments or exams if the student believes it will require too much effort to make up for the 0. Third, it skews the average, making it

TABLE 14.1

Sample Gradebook

Assignment	% of Final Grade for Each Assignment	Student Alpha	Student Beta	Student Delta
Quiz 1	10	90	95	0
Exam 1	25	80	95	0
Quiz 2	10	80	100	95
Exam 2	25	85	95	100
Cumulative Final Exam	30	80	80	100
Final Grade	100%	82.25%	91%	64.5%

an invalid method for a summative grade. In the example in Table 14.1, we can see students Alpha and Beta receive a final grade of B and A, respectively, and we feel this is accurate and representative of their performance throughout the term. But when we add Delta to this scenario, it reflects the unreliability and the unfairness of grading. Delta failed the class even though they outperformed their peers in the last three assessments of the class and received a 100% on an assessment that is supposed to represent cumulative learning over the term. We may think a scenario where a student would get zeros only to turn around and get hundreds in the last few assessments of the class is unlikely, but it does not change the fact that these grading practices are inaccurate and inequitable.

Another unfair and unreliable method is averaging homework, quizzes, and exams attained over the term for a final grade. This is a practice many of us employ, but it does not represent learning or mastery and penalizes students while they are still in the process of learning (Feldman, 2019; Wormeli, 2018). Alternatives to this type of grading are presented in the last section of this chapter.

Subjectivity and Bias

There are multiple ways implicit bias operates in assessment and grading practices. One way is through unconscious tendencies that assess students based on the educator's learning and communication style, strengths, educational background, values, experiences, and practices which could disadvantage some students (Inoue, 2022; Lundquist & Henning, 2020). Evidence has existed for over 100 years on the subjectivity and unreliability of assessment practices in both writing and math (Starch & Elliott, 1912, 1913). When this research was replicated a few years ago, similar results were found, showing evidence of the subjectivity of grading (Brimi, 2011). We can endeavor to be objective, but assessment is a subjective process, and inherently biased, regardless of what is being assessed. "[Educators] create assessments based on their professional judgment of what is to be assessed and how, which is a subjective process. We need to acknowledge this and not apologize for it" (O'Conner, 2022, p. 24).

The Question of Curves and Inflation

The discussion of grade inflation is a common one in academia. According to Muller in *The Tyranny of Metrics,* mistrust of judgment is what drove the development and adherence to metrics (Muller, 2019). When the metrics do not add up, we use a grading curve and adjust student scores to yield a distribution where the majority of students fit within a bell-shaped curve. The use of a bell-shaped curve ". . . portrays a dominant educational discourse that assumes success or failure in learning can be normalized" (Tan Yuen Ling et al., 2020, p. 1). Educators use curves to address grade inflation and deflation, adjust for exams being too easy or difficult, and identify the high-performing students from the low-achieving students (Tan Yuen Ling et al., 2020). Grading curves can be implemented in different ways. One method is throwing out questions that do not perform well psychometrically. This is a practice I used when I administered multiple-choice question exams and accepted that psychometrics was a meaningful way of assessing the reliability of each item. However, the flaw of using psychometrics to assess student learning is that it relies on a comparison of the 'high' vs 'low' performers on an exam. What cannot be accounted for in psychometrics is test-taking skills versus critical thinking or clinical judgment. Another method in which grade curves are used is to give all students the same amount of points to get the highest-scoring student up to 100% (Roell, 2019). This is an unfair practice. A student with a B on the exam may end up with an A after the curve but the student with a failing grade may still have an F. This practice may also create conflict and competition when the highest-scoring student is seen as the individual that threw off the curve for the other students (Roell, 2019). The third method a curve is used for is to adjust all the grades to create a bell-shaped curve, with a normal distribution of As through Fs. Creating a normal distribution of grades means the educator is using a norm-referenced which compares students' performance to one another, rather than a criterion-referenced which assesses students based on pre-set criteria or standards (O'Conner, 2022). A consequence of this grading practice is that it reifies the zero-sum ideology that one person's benefit or success requires another person's failure (O'Conner, 2022). When using curves and other methods of awarding extra points, educators and students are no longer focused on achieving higher levels of learning and shift the focus from learning to grades (O'Conner, 2022; Wormeli, 2018). If we believe our assessments are reliable methods for assessing learning outcomes, then we would not need to utilize grading curves.

GRADING AND ASSESSMENT PRACTICES IN NURSING

Using the NCLEX as a metric for evaluating undergraduate prelicensure programs places pressure on academic leaders and educators to ensure their students pass the test on the first try. Based on the National Council for State Boards of Nursing (NCSBN) guidelines, the Future of Nursing 2020–2030 recommends shifting away from using NCLEX pass rates as a metric for assessing the quality of education in nursing programs and instead focusing on assessments of leadership, faculty, students, curriculum, clinical experiences, and teaching and learning resources (National Academies of Sciences, Engineering, and Medicine (NASEM), 2021; Spector et al., 2020). Nurse educators should not solely use multiple-choice exams in their courses as an obligation to maintain first-time NCLEX pass rates. Dismantling racism and oppression require that we not succumb to coercive systems but collectively push for change and implement recommendations put forth by the Future of Nursing Report and NCSBN.

High-Stakes Testing

Sullivan (2014) provides an in-depth analysis of the concept of high-stakes testing in nursing and explicates the differences between high-stress and high-stakes examinations. A proctored admission essay would be considered high-stress because it may cause anxiety but is not the sole criterion for determining admission into a program. Whereas high-stakes is using an assessment, such as NCLEX, as the only method for obtaining a nursing license. Similarly, in a high-stakes testing environment, students who do not meet a minimum score on exit exams are denied their degrees. With recommendations that these types of exams can be a predictive measure for passing the NCLEX, nursing programs utilize them to prevent students from graduating until they pass the high-stakes exit exams to keep the program's first-time NCLEX pass rates high (Sullivan, 2014). The NCSBN and the National League for Nursing (NLN) have long discouraged the use of high-stakes testing as the sole determinant for graduation or eligibility for NCLEX (NCSBN, 2011; NLN, 2020). Five state boards of nursing (Alabama, Nevada, North Carolina, Oregon, and Texas) ". . . prohibit the use of high-stakes testing as a single measure to stop a nursing student from completion of a program if all other course requirements have been met" (Hunsicker & Chitwood, 2018, p. 185). Research provides evidence of the harm to student's mental health as a result of a high-stakes testing environment (Tagher & Robinson, 2016), indicating that this practice does not support a trauma-informed approach; thus, I would caution against any policy or practice that could potentially cause trauma or re-trauma.

Many educators support the NCLEX and celebrate the Next Gen NCLEX as a way to assess students' professional preparation (Dreher et al., 2019), but we must consider whether these are pathways that support dominant ways of knowing and doing. Disaggregating and explicating national NCLEX results by race and ethnicity may help us better understand the cultural implications and limitations of this standardized test (Muirhead et al., 2022). Following recommendations of changing the academic metrics for accreditation to second- or third-time pass rates (Loftin et al., 2020; Noone et al., 2018) would be a simple first step in mitigating the high-stake component and making these practices more equitable. Muirhead et al. (2022) also recommend adding authentic assessments at a national scale as it best aligns with competency-based education. Authentic assessment requires the students to demonstrate the application of concepts, knowledge, skills, and attitudes outside the classroom and in a real-world context (Maude et al., 2021; Poindexter et al., 2015) and may include performance in mock patient dialogues, clinical simulations, mixed-format exams, and oral or narrative responses (Muirhead et al., 2022).

BUILDING EQUITABLE GRADING AND ASSESSMENT PRACTICES

Although educators have implemented varied ways of assessing students, grades continue to be the method by which students' knowledge and ability are assessed and recognized. Equitable assessment and grading practices require a student-centered and authentic approach. Paolo Freire, a leading advocate on critical pedagogy, believed education should be utilized as a source of liberation through "critical consciousness." According to Freirean philosophy, authentic education is not about educators imposing their worldviews with the purpose of indoctrinating students, and not about passing on 'their knowledge'; rather it is about co-creating and re-creating knowledge through the process of dialoguing (Freire, 2000/1968). This type of dialoguing requires the pedagogical conditions upon which the epistemological curiosity of the teacher empowers students to transform their lived experience in the acquisition of new knowledge, fulfilling the purpose of education, which is to liberate human potential (Freire, 2000/1968). Our current learning and assessment practices leave no room for this emancipatory approach to education. The breakdown of oppressive practices requires the adoption of a Freirean approach to learning (Francis et al., 2020), and the legitimization of students' knowledge and experiences, empowering them to tackle health care's most pressing problems related to equity and justice.

Assessment Practices with Competence-Based Education

The recently released vision statement by the NLN emphasizes the use of criterion-based assessments with the integration of competency-based education (CBE (NLN, 2023). The statement recommends that educators personalize and co-create paths for success, recognizing that each student reaches mastery at a different pace. Other recommendations include using a student-centered approach to competency assessment and formative evaluation with feedback. The NLN vision statement discourages the use of multiple-choice exams and high-stakes testing for CBE assessments, recognizing the difficulty of making high-stakes decisions without adequate psychometric testing of rubrics (NLN, 2023).

My colleagues and I set out to develop reliable and valid rubrics to assess students for summative objective structured clinical examinations (OSCEs) on our campus (Najjar et al., 2016). We learned that the process is time- and resource-intensive, requiring multiple iterations. We were able to achieve high reliability on psychometric skills, but reliability for skills in the affective and cognitive domains was much harder to attain. We developed a training program that is implemented before the administration of each OSCE to maintain reliability among raters. We also had to be purposeful about which courses would have a formative, pass/no pass, or low-stakes summative OSCE (Najjar et al., 2016). Refer to Chapter 16, *Rubric Development*, for more information on developing reliable rubrics.

Developing Student-Centered Approaches through an Equity-Minded Lens

Creating a more equitable and inclusive learning environment requires educators to be equity-minded. Equity-minded educators ". . . question their own assumptions, recognize stereotypes that harm student success, and continually reassess their practices to create change" (University of Southern California Center for Urban Education, n.d.). They apply the critical paradigm to assess and acknowledge the role of power and oppression on policies, practices, and pedagogy that compromise assessment approaches (Montenegro & Henning, 2022). Equity-minded educators include multiple and diverse perspectives from assessment leaders, cultural agents (faculty and staff), and students in articulating learning outcomes and developing culturally responsive assessments, and mitigating inequity in assessments (Montenegro & Jankowski, 2017). Outcomes and assessments written solely from the perspective of educators are a reductionist approach; rather, involving students in this process provides them opportunities to be active agents, clarify the outcomes, and ensure the language is easily understood and realistic to achieve (Lundquist & Henning, 2020).

According to Montenegro and Jankowski (2017), culturally responsive assessments focus on outcomes to improve learning with considerations for varied ways of learning and demonstrating that learning. This requires co-creating assessments with the students while understanding that a person's identity cannot be separated from their experiences or how they create meaning from those experiences (Montenegro & Jankowski, 2017). The authors state, the ". . . English as a second language, first-generation student will experience college, acquire knowledge, and demonstrate knowledge differently than an international English as a second language first-generation student." and still different from a native English-speaking student (Montenegro & Jankowski, 2017, p. 9). Using non-traditional and ungrading practices discussed later in the chapter can be culturally responsive, especially if rubrics and assessments are co-created with students. Also, the Principles of Universal Design provide a framework for implementing culturally responsive assessment practices which is discussed in Chapter 6, *Frameworks to Engage Diverse Learners*.

PATHS TO EQUITABLE GRADING

Ideally, changes to assessment and grading practices occur at the systems level, wherein the field of assessment is aligned with initiatives on diversity, equity, and inclusion. Programs and services focused on this effort at the organizational level help support educators to make changes at the individual level (Lundquist & Henning, 2020). However, institutions that have not committed to decolonizing and dismantling oppressive practices present an additional challenge to nurse educators. Where and when possible, we should push systems to change and, in the same vein, understand that the policies of institutions where we teach and work may limit our ability to make changes. In the following sections, I will provide options to move toward more equitable grading. Table 14.2 presents suggestions if educators are unable to adopt non-traditional grading. I invite you to choose the option or options that are the most comfortable in this season of your career and would be accepted by your institution. One thing to consider as you make changes is that students may arrive in your classroom fully embracing the assessment and grading practices they have experienced. If they have been successful in receiving high marks, they may view deviations from the system as unfair and inequitable. They know 'the formula' for making the grade, and they may experience a loss with the changes to these practices. I would encourage using a trauma-informed approach focused on establishing safety, trust, collaboration, and peer support. Most importantly, and part of the trauma-informed approach, is engaging in wellness and self-care, focusing on self-compassion, and knowing your limitations as an educator. Faculty that have embraced non-traditional grading use a growth mindset recognizing that changing practices may require multiple iterations before finding an approach that

TABLE 14.2

Best Practices in Grading

Consider	Avoid	Rationale
Co-developing performance standards with students	Grading based on student behavior (late submission, absences, and participation)	Co-developing performance standards honors students' diversity and autonomy while maintaining a system based on shared values and expectations without impacting academic grading
Providing additional opportunities for learning or mastery	Extra credit or bonus points	Extra credit reinforces the ideology that learning is about grades, not mastery. This practice is inequitable for students with learning gaps or those that lack time to do 'extra' work
Providing formative feedback for homework	Grading homework	If letter grades or summative assessments are given, they should be post-learning rather than before or during learning
Providing formative feedback during the learning	Giving assignment and exam grades during the term	Penalizing students for attempts at mastering the material during the process of learning. Students should have the full term or semester to demonstrate meeting course outcomes
Giving individual grading or assessments as part of group work	Giving group grades	Group grades do not assess individual learning or achievement and are, therefore, inaccurate. Provide formative feedback for group work and grade individual learning.
Grading structures that support mastery learning by using rubrics with labels such as 'Beginning, Approaching Proficiency, Proficient, Excellent.' If feeling adventurous, try 'Youngling, Padawan, Jedi, Jedi Master.' Using a growth mindset 'Not yet, Almost there, Got it, Wow.'	Using words such as 'exceeds'	Considering the label used in rubrics because students often focus on labels rather than descriptions. Using 'exceeds' communicates that the students must perform beyond what is expected. A non-traditional grading approach would focus on progression throughout the term with the expectation of the last assessment/assignment being closer towards 'Proficient', 'Jedi', or 'Got it', as deserving of an 'A'
Using other measures of central tendency such as mode	Using mean to calculate summative grades and giving zeros	Means are flawed and inaccurate ways of assessing learning. A suggestion would be to use the mode + most recent submissions + professional judgment of educator
Including students in the assessment and grading process	Adopting a faculty-only approach to assessment and grading	Providing students with opportunities to assess their progress on the learning outcomes will enhance self-awareness, self-reflection, and metacognitive skills. The *Successful Learner* graphic created by the Alberta Assessment Consortium is a meaningful and simple example of students monitoring their progress. https://aac.ab.ca/wp-content/uploads/2018/01/Successful_Learners_English.pdf

TABLE 14.2

Best Practices in Grading *(Continued)*

Consider	Avoid	Rationale
Using self-assessment strategies to assess learning and effort	Using hours spent or number of tasks completed to determine effort	The number of hours spent on a task is not indicative of learning. Determining effort is biased and subjective and could potentially punish students for their learning gaps. Instead, consider using a brief reflection with the following prompts: "Explain what you did in this assignment. Describe how you did it. Articulate the lessons you learned and what you would do differently next time."
Provide opportunities for redos and retakes	Using the 100-point scale without opportunities to improve the grade	The 100-point scale is unreliable, unfair, and inaccurate in assessing learning. Using redos and retakes allows for opportunities for growth and teaches perseverance in the face of challenges. A suggestion with redos is asking students to submit a brief reflection using the prompts from the previous strategy.
Provide varied opportunities to demonstrate learning	Using multiple-choice question (MCQs) exams as the sole summative assessment of learning	Using multiple-choice exams (MCQs) as formative or low-stakes assessments and only in combination with other forms of assessments. Developing equitable MCQs requires knowledge of linguistic bias and adequate alignment of each item to course learning outcomes. Utilization of best practice principles of fairness, alignment, importance, and discrimination can promote equity. Item writing and analysis are discussed fully in Chapter 15.

Source: Feldman, J. (2019). *Grading for equity: What it is, why it matters, and how it can transform schools and classrooms* (1st ed.). Corwin, a SAGE publishing company; Wormeli, R. (2018). *Fair isn't always equal: Assessing and grading in the differentiated classroom* (2nd ed.). Stenhouse Publishers; O'Conner, K. (2022). *A repair kit for grading: 15 Fixes for broken grades* (3rd ed.). FIRST Educational Resources, LLC.

works for them and their students (Blum & Kohn, 2020; Ovalle, 2022). Making either incremental changes or rapid transformations of curriculum, courses, and schools will move us in the right direction toward justice.

Upgrading to Motivation 3.0

Motivation 3.0's 'operating system' is powered by intrinsic motivation and supported by science. The way to fuel Motivation 3.0 is through encouraging and facilitating the following: (1) autonomy by offering voice and choice, (2) mastery with clearly established goals and providing immediate feedback and challenges well matched with ability, and (3) purpose that is connected to the greater good (Pink, 2012). Upgrading to Motivation 3.0 requires shifting from traditional to non-traditional grading practices. This will not be easy, and it is normal to encounter resistance within ourselves and others.

Non-traditional Grading Practices

Exams are considered traditional assessments, but educators can begin to shift their grading to non-traditional assessments. Adopting non-traditional assessment practices may address some of the inequities in the learning environment by providing voice and choice. Diversification assessment is when faculty change their assessment practice to an alternative or non-traditional assessment; for example, changing the end-of-term exam to a presentation, project, or reflective writing (O'Neill & Padden, 2022). With this method, students can select between two or more ways to demonstrate learning, for example, choosing between a poster or a presentation. Research indicates that diversification and choice of assessment empower and accommodate the learning needs and strengths of students (O'Neill & Padden, 2022). Educators may also prefer to utilize a more structured approach, such as alternative assessment techniques. These types of assessments, sometimes called authentic assessments, promote creativity, autonomy, motivation, higher order, and critical thinking skills and include problem-based assignments, presentations, reports, reflective writing, concept maps, case-based scenarios, critical analyses, infographics, podcasts, blogs/vlogs, and portfolios (Elkhoury, 2020; Villarroel et al., 2018). Resources for alternative assessments are available in Table 14.3.

O'Neill (2022) suggests a seven-step process for implementing alternative assessments: (1) consider the course, (2) consider the diverse choices ensuring that they cater to different strengths, (3) develop equity or fairness between choices, (4) make standards explicit by providing examples and rubrics, (5) provide a rationale for choosing the assessment methods to ensure students make an informed decision (one assessment method could be the default if students do not select one in the time allotted), (6) support the process by offering time and opportunities for discussing the choices early in and throughout the process, and (7) evaluate by gathering students feedback (O'Neill, 2022). Educators can utilize a template to outline the assessment choices, details and weight of assessment, learning outcomes, equity markers, expected student workloads, and exemplars of the choices in case students are not familiar with the type of assessment offered (O'Neill, 2011). Students would be required to sign and submit to the template indicating what they chose. Evidence indicates that offering students to choose from more than two to three choices can be overwhelming (Montenegro & Jankowski, 2017; O'Neill & Padden, 2022).

Flexible Assessment for Student-Centered Approaches

Another inclusive, student-focused, transparent, and shared approach is called flexible assessment (see Table 14.4). Wanner et al. (2021) used a mixed-methods approach to evaluate a flexible assessment practice implemented in undergraduate and graduate courses. They found that using flexible assessments allowed students to capitalize on

TABLE 14.3	
Resources for Grading Practices	
Non-Traditional Grading Practice	**Link to Resource**
Alternative Assessment Tools	https://www.yorku.ca/bold/wp-content/uploads/sites/393/2020/11/Guide_Alternative_Assessments.pdf
	https://www.ucd.ie/teaching/t4media/choice_of_assessment.pdf
	https://www.ucd.ie/teaching/resources/assessmentfeedback/
	https://www.torontomu.ca/content/dam/mental-health-wellbeing/Documents/Flex-Learning-Res-Full.pdf
	https://heqco.ca/pub/differentiated-evaluation-an-inclusive-evaluation-strategy-aimed-at-promoting-student-engagement-and-student-learning-in-undergraduate-classrooms/
Labor-Based Grading	https://wac.colostate.edu/books/perspectives/labor/
	https://asaobinoue.blogspot.com/p/labor-based-grading-contract-resources.html
Specification Grading	https://www.insidehighered.com/views/2016/01/19/new-ways-grade-more-effectively-essay
	https://ii.library.jhu.edu/wp-content/uploads/sites/31/2019/03/Kelly-Making-Grades-Meaningful-with-Specs-Grading.pdf
	https://higheredpraxis.substack.com/p/tip-specs-grading
	http://matthematics.com/standards-based-grading-my-implementation/

their strengths; increase feelings of empowerment, control, motivation, and responsibility; and improve their ability to manage their course load with other courses. Schwartz et al. (2016) suggest that a path to learning and well-being in the educational setting is through flexibility, reminding us that high stress and anxiety are impediments to the cognitive process and learning. Students reported that this approach works best with the guidance and support of motivated educators (Wanner et al., 2021). Other flexible methods include the Bento and Buffet Approaches. Research is not available on the efficacy of these two approaches; however, in course evaluations, students seem to prefer the Buffet. According to Didicher, the Buffet is easier to implement, improves student engagement, and reduces stress (Didicher, 2016).

Table 14.4 provides examples of flexible learning with advantages and disadvantages to these approaches. The recommendation is to adopt the strategy that best meets the needs of the educator and students with considerations for pedagogical aspects such as content, topics, and other logistics.

Ungrading and Labor-Based Grading

The book *Ungrading: Why Rating Students Undermines Learning (and What to Do Instead)* provides readers with multiple approaches to ungrading or partial ungrading (Blum & Kohn, 2020), some of which are described in Table 14.5. Feedback on these

TABLE 14.4

Flexible Approach to Summative Assessments

Approach	Description	Advantages and Disadvantages
Flexible & Personalized (Wanner et al., 2021)	Undergraduate courses: ➤ Choose either an essay or report ➤ Choose submission days for all assignments (except take-home exam) ➤ Adjust pre-set weighting of assignments within 10% range up or down (i.e., choose to change the essay or report from the pre-set weight of 40% to either 30%–50% of the course grade) ➤ Choose how they wanted to receive feedback (written, audio, video, or personal consultation) ➤ All students had to submit learning journal and take-home exam Graduate courses: ➤ Choose to weight two tasks (group research presentations and individual research proposal) ➤ Choose the research topic and date of submission ➤ Students received formative feedback over a 6-week period	Advantages ➤ Students could capitalize on their strengths ➤ Choosing dates of submission reduced stress because it allowed them to coordinate with assignments in other courses ➤ Flexibility facilitated learning, improved motivation and accountability ➤ Transforms power relations and shifts power to students regarding assessment choice Disadvantages ➤ Having to make choices can be stressful ➤ Students regretted choices where they did better on lower-weight assignments ➤ Concerns over teaching duties transferred to students or not having teacher support ➤ Concerns over not having peer support with the flexibility to choose any topic of interest ➤ Increase workload for faculty to set up personalized assessment tasks in the learning management system
Bento Approach (Didicher, 2016)	Choose the weight of each assessment at the beginning of each term Or Choose between four different grading schemas with an option to omit one assignment (other assignments would have the added weight of the eliminated assignment)	Advantages ➤ Encourage self-reflection of strengths ➤ Reduce anxiety ➤ Omitting assignments reduced the workload on students and educator ➤ Can add a formative assessment to mitigate poor choices Disadvantages ➤ Students may make poor choices, and learning will suffer ➤ Personalizing choices can decrease engagement

TABLE 14.4

Flexible Approach to Summative Assessments *(Continued)*

Approach	Description	Advantages and Disadvantages
Buffet Approach (Didicher, 2016)	Students choose from a menu of assessments and select weights and due dates The agreement form is completed by a specified date Cannot choose an assignment more than once Can add assignments if they do not score well on an assignment Formative assessments are permissible in the form of drafts	Advantages ‣ Students focus on interests and skills ‣ Students can try a new skill/challenge and minimize the weight to decrease the risk of impacting their grade Disadvantages ‣ May increase workload for educators and students ‣ Students may procrastinate, which impacts learning and grades ‣ Students may make poor choices, and learning will suffer

promising practices includes students reporting less stress and more motivation and educators reporting better communication with students, less stress, and increase focus on teaching than grading (Blum & Kohn, 2020).

Another approach that is gaining traction in higher education is labor-based grading, where a grade is determined based on the 'labor' or work completed rather than grades awarded on individual assignments, papers, or activities. In this type of grading system, students completing all the work for the course will receive a B. Educators have implemented a variety of methods with labor-based grading with considerations to class participation or presence, number of assignments submitted, late submissions, process, and other elements including providing details for how students can 'labor' more to achieve an A or 'labor' less for a C. Educators state this system decentralizes grades, mitigates bias existing in writing and grading, co-creates language for a shared standard, and diminishes teacher and institutional power (Inoue, 2022; Ovalle, 2022). One critique of this approach is grading on effort. Feldman (2019) discourages grading based on effort since this process can be fraught with bias and leads to an inequitable practice. If you are considering this approach, I would recommend reading the e-book by Asao Inoue where he provides a thoughtful analysis of the words labor, empathy, and compassion (Inoue, 2022). Links to the e-book and resources are provided in Table 14.3.

Specifications Grading

Nilson (2015) identifies multiple problems with the current grading system and states that grades are not correlated with future success or achievement in employment. She offers a different alternative called specifications, or specs, grading. This grading system builds on competency-based education and mastery learning and includes three

TABLE 14.5

Ungrading and Partial Ungrading Approaches

Approach	Description
Ungrading Stommel (Chapter 1) Course: Writing/ Digital Rhetorics	1. Sets trajectories for learning (rather than learning outcomes) and co-creates *emergent outcomes* with students early in the term 2. Project: students work on a project during the term. They can choose whether they want to do this independently or in a group 3. Self-evaluation: students submit two to three/term. The first requires students to answer specific questions, and the last is more reflective 4. Process letters: this could be in written format or digital using voice or film. Students are required to describe their learning and its evolution over time 5. Peer assessments: students either evaluate each other through a formal process or engage in each other's work and provide feedback in an informal way 6. Grade: students are asked to grade themselves, with the educator reserving the right to change a grade. Most of the time, if the grade is changed, it's to give a higher grade. Sample syllabus: https://www.jessestommel.courses/dgst395/
Ungrading Blum Chapter 3 Course: Linguistic Anthropology	1. Decenter grading: focused on goals with no point breakdowns for work/assignments. Meets three times with students for approximately five-minute sessions over the term. The first meeting is to establish individualized learning goals (using Universal Design Principles); the second is to assess progress and adjust using their portfolios; and the third is an evaluation of the term. 2. Portfolio: represent learning during the term and contains self-assessments, specific activity, general reflection, feedback 3. Self-assessments: reflections on each assignment focused on what they learned, success in learning, and lessons learned 4. Specifics: students answer questions pertaining to topics throughout the term 5. General reflection: students reflect on eleven questions related to their learning and growth over the term 6. Feedback: students provide feedback on their experience in the course by answering a set of questions. They also provide data on how much of the readings and work they complete over the term. 7. Grade: student determines their grade at the end of the term and provides a rationale for their grade
Critique-driven gradeless Riesbeck (Chapter 8) Course: Artificial Intelligence Programming	1. Mastery: students focus on skill building through mastery, where they submit exercises, receive feedback (critique), and then revise. They continue to revise the exercises until they reach mastery. 2. Assignment: the expectation is that students complete three new exercises a week and revisions for previous exercises. 3. Critique: students do not receive a grade for any of their submissions. Instead, a single-point rubric is used where either the criteria are met or not. The criteria include specifications (of the computer program), readability, and reusability. If the students do not meet the criteria, they are given a critique and can revise and resubmit

TABLE 14.5

Ungrading and Partial Ungrading Approaches *(Continued)*

Approach	Description
	4. Grade: students are graded only at the end of the term on progress (assessment of progress for each exercise, whether they progressively selected harder exercises, etc.), quality (how good they were coding by the end of the course based on the level of critiques they were getting), and effort (submitted exercises steadily including revisions and level of individualized growth/learning over the term)
Grade Anarchy Schultz-Bergin (Chapter 11) Course: Philosophy of Law	1. Collaborative learning approach: on the first day of the class, students and educators co-create learning outcomes. Based on this work, the educator will develop a syllabus and presents the argument for the Grade Anarchy approach. 2. Attendance and participation: attendance and participation are encouraged but not mandatory. The educator has not seen a difference between both from other graded courses. In general, students do the readings and prepare for class discussion by having a summary of questions. 3. Buffet of learning: students were provided a selection of learning opportunities they could complete at their discretion. They could establish their own assignment schedule and determine what they wanted to complete based on their learning goals. Some of these assignments included argumentative summaries, summarizing key arguments to lead a discussion, papers, projects such as written debates or response 4. Required elements: students were required to submit three learning reflections spread throughout the term (beginning, middle, and final). These reflections focused on student goals, how they achieved their goals, and any modifications they wanted to make 5. Two learning conferences: students were required to meet with the educator at midterm and end of the semester to discuss learning reflections and portfolio 6. Midterm adjustments: the educator made some adjustments with students who had shown little effort to complete any assignments by providing either a suggested schedule, offering ungraded midterm exam questions (short answer and essay), or paper 7. Revisions: in future iterations, the educator would eliminate the buffet option and have a precise assignment schedule. They would require students to create a *portfolio* of their work that would represent their learning and growth so as to not be punitive if an assignment is missed. Students would also be able to negotiate for changes in the assignments or schedule.

Note: All ungrading practices in the table above are from the book *Ungrading: Why Rating Students Undermines Learning (and What to Do Instead)*. The educator's last name and the corresponding chapter have been listed, as well as the course they were teaching. This is not a comprehensive list but should provide a sample of the types of ungrading and partial ungrading practices currently being utilized by educators teaching in post-secondary or higher education institutions.

Source: Blum, S. D., & Kohn, A. (Eds.). (2020). *Ungrading: Why rating students undermines learning (and what to do instead)* (1st ed.). West Virginia University Press.

components: clear assignment specifications, bundles of assignments, and tokens. The educator should outline clear specifications (or expectations) of the requirements of each assignment to meet course outcomes. In specs grading, students receive either satisfactory/unsatisfactory or pass/fail, freeing the educators from perseverating over point allocation for assignments. The specs rubric should be written with a clear description of what is expected and provide exemplars. Based on educator discretion, students are allowed to resubmit their work. In specs grading, course grades are based on bundles where students can choose the bundle of assignments they want to complete and the final course grade they want to earn (Nilson, 2015). For more information, online resources are available in Table 14.3.

Faculty who use specs grading report that their experience with this type of grading frees them to focus more on feedback and mastery learning than grades (Jones, 2016; Mittel, 2016). The advantage of using specs is that it supports the trauma-informed principle of empowerment by giving choice. Providing feedback and options for choosing a grade is collaborative; however, shifting to a more culturally responsive approach would require co-creating rubrics and assignments. Opportunities for inequities may persist if academic learning gaps are not accounted for in this type of grading system.

Pass/No Pass or Satisfactory/No Credit

The use of summative grading is a barrier to learning. Methods such as contract, labor, specifications, and flexible grading practices provide students with autonomy and choice, but these approaches continue to tether learning to grades and potentially create inequities. Shifting our courses, curriculum, and programs to pass/no pass or satisfactory/no credit will provide educators with minimal constraints in making changes. Some higher education institutions have transitioned either optionally or entirely to grade-free; some such have shifted to satisfactory/no credit; and many medical schools across the US have transitioned to pass/fail (Blum, 2020).

CHAPTER SUMMARY

The educational system has created a pedagogical distraction in the form of grading, with faculty more focused on grading than teaching and students more focused on grades than learning. The transition to CBE is the ideal time to transform our assessment and grading practices.

Connecting with students and respecting their diversity (more specifically, their diversity and individuality in learning) by co-creating outcomes and assessments improves their confidence, motivation, performance, and behavior (Wormeli, 2018). I hear the words 'how can we make our learning environments safe' and 'how can we improve the sense of belonging' reverberate through the walls (and virtual spaces) of academia. My answer is, first and foremost, to evaluate and change assessment and grading practices. Are those well aligned with our messages regarding growth mindset, innovation, leadership, diversity, and equity? We must ask ourselves where quantitative grades and assessments belong in a trauma-informed and inclusive educational environment. We need to work collectively with our board-certifying institutions to ensure that they are considering the most equitable metrics. It is not enough to align our social justice ideals in mission and vision statements or even in class dialogue and discussion; rather, we should embed these ideals in our grading and assessment practices.

References

Baran, L., & Jonason, P. K. (2020). Academic dishonesty among university students: The roles of the psychopathy, motivation, and self-efficacy. *PLoS ONE, 15*(8), e0238141. https://doi.org/10.1371/journal.pone.0238141

Baygi, A. H., Ghonsooly, B., & Ghanizadeh, A. (2017). Self-fulfillment in higher education: Contributions from mastery goal, intrinsic motivation, and assertions. *The Asia-Pacific Education Researcher, 26*(3–4), 171–182. https://doi.org/10.1007/s40299-017-0338-1

Biggs, J. B., & Tang, C. S. (2011). *Teaching for quality learning at university: What the student does* (4th ed.). McGraw-Hill, Society for Research into Higher Education & Open University Press.

Biggs, J. B., Tang, C. S., & Kennedy, G. (2022). *Teaching for quality learning at university* (5th ed.). Open University Press.

Blum, S. D. (2020). Why ungrade? Why Grade? In *Ungrading: Why rating students undermines learning (and what to do instead)* (1st ed., pp. 1–22). West Virginia University Press.

Blum, S. D., & Kohn, A. (Eds.). (2020). *Ungrading: Why rating students undermines learning (and what to do instead)* (1st ed.). West Virginia University Press.

Brimi, H. M. (2011). Reliability of grading high school work in English. *Practical Assessment, Research & Evaluation, 16*(17), 1–12. https://doi.org/10.7275/J531-FZ38

Carleton, D. (2009). Horace Mann. In *The First Amendment encyclopedia*. Middle Tennessee State University. Retrieved from https://www.mtsu.edu/first-amendment/article/1283/horace-mann

Didicher, N. (2016). Bento and Buffet: Two approaches to flexible summative assessment. *Collected Essays on Learning and Teaching, 9,* 167–174. https://doi.org/10.22329/celt.v9i0.4435

Dreher, H. M., Smith Glasgow, M. E., & Schreiber, J. (2019). The use of "high-stakes testing" in nursing education: Rhetoric or rigor? *Nursing Forum, 54*(4), 477–482. https://doi.org/10.1111/nuf.12363

Dweck, C. S. (2006). *Mindset: The new psychology of success.* Ballantine Books.

Elkhoury, E. (2020). *A guide to alternative assessments (Version 1.0; Teaching Commons).* York University. Retrieved from https://www.yorku.ca/bold/wp-content/uploads/sites/393/2020/11/Guide_Alternative_Assessments.pdf

Espinola, M. (2017). History of the college grading scale. *GradeHub.* Retrieved from https://gradehub.com/blog/college-grading-scale/

Feldman, J. (2019). *Grading for equity: What it is, why it matters, and how it can transform schools and classrooms* (1st ed.). Corwin, a SAGE publishing company.

Francis, P., Broughan, C., Foster, C., & Wilson, C. (2020). Thinking critically about learning analytics, student outcomes, and equity of attainment. *Assessment & Evaluation in Higher Education, 45*(6), 811–821. https://doi.org/10.1080/02602938.2019.1691975

Freire, P. (2000). *Pedagogy of the oppressed* (M. Ramos, Trans.; 30th anniversary ed.). Continuum. (Original work published 1968).

Gajda, A., Karwowski, M., & Beghetto, R. A. (2017). Creativity and academic achievement: A meta-analysis. *Journal of Educational Psychology, 109*(2), 269–299. https://doi.org/10.1037/edu0000133

Garrison, M. J. (2020). Standardized testing, innovation, and social reproduction. In M. A. Peters, & R. Heraud (Eds.), *Encyclopedia of educational innovation* (pp. 1–7). Springer Singapore. https://doi.org/10.1007/978-981-13-2262-4_118-2

Giroux, H. A. (2005). *Border crossings: Cultural workers and the politics of education* (2nd ed). Routledge.

Hartmann, T. (2000). *Thom Hartmann's complete guide to ADHD: Help for your family at home, school and work* (1st ed.). Underwood Books.

Hunsicker, J., & Chitwood, T. (2018). High-stakes testing in nursing education: A review of the literature. *Nurse Educator*, *43*(4), 183–186. https://doi.org/10.1097/NNE.0000000000000475

Inoue, A. B. (2022). *Labor-based grading contracts: Building equity and inclusion in the compassionate writing classroom* (2nd ed.). The WAC Clearinghouse; University Press of Colorado. (Originally published in 2019.)

Jones, J. B. (2016, March 23). *Experimenting with specifications grading*. The Chronicle of Higher Education. Retrieved from https://www.chronicle.com/blogs/profhacker/experimenting-with-specifications-grading

Lehigh University. (2013, October 18). *History of standardized testing*. Lehigh University College of Education. Retrieved from https://ed.lehigh.edu/news-events/news/history-standardized-testing

Loftin, C., Reyes, H., Hartin, V., & Rice, L. (2020). A closer look at first-time pass rates as the primary measure of program quality. *Journal of Professional Nursing*, *36*(6), 707–711. https://doi.org/10.1016/j.profnurs.2020.09.011

Lundquist, A., & Henning, G. (2020). From avoiding bias to social justice: A continuum of assessment practices to advance diversity, equity, and inclusion. In A. D. Spicer-Runnels, & T. E. Simpson (Eds.), *Advances in Educational Marketing, Administration, and Leadership*. IGI Global. https://doi.org/10.4018/978-1-7998-4108-1

Maude, P., Livesay, K., Searby, A., & McCauley, K. (2021). Identification of authentic assessment in nursing curricula: An integrative review. *Nurse Education in Practice*, *52*, 103011. https://doi.org/10.1016/j.nepr.2021.103011

McFadden, C. (2017, May 22). *The origins and history of IQ tests*. Interesting Engineering. Retrieved from https://interestingengineering.com/science/the-origins-and-history-of-iq-tests

Mittel, J. (2016, February 16). Rethinking grading: An in-progress experiment. *Just TV*. Retrieved from https://justtv.wordpress.com/2016/02/16/rethinking-grading-an-in-progress-experiment/

Montenegro, E., & Henning, G. (2022). Why the intersection of assessment and equity? In G Henning, G. R. Baker, N. A. Jankowski, A. E. Lundquist, & E. Montenegro (Eds.), *Reframing assessment to center equity: Theories, models, and practices* (1st ed., pp. 3–17). Stylus Publishing, LLC.

Montenegro, E., & Jankowski, N. A. (2017). Equity and assessment: Moving towards culturally responsive assessment. *National Institute for Learning Outcomes Assessment (NILOA)*, Occasional Paper #29. Retrieved from https://www.learningoutcomesassessment.org/wp-content/uploads/2019/02/OccasionalPaper29.pdf

Muirhead, L., Cimiotti, J. P., Hayes, R., Haynes-Ferere, A., Martyn, K., Owen, M., & McCauley, L. (2022). Diversity in nursing and challenges with the NCLEX-RN. *Nursing Outlook*, *70*(5), 762–771. https://doi.org/10.1016/j.outlook.2022.06.003

Muller, J. Z. (2019). *The tyranny of metrics*. Princeton University Press.

Najjar, R. H., Docherty, A., & Miehl, N. (2016). Psychometric properties of an objective structured clinical assessment tool. *Clinical Simulation in Nursing*, *12*(3), 88–95. https://doi.org/10.1016/j.ecns.2016.01.003

National Academies of Sciences, Engineering, and Medicine (NASEM). (2021). *The future of nursing 2020–2030: Charting a path to achieve health equity*. The National Academies Press. https://doi.org/10.17226/25982

National Council of State Boards of Nursing (NCSBN). (2011, October). *Understand the NCLEX examination through the core values of NCSBN*. Retrieved from https://www.ncsbn.org/public-files/NCLEX_Core_Values.pdf

National League for Nursing (NLN). (2020). *Fair testing guidelines for nursing education (NLN Vision #18; NLN Vision Series)*. Retrieved from https://www.nln.org/docs/default-source/uploadedfiles/advocacy-public-policy/fair-testing-guideline-s2e88cc5c78366c709642ff00005f0421.pdf?sfvrsn=bebea00d_0

National League for Nursing (NLN). (2023). *NLN Vision Statement: Integrating Competency-Based Education in the nursing curriculum (NLN Vision # 21; Vision Series)*.

Retrieved from https://www.nln.org/docs/default-source/default-document-library/vision-series_integrating-competency-based-education-in-the-nursing-curriculum.pdf?sfvrsn=99344133_3

Nilson, L. B. (2015). *Specifications grading: Restoring rigor, motivating students, and saving faculty time*. Stylus Publishing.

Noone, J., Ingwerson, J., & Kunz, A. (2018). Analysis of licensure testing patterns of RN graduates in Oregon. *Journal of Nursing Education*, *57*(11), 655–661. https://doi.org/10.3928/01484834-20181022-05

O'Conner, K. (2022). *A repair kit for grading: 15 Fixes for broken grades* (3rd ed.). FIRST Educational Resources, LLC.

O'Neill, G. (2011). *A practitioner's guide to choice of assessment methods within a module*. UCD Teaching and Learning. Retrieved from https://www.ucd.ie/teaching/t4media/choice_of_assessment.pdf

O'Neill, G. (2022). Student choice of assessment methods. In R. Ajjawi, J. Tai, D. Boud, & T. Jorre de St Jorre (Eds.), *Assessment for inclusion in higher education* (1st ed., pp. 199–210). Routledge. https://doi.org/10.4324/9781003293101-22

O'Neill, G., & Padden, L. (2022). Diversifying assessment methods: Barriers, benefits and enablers. *Innovations in Education and Teaching International*, *59*(4), 398–409. https://doi.org/10.1080/14703297.2021.1880462

Ovalle, P. P. (2022). Strategic vulnerability and antiracist pedagogies. *The Journal of Cinema and Media Studies*, *62*(6). Retrieved from https://quod.lib.umich.edu/cgi/t/text/idx/j/jcms/18261332.0062.606/–strategic-vulnerability-antiracist-pedagogies?rgn=main;view=fulltext

Pink, D. H. (2012). *Drive: The surprising truth about what motivates us* (Reprint, paperback ed). Riverhead Books.

Poindexter, K., Hagler, D., & Lindell, D. (2015). Designing authentic assessment: Strategies for nurse educators. *Nurse Educator*, *40*(1), 36–40. https://doi.org/10.1097/NNE.0000000000000091

Roell, K. (2019, July 22). *What is grading on a curve?* ThoughtCo. Retrieved from https://www.thoughtco.com/grading-on-a-curve-3212063

Rosales, J., & Walker, T. (2021, March 20). *The racist beginnings of standardized testing*. NEA News. Retrieved from https://www.nea.org/advocating-for-change/new-from-nea/racist-beginnings-standardized-testing

Schwartz, M., Roach, S., Anwar, S., Tanner, J., & Thistle, R. (2016). *Flexible learning resource (Ryerson Mental Health & Wellbeing Committee)*. Ryerson University. Retrieved from https://www.torontomu.ca/content/dam/mental-health-wellbeing/Documents/Flex-Learning-Res-Full.pdf

Spector, N., Silvestre, J., Alexander, M., Martin, B., Hooper, J. I., Squires, A., & Ojemeni, M. (2020). NCSBN regulatory guidelines and evidence-based quality indicators for nursing education programs. *Journal of Nursing Regulation*, *11*(2), S1–S64. https://doi.org/10.1016/S2155-8256(20)30075-2

Starch, D., & Elliott, E. C. (1912). Reliability of the grading of high-school work in English. *The School Review*, *20*(7), 442–457. https://doi.org/10.1086/435971

Starch, D., & Elliott, E. C. (1913). Reliability of grading work in mathematics. *The School Review*, *21*(4), 254–259.

Sullivan, D. (2014). A concept analysis of "high-stakes testing." *Nurse Educator*, *39*(2), 72–76. https://doi.org/10.1097/NNE.0000000000000021

Tagher, C. G., & Robinson, E. M. (2016). Critical aspects of stress in a high-takes testing environment: A phenomenographical approach. *Journal of Nursing Education*, *55*(3), 160–163. https://doi.org/10.3928/01484834-20160216-07

Tan Yuen Ling, L., Yuen, B., Loo, W. L., Prinsloo, C., & Gan, M. (2020). Students' conceptions of bell curve grading fairness in relation to goal orientation and motivation. *International Journal for the Scholarship of Teaching and Learning*, *14*(1), 1–9. https://doi.org/10.20429/ijsotl.2020.140107

Tugend, A. (2019, October 9). *Questioning their fairness, a record number of colleges stop requiring the SAT and ACT*. The Hechinger Report. Retrieved from http://hechingerreport.org/questioning-their-fairness-a-record-number-of-colleges-stop-requiring-the-sat-and-act/

University of Southern California Center for Urban Education. (n.d.). *Equity mindedness*. Retrieved from https://cue.usc.edu/equity/equity-mindedness/

Villarroel, V., Bloxham, S., Bruna, D., Bruna, C., & Herrera-Seda, C. (2018). Authentic assessment: Creating a blueprint for course design. *Assessment & Evaluation in Higher Education*, *43*(5), 840–854. https://doi.org/10.1080/02602938.2017.1412396

Wanner, T., Palmer, E., & Palmer, D. (2021). Flexible assessment and student empowerment: Advantages and disadvantages—research from an Australian university. *Teaching in Higher Education*, 1–17. https://doi.org/10.1080/13562517.2021.1989578

Wormeli, R. (2018). *Fair isn't always equal: Assessing and grading in the differentiated classroom* (2nd ed.). Stenhouse Publishers.

Yu, H., Glanzer, P. L., Sriram, R., Johnson, B. R. & Moore, B. (2017). What contributes to college students' cheating? A study of individual factors. *Ethics & Behavior*, *27*(5), 401–422. https://doi.org/10.1080/10508422 2016.1169535

15

Item Writing and Analysis

Joanne Noone, PhD, RN, CNE, FAAN, ANEF

CHAPTER OVERVIEW

Best practices in item writing are reviewed with a focus on developing multiple-choice items. Strengths and weaknesses of various item formats will be reviewed. Topics include the principles of item writing: alignment, importance, differentiation, and fairness. Concepts reviewed include reducing linguistic bias, alignment with course content and outcomes, and Next-Gen NCLEX testing. An overview of item and test analysis is presented.

THE PURPOSES OF TESTS

In this chapter, the terms *test, quiz,* or *examination* are used interchangeably to all mean the same: an intended measurement of learning. Tests provide information about students and their ability to retrieve and apply knowledge. As such, tests can be oral, written, or practical. They can be used for formative or summative assessments. They can be used for admission or progression purposes. It is very helpful to consider the purpose of the test as you are designing it to develop a test that best matches its intended purpose. According to Oermann and Gaberson (2021, p. 49), "The *purpose* for the test involves why it is to be given, what it is supposed to measure, and how the test scores will be used." In thinking about the purpose of a test, it is helpful to review Chapter 3, *The Science of Learning* and some of the best practice principles discussed there. As you may recall, testing is primarily used as a form of *summative* assessment, with a grade attached to it. Testing can and should be used to provide information for and about learning and used for formative assessment. Benefits of testing for formative assessment include to:

> identify gaps in students' knowledge
> determine if learners have the necessary foundational knowledge for current learning
> strengthen learning and memory through information retrieval
> provide an opportunity for learners to gain skill in test-taking
> identify instructional and curriculum gaps

When tests are used primarily for *formative* assessment, assessment typically occurs before and during the learning process to better understand prior learning and skills as well as to identify learning progress or problems. This type of testing can provide feedback that guides the teacher to identify what to focus on for further learning. These examples of formative assessment are typically not graded, or a grade is assigned based on participation, or given a score that makes the test a low-stakes assessment.

We most commonly recognize and use testing as *summative* assessment, primarily used after teaching has occurred to determine what the student has learned and how well they can apply new knowledge to nursing practice. For tests to be an effective summative assessment, they should be linked to unit or course outcomes. Use of the best practices recommended in this chapter will aid in an optimal design of a reliable and valid test that provides meaningful information about learner achievement. As discussed in Chapter 3, *The Science of Learning,* even summative examinations can be learning opportunities for students when review with rationale for correct and incorrect answers are provided.

ANATOMY OF A TEST QUESTION

We begin with a review of terminology used in developing test *questions*, also known as *items*, and we use the framework of multiple-choice questions to define these terms. The *stem* is the question being asked, or statement used to elicit the correct response. Phrasing the stem in the form of a question is best practice and will be discussed in a later section of this chapter. Sometimes the stem contains a scenario or case study, which is additional information that should be relevant to answering the question. In the multiple-choice question example in Table 15.2 later in this chapter, the scenario is "A client who is admitted directly from a private medical office to the hospital for treatment of pneumonia has all of the following orders" and the stem is "Which should the nurse implement **FIRST?**" The choices are called *options,* with the correct option termed the *key* and the incorrect options called the *distractors*. In that example in Table 15.2, all four choices are options. The *key*, or correct answer, is "O2 by nasal cannula 2–3 l/min to keep O2 saturation above 92%" and the other three choices are the *distractors*, or incorrect answers.

TYPES OF QUESTIONS

The focus of this chapter will be on best practices in writing multiple-choice questions (MCQs) since these types of questions predominate in health profession examinations. A brief overview of commonly used question formats, their strengths and weaknesses, and recommendations for use are provided. Newer question formats that are being used to assess for clinical judgment (commonly referred to as Next Generation or Next-Gen NCLEX Testing) are discussed. Ample descriptions of best practices to use in creating and administering exams predominantly containing MCQs in the healthcare professions are available (Rudolph et al., 2019). Although there is limited information available about nurse educator testing practices, a survey of 200 nurse educators in New York State identified that standard four-option MCQs comprised 81% of items in examinations these nurse educators used and 65% of respondents reported that such examinations contributed to at least 80% of the course grade (Birkhead et al., 2018).

Test items are generally characterized by the type of response required by the test-taker and how the items are scored. "Selected-response" item formats most commonly include matching, true-false statements, multiple-choice, and multiple-response items. In these formats, test-takers select from the options provided by the test developer. These items are typically objectively scored; that is, there is a correct answer key. This eases the burden of scoring for faculty. Newer items, such as drag and drop and drop-down question formats used in the Next Generation NCLEX Project, optimally require electronic testing for best use (Billings, 2020). "Constructed-response" items include fill-in-the-blank, essay questions (either short answer or longer), and hot-spot testing in which a graphic is provided and the tester is asked to locate the area on the graphic in response to the question. Test-takers are required to provide a response and there may be more subjectivity and faculty burden in scoring, particularly for essay questions. If fill-in-the-blank or essay questions are used, a model response or rubric is recommended to facilitate scoring and reduce variability among raters (Oermann & Gaberson, 2021). Hot-spot testing is most effectively used in electronic testing situations although there is limited knowledge about best practice use of these items (Billings, 2020; Rudolph et al., 2019).

Deliberation about which item formats to use ideally should include consideration of test purpose, the learning outcomes under assessment, and how this knowledge will be used in clinical practice (McDonald, 2018). It may be difficult to assess higher ordered thinking in certain formats, such as matching and true-false items. However, these methods may be best suited for pre-assessments and information retrieval situations for formative assessments as discussed in Chapter 3, *The Science of Learning*, since they tend to better assess knowledge recall and comprehension. Items that can best test higher-ordered thinking, including aspects of assessing for clinical judgment and reasoning, need to be clearly written using the principles delineated in this chapter to be most effective. When choosing a format, consider how this knowledge will be used in clinical practice and select a format that best aligns with the knowledge the learner should be applying. For example, hot-spot testing may be best associated with physical assessment or diagnostic interpretation tests and fill-in-the-blank questions with mathematic calculations since these methods most closely align with how this knowledge is used in clinical practice. Many of the best practice principles we discuss in this chapter apply to these various item formats. Table 15.1 provides a description, an assessment of strengths and weaknesses, and recommendations for use of various item formats. Examples of item formats are provided in Table 15.2.

PRINCIPLES OF ITEM-WRITING

Sutherland et al. (2012) identify four best practice principles for item writing that are defined first and specific tips for each principle are reviewed in subsequent sections. Their four principles are:

> Alignment: The concept of alignment in any assessment is that the assessment directly measures the course and unit outcomes. According to Sutherland et al. (2012, p. 35) "alignment is the extent to which each test item corresponds to

TABLE 15.1

Description and Evaluation of Item Types

Type	Description	Strengths	Weaknesses	Recommendations
Selected-Response Item Formats				
True-false	A statement is provided and the tester needs to decide if the statement is true or false.	Easy to score Testers can complete faster than other formats so can test a wide range of information	Tends to test lower-ordered thinking, such as recall and comprehension	Best used for pre-assessments and information retrieval practice. Avoid testing meaningless or irrelevant information. Best used to test only one idea.
Matching	Two columns are provided: one column has the problem to be answered and the other column has the answer. Testers answer according to directions provided regarding making the match.	Easy to score Testers can complete faster than other formats so can test a wide range of information	Tends to test lower-ordered thinking, such as recall and comprehension	Best used for pre-assessments and information retrieval practice. Avoid testing meaningless or irrelevant information. Group matching items that are similar in content. Limit a matching exercise to no more than 10 sets.
Multiple choice	A question consisting usually of a scenario, a stem (question or direction for answering), and three to four options with usually one right answer.	Easy to score Can test higher ordered thinking	Has limits in assessing practice-based application of knowledge and clinical judgment	Needs to be well written according to standards to be optimally effective
Multiple response	Similar to a multiple-choice question with a scenario, stem, and usually 5 to 6 options; more than one option is correct. Directions include "Select all that apply."	Easy to score Can test higher ordered thinking	Has limits in assessing practice-based application of knowledge and clinical judgment	Decide whether partial credit is given if not all correct options are chosen Needs to be well written according to standards to be optimally effective
Drag and drop	A question consisting usually of a scenario, a stem (question or direction for answering), and multiple options provided. Directions include moving selected options to a response area to answer the question. Directions may include ranking or ordering the responses. Also known as "ordered response."	Can test higher ordered thinking	Ideally need electronic testing feature for optimal effectiveness Paper and pencil version may limit effectiveness	Decide whether partial credit is given if not all correct options are chosen Best used to assess prioritization and procedural knowledge

TABLE 15.1

Description and Evaluation of Item Types *(Continued)*

Type	Description	Strengths	Weaknesses	Recommendations
Drop-down	An item consisting usually of a scenario and statement with multiple options provided in a drop-down menu to complete the statement. May have more than one drop-down feature in one statement. Also known as "Cloze."	Can test higher ordered thinking	Ideally need electronic testing feature for optimal effectiveness Paper and pencil version may limit effectiveness	If multiple drop-downs are in one item, decide whether partial credit is to be given if not all correct options are chosen.
Constructed-Response Item Formats				
Fill-in-the-blank	The tester supplies a written answer (usually a word, phrase, or sentence) to a question or incomplete sentence.	Tester constructs response so less likelihood of guessing	Time-consuming to grade There can be increased subjectivity in grading Tends to assess lower ordered thinking	Model answers may help improve objectivity in grading Most effectively used in mathematic calculations
Essay	The tester supplies an expanded written response to a question.	Tester constructs response so less likelihood of guessing. Can test higher ordered thinking	Time-consuming to grade Limited ability to test a wide content area	Model answers or rubric may help improve objectivity in grading
Hot-spot	A graphic is provided and the tester is asked to locate the area on the graphic in response to the question.	Can test higher ordered thinking	Ideally need electronic testing feature for optimal effectiveness Paper and pencil version may limit effectiveness	Best used in physical assessment or procedural skill situations

the specific statement, skill, or objective it is intended to measure. An item inadequately aligned with the intended skill cannot adequately define the examinee's proficiency in that skill."

▸ Importance: The test item should assess relevant and important information to determine minimal expected competency in meeting the learning outcomes. Avoiding trivial concepts and writing higher-level thinking questions can help to focus on important concepts.

TABLE 15.2

Item Type Examples

Format	Example
True-false	True or False: Death rates from unintentional injuries decline in middle-aged adults.
Matching	Match the following epidemiological terms in the left column with the best definition provided in the right column (Centers for Disease Control and Prevention, 2015). ___ 1. Sensitivity ___ 2. Specificity ___ 3. Incidence ___ 4. Prevalence ___ 5. Odds Ratio a. A measure of the frequency with which an event, such as a new case of illness, occurs in a population over a period of time. b. The number or proportion of cases or events or conditions in a given population. c. The proportion of persons without disease who are correctly identified by a screening test or case definition as not having disease. d. A measure of association, which quantifies the relationship between an exposure and health outcome from a comparative study. e. The proportion of persons with disease who are correctly identified by a screening test or case definition as having disease
Multiple choice	A client who is admitted directly from a private medical office to the hospital for treatment of pneumonia has all of the following orders. Which should the nurse implement **FIRST**? a. Draw blood cultures and routine admission bloodwork b. Establish IV and infuse normal saline at 125 mL/hr c. Administer Azithromycin 500 mg IV once daily d. O2 by nasal cannula 2–3 L/min to keep O2 saturation above 92%
Multiple response	You are screening a new client for an annual health check. The client is a 68-year-old female, who is a retired office assistant, with a history of hypertension. There are no other medical conditions. The client brings documentation of up-to-date Covid vaccinations but there is no documentation of other vaccinations. Based on this history, what vaccinations are recommended? SELECT ALL THAT APPLY. ❑ Influenza ❑ TDaP ❑ Varicella ❑ MMR ❑ Zoster ❑ Pneumococcal
Drag and drop	Order the three stages of backward design approach to curriculum development: 1 Identify desired learning outcomes 2 Develop learning assessments 3 Determine learning activities

TABLE 15.2

Item Type Examples *(Continued)*

Format	Example
Fill-in-the-blank	The recommended safe dose of an oral drug for a child is 20–40 mg/kg/day. The child weighs 22 lb. The maximum safe daily dosage of medicine for this client is _____:
Essay	Select three classifications of antihypertensives and describe their mechanism of actions.
Drop-down	**Choose the correct answer in the drop-down list.** In evaluating a client with uncompensated respiratory acidosis, the nurse should anticipate the pH to be:

-Select-	↓
within normal range	
below normal range	
above normal range	

Hot-spot:

The nurse is performing a physical assessment on an adult. Identify the area on the chest where the nurse would BEST palpate the point of maximal impulse.

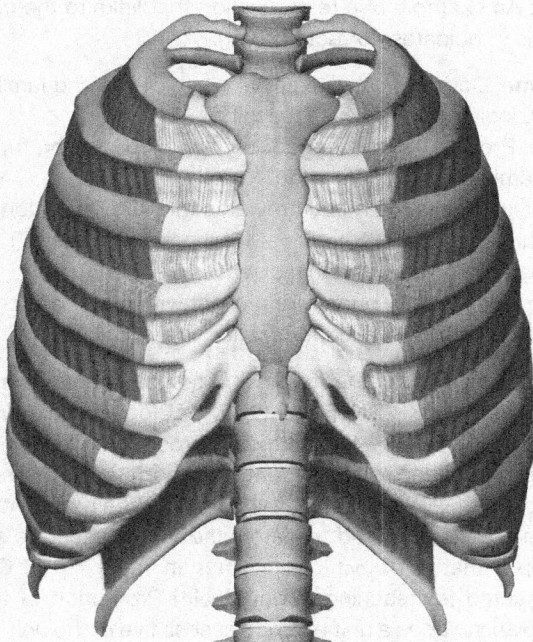

▷ Differentiation: This principle refers to the test item's ability to measure student's knowledge and ability related to the content and concepts under assessment. While this principle is best assessed after using the test items and evaluating the item analysis, questions that are too easy or too hard and trick questions do not contribute to differentiating students' ability in understanding the content being assessed.

▷ Fairness: This principle refers to writing questions clearly that avoids cultural or linguistic bias, which may advantage certain testers over others. "Test items must be appropriate and applicable to all examinees, including minority, nonnative English-speaking, and international examinees" (Sutherland et al., 2012, p. 35). Poorly written questions tend to assess student's ability to take an exam or interpret irrelevant cultural information. For example, referring to a Twinkie will only be understandable to a select group of learners familiar with this snack popular in the previous century. Such a reference distracts from determining mastery of the content the teacher aims to assess.

ALIGNMENT

Alignment is best achieved by mapping or "blueprinting" test questions to the course outcomes or, ideally, unit objectives. Developing clear unit, or module, objectives, as discussed earlier in Chapter 7, *Backward Design: Aligning Outcomes, Assessments, and Activities*, are a recommended best practice to link specific course content to overall course outcomes. An example of a test question that links to the course outcome and module objective is (* indicates correct answer):

Course Outcome: Communicates effectively with clients and families to provide accurate and individualized health teaching.
Unit Objective: Provide recommended nutritional counseling for clients with common vitamin and mineral needs.
Item: In which situation is the nurse providing the BEST nutritional counseling?
   A. Recommending a spinach omelet for a pregnant client (*)
   B. Encouraging a client with renal disease to eat bananas
   C. Advising a veggie soy burger for a client with hypertension
   D. Counseling a client with kidney stones to avoid yogurt

There are various renditions in the literature of test blueprints—for example, tests can be blueprinted to the NCLEX—RN Test Plan or to Bloom's Taxonomy. These types of blueprints help with importance—testing higher-ordered thinking that is relevant to the practice of nursing. Test blueprinting to content and unit objectives can help to ensure alignment of assessment with outcomes (Billings, 2020). The blueprint is then reviewed to assess for gaps in assessment and to determine that the test as a whole collectively assesses the subject matter (Tarrant & Ware, 2012). In Table 7.6 of Chapter 7, a unit of instruction is presented for teaching about Health Promotion of the Adolescent and Young Adult. The plan includes a unit exam to assess five of the unit objectives. The faculty creates a 10-item exam and blueprints the exam items to the content areas and unit objectives. Table 15.3 provides an example of a test blueprint for unit objectives and course content for this unit of instruction. In reviewing the test blueprint, it is identified that more questions are needed to assess content area D and the last unit objective.

TABLE 15.3

Test Blueprint for Unit Objectives and Course Content

Unit Objectives	Content Area A	Content Area B	Content Area C	Content Area D
Apply developmental concepts for adolescents and young adults into health history and assessment techniques.	Question 1, 10	Question 4		
Integrate identification of unique health needs of adolescents and young adults into counseling for risk reduction.	Question 2		Question 3	
Explain legal and ethical issues related to confidentiality in the treatment of minors and public health reporting.		Question 6		Question 5
Demonstrate professional communication techniques in completing a health history on an adolescent client.			Question 7, 8	
Develop and implement an evidenced-based birth control teaching plan for a young adult.		Question 9		

IMPORTANCE

In Chapter 7, *Backward Design: Aligning Outcomes, Assessments, and Activities*, we discuss that when designing units of instruction, to meet educational standards the teacher should consider the priorities for learning and identify what learners need to be able to know and do to be successful in meeting course outcomes. Similarly, when developing test items, we recommend designing exams to test important concepts and to avoid trivial or meaningless test items. Sutherland et al. (2012) recommend when developing a test item to ask what is something important students should know

Writing higher-level thinking items at the application level and above according to Bloom's taxonomy can assist with developing items that test important concepts used by nurses in practice, particularly since nursing is a practice-based profession. Writing test-items within a clinical scenario can assist with writing higher level items

(Tarrant & Ware, 2012) and can minimize the chances of writing knowledge recall items. Consider these items for a health promotion exam (* indicates correct answer):

Item A: The expected normal visual acuity for a four-year-old is:
   a.   20/20
   b.   20/30
   c.   20/40*
   d.   20/50

Revised Item A: The nurse is screening clients at a health fair. Which finding requires referral?
   a.   Visual acuity screening of 20/30 in a 4-year-old boy.
   b.   A 58-year-old man who has not had the pneumococcal vaccine.
   c.   A 48-year-old woman with a blood pressure of 96/56.
   d.   Lateral spinal deviation on a 14-year-old girl upon bending at the waist.*

Item A is an example of a knowledge recall question that has no clinical context. While assessing visual acuity in a toddler may be an important concept, the item's importance can be strengthened by incorporating clinical scenarios and revising the item to test at a higher level. Revised Item A is asking the learner to analyze and interpret data and tests understanding of four different concepts rather than one.

DIFFERENTIATION

All items in a test should ideally provide information about students' ability in the content area under assessment. We will revisit this principle in the section on item analysis, which can provide information about how easy or difficult a question is and how the distractors in a question contribute to assessment. However, when writing an item, there are certain recommendations that can enhance the principle of differentiation. All distractors, or the incorrect answers, should be plausible and valid. In considering the principle of differentiation, Sutherland et al. (2012) recommend, when developing a test item, to ask, "What are some things a student would think if they did not know the correct answer?" Consider the most common misunderstandings as you create distractors.

A key recommendation to writing a clear item that incorporates the principle of differentiation is to avoid the influence of invalid moderators, or something other than content that influences student's selection of an answer. Recommendations to improve the validity of distractors include:

➤ There should be only one correct answer in an MCQ. If you have more than one correct answer, switch the question to a multiple-response question, using the terminology "Select all that apply" as shown in the example in Table 15.2. Avoid "all" or "none of the above" options. Use a three-option question if a valid fourth option is difficult to come up with. Tarrant and Ware (2010) compared the performance of three-option and four-option multiple-choice questions and identified that clearly written three-option questions can perform as well as four-option items, especially since the use of implausible distractors are decreased.

➤ Avoid repetitious wording in the stem and key or in the key and one of the distractors. An example of repetitious wording is if the question and right answer both say "hypertension" and "hypertension" doesn't appear anywhere else. If repetitious wording appears in the correct option and the exact opposite in another distractor, students will eliminate the other choices as an option, reducing their effectiveness. If one option is high potassium and the other is low potassium, students will eliminate the other two options as distractors.

➤ Use consistent spacing and punctuation. Avoid negative phrasing in the stem or options. For example, instead of asking "Which of the following should the patient not do?" ask, "Which action is BEST to avoid?" Avoid absolutes, such as "always" or "never." All options should be the same general length and amount of information. The key should not be longer in length or amount of information.

➤ Vary the correct option throughout exam except for numerical options, which should be written in ascending or descending order (Krantz et al., 2019). If using electronic testing software, employ the feature of randomization.

FAIRNESS

The principle of fairness is best achieved through writing clear test items that avoid cultural and linguistic bias. In items that have linguistic or cultural bias, students' cultural knowledge and English proficiency are being tested, which interferes with assessment of content knowledge. Linguistic and cultural bias in test items refers to cultural and language knowledge that is unnecessary and is not available to all test-ers (Bosher, 2003). As a result, some testers are unfairly disadvantaged and perform differently on an exam (Hicks, 2011). Applying such recommended practices is termed *linguistic modification*, which refers to decreasing the linguistic and cultural complex-ity of a test item. Multiple studies have shown the benefit of incorporating these modi-fications towards the academic success of culturally and linguistically diverse (CALD) nursing students. Linguistic modification of items is associated with better under-standing of test items and reduced time in testing for CALD students (Lewis & Bell, 2020; Moore & Clark, 2016; Moore & Waters, 2020). Recommendations to improve the fairness of items include:

➤ To reduce testing knowledge of the dominant culture, avoid uncommon words, colloquialisms, slang, and euphemisms. For example, use the term "home" instead of "abode." Avoid phrases such as "temper tantrum" which may not be understood by students from other cultures; instead describe the behavior being observed.

➤ Avoid unnecessary phrases or wordiness. For example, ask "Which" instead of "Which of the following." The more words you put in the stem, the more complex it becomes. If a sentence becomes too wordy, consider breaking it into two sentences.

➤ The stem should be in the form of a question instead of a phrase. In a study by Bosher and Bowles (2008) of the comprehensibility of items by CALD students, students reported items in a question format to be easier to understand. In the example above in the Importance section, the stem in Item A is in the form of a phrase: "The expected normal visual acuity for a four-year old is." The item was revised into a question and broken into two sentences to reduce complexity: "The nurse is screening clients at a health fair. Which finding requires referral?"

➤ Avoid use of modal verbs "may", "should", or "would" in the stem as that may be interpreted as a moral obligation to do something in some cultures or that the nurse has the discretion to do something different than expected (Bosher, 2003; Hicks, 2011). For example, instead of asking "Which of the following symptoms should the nurse immediately report to the physician?", a stem that incorporates this recommendation is revised to "Which symptom requires immediate reporting to the physician?." Also note that wordiness was reduced in this revision through eliminating "of the following."

➤ In questions that are asking for the best answers in situations where all options may be correct, it is recommended to capitalize, bold, or underline important words such as **FIRST, BEST, MOST IMPORTANT** for clarity in calling out key words for prioritization. The example provided in the Alignment section above utilizes this recommendation: "In which situation is the nurse providing the BEST nutritional counseling?"

NEXT GENERATION TESTING ITEM GENERATION

The National Council of State Boards of Nursing (NCSBN) has adopted a clinical judgment framework for evaluating prelicensure candidates' ability to provide safe nursing care that consists of six iterative processes, or cognitive functions, to be measured through testing (Dickison et al., 2019). This revised testing format is referenced to as Next Generation NCLEX, or NGN, testing. Silvestri (2019, p. 4) defines these cognitive functions or skills and links them to the nursing process:

➤ **Recognize cues**—identifying significant data from many sources (assessment)

➤ **Analyze cues**—connecting the data to the client's presentation—is this data expected? Unexpected? What are the concerns? (analysis)

➤ **Prioritize hypotheses**—rank the hypotheses, concerns, client needs (analysis, diagnosis)

➤ **Generate solutions**—use hypotheses to determine interventions for an expected outcome (planning)

➤ **Take actions**—implement the generated solutions addressing the highest priorities or hypotheses (implementation)

➤ **Evaluate outcomes**—compare observed outcomes with expected ones (evaluation)

Revised testing processes include developing case studies or scenarios that include expanded clinical information, such as client history of a disease or condition, shift reports, current medications, lab results, clinical notes from interprofessional team members, or interactions with the client or family members (Betts et al., 2019; Poorman & Mastorovich, 2020). Alternative test items for NGN testing include (NCSBN, 2022):

➤ Extended Multiple Response items allow candidates to select one or more answer options at a time. This item type is similar to the current NCLEX multiple response items with more options and using partial credit scoring.

➤ Extended Drag and Drop items allow candidates to move or place response options into answer spaces. This item type is like the current NCLEX ordered

			Potential Additional			
	Current	**Current Cognitive**	**Cognitive Functions**	**Additional Information**	**Potential Revised**	**Revised**
Current Item	**Item Format**	**Function**	**Measured**	**Needed**	**Format**	**Question**
Insert current item here.	E.g., Multiple choice	E.g., Recognize cues	E.g., Analyze cues	E.g., Add lab results and current medications	E.g., Revise to cloze, drop-down	Insert revised item here.

TABLE 15.4

Next Generation NCLEX Blueprint Template

response items but not all of the response options may be required to answer the item. In some items, there may be more response options than answers spaces.

➤ Cloze (Drop–Down) items allow candidates to select one option from a drop-down list. There can be more than one drop-down list in a cloze item. These drop-down lists can be used as words or phrases within a sentence, tables, and charts.

➤ Enhanced Hot Spot (Highlighting) items allow candidates to select their answer by highlighting pre-defined words or phrases. Candidates can select and deselect the highlighted parts by clicking on the words or phrases. These types of items allow an individual to read a portion of a client medical record, (e.g., a nursing note, medical history, lab values, medication record, etc.) and then select the words or phrases that answer the item.

➤ Matrix/Grid items allow the candidate to select one or more answer options for each row and/or column. This item type can be useful in measuring multiple aspects of the clinical scenario with a single item.

As faculty consider how to prepare learners for this new form of testing, recommended strategies incorporate some of these revisions into current testing practices. Recommendations include considering how to categorize current items according to the clinical judgment framework, identifying if additional information needs to be added to create a case study or scenario, and evaluating if the item can be revised to test additional processes of clinical judgement and to an alternative format (Poorman & Mastorovich, 2020; Silvestri, 2019). Silvestri (2019) suggests developing an NGN test blueprint to facilitate revision of items into an NGN format (see Table 15.4 for a recommended blueprint template).

ITEM ANALYSIS

An item analysis report evaluates information about the overall test results and individual items and is an integral component of test administration to improve the quality of test items. According to McGahee and Ball (2009, p. 166), "Item analysis is a process of statistically examining both the test questions and the students' answers to assess the quality of the questions and the test as a whole." Examining test results through this process facilitates achievement of the best practice principle of differentiation in helping to understand if the items and their components are providing information about students' ability and knowledge of topics under assessment. A test analysis can also provide information about the principle of alignment and if the test is assessing what you want it to assess. So test results can be analyzed at an aggregate level and at an individual item level to determine:

> Are there areas for further student learning?
> Are the test items developed fundamentally sound?
> Are there areas for test item improvement?

Test-scoring statistical scoring machines are available for paper and pencil examinations–Scantron® being one of the most common products. These aggregate results of an exam can be saved electronically for review, analysis, and interpretation. Electronic testing software, such as ExamSoft®, or those within a Learning Management System also provide an analysis of test results. It is important to familiarize oneself with the statistical analyses provided by the scoring product used as they may differ in what results are provided.

Aggregate Exam Results

Common aggregate test results provided in an item analysis include the number of questions and participants being scored; measures of central tendency, such as the mean or median; the standard deviation, or the average number of points that testers vary from the mean; and, the range of highest and lowest raw scores. There is also a reliability coefficient reported which is the amount of measurement error associated with an exam score or the internal consistency of scores. Most commonly reported is a Kuder-Richardson formula 20 (KR 20), the measure of reliability most appropriate for multiple-choice exams. The range of a Kuder-Richardson is from 0.0 to 1.0. The higher the value, the more reliable the overall exam score is. There are variations of acceptable ranges for this result although the consensus is that a minimum result of .6 or greater is acceptable reliability (Magaldi et al., 2019; Rudolph et al., 2019). This indicates how well the items are correlated with one another and how well they measure similar constructs. The reliability of an exam is influenced by a number of factors, including:

> The number of items on the test and the number of testers. Reliability improves with variability so increasing the number of items, generally to at least 40 (McDonald, 2018), is recommended. Determining a reasonable number of questions to assess knowledge within the testing period needs to be considered. It is recommended allotting 90 seconds per test question; or about 60 questions for a 90-minute testing period. Increasing the number of testers also improves reliability of the exam; however, this may not be a feasible solution unless there are multiple sections of a course where the test results can be combined.

> The quality of the test items. Improving the quality of test items improves reliability of the exam. We will review these concepts in the next section.

TABLE 15.5

Sample Overall Examination Statistics

Exam Takers	Total Points	Mean	Median	Standard Deviation	Highest Score	Lowest Score	KR 20
30	64	49.50 (77.34%)	50.50	6.69	63	34	.81

▸ The homogeneity of the content being assessed. Consistent test content improves reliability since similar constructs are being assessed. This is generally not an issue in a nursing exam since like constructs related to health conditions are being tested.

▸ Heterogeneity of the test group, or a range of abilities, can improve reliability since this facilitates variation. Again, this is generally not something that may be within the control of the faculty creating the exam.

Table 15.5 provides an example of an item analysis with aggregate test results for a 64-question examination in which there were 30 testers. The KR 20 of .81 demonstrates good reliability.

Evaluating Individual Items

There are typically three areas of focus on evaluating individual item statistics on an item analysis. The first two assess: *item difficulty,* which is a report of how many people answered the item correctly and *item discrimination,* which evaluates how well testers did on the item in relation to their performance on the total exam. Then, the distractors can be reviewed to evaluate how well they contribute to learner assessment and is called *distractor efficiency.*

Item difficulty, commonly referred to as a *p* value, is the percentage or proportion of testers who answered the question correctly. Depending on how this is reported, values may appear with a range of a percentage from 0% to 100%, or can be written as a proportion of 0.0 to 1.00. The higher the value, the easier the item. Since, in a four-option item, a tester has a 25% chance of getting an item right by guessing, it is usually recommended that item difficulty be in the range of 30% to 80% (McDonald, 2018; Tarrant & Ware, 2012). An item less than 30% is considered too difficult and the item should be evaluated if it was keyed correctly, too confusing, or if additional teaching may be needed. An item difficulty above 80% is considered too easy and does not discriminate between high and lower achieving testers. Poor distractors may contribute to a high *p* value if they are so implausible they are not chosen.

Item discrimination refers to how high- and low-ability students perform on the item. Students who score high on a test (top 27%, high ability) should tend to get items correct more frequently and students who score low on a test (bottom 27%, low ability) should tend to get items wrong more frequently. There are two different measures of item discrimination: the point-biserial index and the discrimination index. Some test scoring products report both.

The point-biserial index, or pbi, is the most commonly reported measure of item discrimination. The pbi is a correlation of a discrimination value of students' responses to one item with their overall test score. The range is from –1.00 to 1.00. The higher the value, the more discriminating the item. A highly discriminating item indicates that the students who had high exam scores got the item correct whereas students who had low exam scores got the item incorrect. An acceptable pbi is +0.15 to +.20, with recommended pbi at or above +.40 (McDonald, 2018; McGahee & Ball, 2009, Rudolph et al., 2019, Tarrant & Ware, 2012).

A second measure that may also be reported is the discrimination index. This is a more simple calculation, which reports the fraction of people with high exam scores who answered the item correctly and the fraction of people with low exam scores who answered the item correctly. The discrimination index is a ratio of the fraction of people with higher exam scores who answered the item correctly minus the fraction of people with lower scores who answered the item correctly. For example, if 100% of the top performers got the item right and 50% of the low performers got item right, the discrimination index is .5. Recommended results are similar to the pbi (Rudolph et al., 2019, Tarrant & Ware, 2012).

Lastly, review distractors to make sure each distractor contributes to student assessment. Acceptable distractors are those that are selected by greater than 5% of testers (Tarrant & Ware, 2012). Distractors that are selected by less than 5% of testers are called *nondistractors*, since they are not functioning as intended. Nondistractors should be evaluated if they are too easy or too implausible to be chosen. These should be flagged for revision in future examinations.

Let's look at some examples in Table 15.6 of item results to analyze from the test administered in Table 15.5. In this item analysis, the *p*-value is reported as a proportion

TABLE 15.6

Sample Item Analysis

Item	p-Value	pbi	Upper Correct Reponses	Lower Correct Reponses	Frequency of Responses (* correct answer)			
					A	B	C	D
1	.70	.36	88.89%	50%	4 (13.33%)	3 (10%)	2 (6.67%)	21* (70%)
2	.93	.52	100%	75%	28* (93.33%)	0 (0%)	0 (0%)	2 (6.67%)
3	.30	.42	55.56%	0%	2 (6.67%)	9* (30%)	2 (6.67%)	17 (56.67%)
4	.67	.10	66.67%	62.5%	1 (3.33%)	0 (0%)	20* (66.67%)	9 (30%)
5	.47	.04	44.44%	50%	4 (13.33%)	12 (40%)	14* (46.67%)	0 (0%)

(from 0–1.0) and the point-biserial index is the measure used to assess item discrimination. To recap: we will evaluate:

▸ Is the *p*-value between 30% to 80% (or .3–.8)?
▸ Is the pbi or discrimination index above +.20?
▸ Do all moderators assess learning (at least 5% of testers choosing each option)?

Item 1 is an example that meets all the criteria. Seventy percent of the learners scored correctly with high achievers performing better than low achievers as represented by the pbi of +.36. All the distractors participated in assessing learners with at least 5% of testers choosing each distractor. Item 2 is an example of results that may be seen if the question is too easy. Even though the item discriminates between high and low achievers (with a pbi of +.52), 93% of testers scored correctly, which is above the 80% threshold. Distractors B and C are nondistractors; no one chose them. The item should be reviewed for item difficulty and plausibility of distractors and flagged for future revision. Item 3 is an example of results that may be seen if the question is too hard. This question barely meets the minimum *p*-value with 30% of testers scoring correctly. While the item has good discrimination with a pbi of +.42, none of the low achievers scored correctly. The distractors all functioned correctly, with at least 5% of testers choosing them. This item should be reviewed for difficulty and potentially be moved to a more advanced course or later in the program of study.

Two-thirds of testers scored item 4 correctly, which is within the range of acceptability of *p*-values although the item does not discriminate well between high and low achievers, with a pbi of +.10. In looking at the distractors, options A and B are considered nondistractors; revision of these distractors could potentially improve the discrimination of this item. In item 5, while the item meets the criteria for item difficulty with a *p*-value of .47, the item does not discriminate with a pbi of .04 and more low achievers getting it correct than high achievers. In reviewing the distractors' performance, option D should be flagged for review if it is too easy or implausible. It is noteworthy that almost as many testers chose option B as the correct option C. Option B should be reviewed to evaluate whether this choice may also be correct.

What to Do with Test Results

In general, determining what to do with test results fall into two categories: (1) what changes to make regarding the current test scores, and (2) flagging items for revision for future use. Current test scores should certainly be adjusted if an item is miskeyed or, upon review, a second option is determined to also be correct. Since most health care examinations contain flawed items, deleting items and adjusting scores should be done sparingly (Rudolph, 2019). Awarding everyone points for a question is not recommended as that does not contribute to assessment of students' knowledge. Deleting a flawed item, especially one with a low *p*-value and low discrimination, and lowering the total number possible points seems the most psychometrically sound solution although it may result in lower scores for those who scored the item correctly. Justifying decisions about scoring from an item analysis and implementing such decisions as a standard programmatic approach is recommended as well as creating a system to capture suggested changes to improve items for future use (Magaldi et al., 2019; McDonald, 2018).

CHAPTER SUMMARY

Table 15.7 summarizes the key questions to ask regarding each principle to suppor best practices. In addition, such strategies can best be maximized when all faculty in a program have this shared understanding and implement these best practices into thei courses. Hijji (2017) and Bristol et al. (2018) describe the problems that can result from lack of faculty training and use of standard best practices: flawed test items and poten tially inaccurate and inequitable assessment of learners. Schroeder (2013) reported tha licensure pass rates improved after implementing faculty development on item writ ing and a standard approach to item writing and analysis. Some recommendations to implement to support infusion of best testing practices are:

> Ensure faculty use a test blueprint to align items with learning outcomes and to identify cognitive level of the item.

> Encourage peer review of test items to assess adherence to best practices

> Perform a post-test administration item analysis to further refine items

TABLE 15.7

Summary of Principles of Item Writing

Principle	Questions
Alignment	❑ Does item assess a learning outcome? ❑ Do the items on the test assess all the intended outcomes?
Importance	❑ Does the item test an important concept? ❑ Does the item avoid testing trivial or meaningless facts? ❑ Are the majority of test items written at the application level or above?
Differentiation	❑ Are all distractors plausible and valid? ❑ Is there only one correct answer? ❑ Are options such as "all" or "none of the above" avoided? ❑ Is repetitious wording minimized to avoid cuing? ❑ Is there consistent spacing and punctuation? ❑ Is negative wording avoided? ❑ Are absolutes, such as "always" or "never" in options avoided? ❑ Are all options the same general length and amount of information? ❑ Is the correct answer varied throughout the exam? ❑ Are numerical options written in ascending or descending order?
Fairness	❑ Are uncommon words, colloquialisms, slang, euphemisms avoided? ❑ Are unnecessary words or phrases eliminated? ❑ Is the stem in a form of a question? ❑ Are modal verbs "may", "should", or "would" eliminated from the stem? ❑ Are important words in the stem, such as **FIRST, BEST, MOST IMPORTANT** capitalized, bolded, or underlined?

▶ Create standard processes for item development and analysis within a program to promote fairness and evidence-based testing practices.

Best practices in testing include application of the recommendations provided in Chapter 3, *The Science of Learning* to promote incorporation of learning into assessment through testing. Specifically, we recommend the use of quizzing for formative assessment and the importance of reviewing tests and providing correct rationale for the correct answers. Providing opportunities for learners to better understand their test-taking study habits through using exam wrappers, as discussed in Chapter 3, *The Science of Learning*, is recommended to promote self-knowledge of study habits and testing practices.

References

Betts, J., Muntean, W., Kim, D., Jorion, N., & Dickison, P. (2019). Building a method for writing clinical judgment items for entry-level nursing exams. *Journal of Applied Testing Technology*, 20(S2), 21–36.

Billings, D. (2020). Developing and using multiple-choice and alternate format tests. In Billings, D. M. G., & Halstead, J. A. (Eds). *Teaching in nursing: A guide for faculty* (6th ed.). Saunders.

Birkhead, S., Kelman, G., Zittel, B., & Jatulis, L. (2018). The prevalence of multiple-choice testing in registered nurse licensure-qualifying nursing education programs in New York State. *Nursing Education Perspectives*, 39(3), 139–144. https://doi.org/10.1097/01.NEP.0000000000000280

Bosher, S. (2003). Barriers to creating a more culturally diverse nursing profession: Linguistic bias in multiple-choice nursing exams. *Nursing Education Perspectives*, 24(1), 25–34.

Bosher, S., & Bowles, M. (2008). The effects of linguistic modification on ESL students' comprehension of nursing course test items. *Nursing Education Perspectives*, 29(3), 165–172.

Bristol, T. J., Nelson, J. W., Sherrill, K. J., & Wangerin, V. S. (2018). Current state of test development, administration, and analysis: A study of faculty practices. *Nurse Educator*, 43(2), 68–72. https://doi.org/10.1097/NNE.0000000000000425

Centers for Disease Control and Prevention. (2015). *Epidemiological Glossary*. Retrieved from https://www.cdc.gov/reproductive-health/data_stats/glossary.html

Dickison, P., Haerling, K., & Lasater, K. (2019). Integrating the National Council of State Boards of Nursing clinical judgement model into nursing. *Journal of Nursing Education*, 58(2), 72–78. https://doi.org/10.3928/01484834-201901220

Hicks, N. A. (2011). Guidelines for identifying and revising culturally biased multiple-choice nursing examination items. *Nurse Educator*, 36(6), 266–270. https://doi.org/10.1097/NNE.0b013e3182333fd2

Hijji, B. M. (2017). Flaws of multiple choice questions in teacher-constructed nursing examinations: A pilot descriptive study. *Journal of Nursing Education*, 56(8), 490–496. https://doi.org/10.3928/01484834-20170712-08

Kranz, C., Love, A., & Roche, C. (2019). How to write a good test question: Nine tips for novice nurse educators. *The Journal of Continuing Education in Nursing, 50*(1), 12–14.

Lewis, L. S., & Bell, L. M. (2020). Academic success for culturally and linguistically diverse nursing students: An integrative review. *Journal of Nursing Education*, 59(10), 551–556. https://doi.org/10.3928/01484834-20200921-03

Magaldi, M., Kinneary, P., Colalillo, G., & Sutton, E. (2019). A guide to postexamination analysis: Utilizing data to increase reliability and ensure objectivity. *Nurse Educator*,

44(2), 61–63. https://doi.org/10.1097/NNE.0000000000000612

McDonald, M. E. (2018). *The nurse educator's guide to assessing learning outcomes* (4th ed.). Jones & Bartlett.

McGahee, T. W., & Ball, J. (2009). How to read and really use an item analysis. *Nurse Educator, 34*(4), 166–171. https://doi.org/10.1097/NNE.0b013e3181aaba94

Moore, B. S., & Clark, M. C. (2016). The role of linguistic modification in nursing education. *Journal of Nursing Education, 55*(6), 309–315. https://doi.org/10.3928/01484834-20160516-02

Moore, B., & Waters, A. (2020). The effect of linguistic modification on English as a second language (ESL) nursing student retention. *International Journal of Nursing Education Scholarship, 1*, 1–9. https://doi.org/10.1515/ijnes-2019-0116

NCSBN. (2022). *NGN facts for candidates.* Retrieved from https://www.ncsbn.org/11436.htm.

Oermann, M. H., & Gaberson, K. B. (2021). *Evaluation and testing in nursing education* (6th ed.). Springer Publishing Company.

Poorman, S. G., & Mastorovich, M. L. (2020). Constructing Next Generation National Council Licensure Examination (NCLEX) (NGN) style questions: Help for faculty. *Teaching & Learning in Nursing, 15*(1), 86–91. https://doi.org/10.1016/j.teln.2019.08.008

Rudolph, M. J., Daugherty, K. K., Ray, M. E., Shuford, V. P., Lebovitz, L., & DiVall, M. V. (2019). Best Practices Related to Examination Item Construction and Post-hoc Review. *American Journal of Pharmaceutical Education, 83*(7), 7204. https://doi.org/10.5688/ajpe7204

Schroeder, J. (2013). Improving NCLEX-RN pass rates by implementing a testing policy. *Journal of Professional Nursing, 29*(2 Suppl 1) S43–S47. https://doi.org/10.1016/j.profnurs.2012.07.002

Silvestri, L. A. (2019). *White paper: Higher-cognitive level test questions: A starting point for creating Next Generation NCLEX® (NGN) test items.* Elsevier Inc. Retrieved from https://evolve.elsevier.com/education/expertise/next-generation-nclex/higher-cognitive-level-test-questions-a-starting-point-for-creating-next-generation-nclex-ngn-test-items/

Sutherland, K., Schwartz, J., & Dickison, P. (2012). Best practices for writing test items. *Journal of Nursing Regulation, 3*(2), 35–39. https://doi.org/10.1016/S2155-8256(15)30217-9

Tarrant, M., & Ware, J. (2010). A comparison of the psychometric properties of three- and four-option multiple-choice questions in nursing assessments. *Nurse Education Today, 30*(6), 539–543. https://doi.org/10.1016/j.nedt.2009.11.002

Tarrant, M., & Ware, J. (2012). A framework for improving the quality of multiple-choice assessments. *Nurse Educator, 37*(3), 98–104. https://doi.org/10.1097/NNE.0b013e31825041d0

16

Rubric Development

Kathie Lasater, EdD, RN, FAAN, ANEF

CHAPTER OVERVIEW

This chapter reviews how to construct rubrics for the assessment of learning in the classroom and in clinical settings. The purpose of rubrics will be presented and various ways rubrics can be used for assessment will be presented. The main parts of a rubric will be reviewed as well as steps in rubric construction

INTRODUCTION

Although there is no known research, it is highly likely that for most, grading (or marking) is our least favorite part of the nurse educator role. There are many reasons why this is so, some of which include the length of time it takes to read, grade, and give feedback for each assignment, multiplied by how many submissions there are; the worry of not giving equal effort to each submission due to fatigue or multiple interruptions from colleagues, family, or pets; the monotony of giving the same feedback repeatedly; the ambiguous criteria for the assignment which can lead to wonder about subjectivity or worse; and a struggle to give helpful feedback. Then there are the niggly issues of acknowledging our own unconscious biases and of students misunderstanding the expectations for an assignment and the resulting confusion that may lead to extra work to give the student the benefit of the doubt. There is the dubious perception of the feedback—do students actually read and incorporate it? A related issue is the pressure students communicate to make good grades for admission to graduate school, to satisfy family, or to keep their loans or scholarships. Experienced educators likely can identify with most, if not all, of these grading issues.

Yet, as educators, our responsibility is to assess, both formatively and summatively, and provide feedback as part of the educational process so our graduates become safe, competent practitioners. Research informs us that students want and need clear, concise, objective feedback (Cockett & Jackson, 2018; Fink, 2013; Wiggins & McTighe, 2005) and benefit from knowing expectations for assessment (Cheng & Chan, 2019). As our student bodies become increasingly diverse, educators must adapt to provide an assessment of a broader range of students whose lives and educational experiences may be very dissimilar to their peers or their educators (Lasater et al., 2019). Rubrics may provide a helpful solution to benefit educators and students alike. This chapter presents the construction of rubrics for assessment of learning in classroom and clinical settings, as well as the development of skills nurses need, such as reflection (Cheng & Chan, 2019), clinical judgment (Lasater, 2011), and leadership. Consideration of the benefits and limitations of rubrics along with some examples of different types of rubrics and the steps involved in constructing a rubric are explained.

Pedagogically speaking, a rubric is simply "a scoring tool that lays out the specific expectations for an assignment" (Stevens & Levi, 2013, p. 3). Further, a rubric can also be a guide for development of a skill over a period of time, such as a semester or the length of a program, communicating a trajectory of development (Lasater, 2011).

BEST REASONS TO USE RUBRICS

As a first-generation college student, I can attest that academe uses a different language than everyday communication. With an influx of students from other countries and languages, many of whom are first-generation college students, it is critical to their success to communicate clearly and equitably. There is evidence to indicate that rubrics do produce higher levels of learning (Howell, 2014; Jonsson, 2014). In addition, Stevens and Levi (2013) have identified a number of other excellent reasons to use rubrics. Here are some of their best reasons as well as some from my own experience:

> Rubrics save educator time. If the criteria for success are clearly laid out in the form of a rubric, the educator does not need to repeat or rewrite the expectations for an assignment or competency performance. A few additional words may be necessary on occasion, but the feedback is usually already there in black and white; it just needs to be indicated for the student's benefit. There is no question that some upfront time is required to construct or modify a well-designed rubric, but once constructed, the grading becomes easier and far less time-consuming.

> Rubrics can provide more timely feedback. We sometimes wonder if students actually read the feedback we work so hard to provide. There is evidence (Black & Wiliam, 1998; Rucker & Thomson, 2003) that feedback given sooner is more effective for learning impact than feedback given later. This also means that the time spent by educators to provide feedback is better spent and more likely to be meaningful. Rubrics offer educators the opportunity to more efficiently grade assignments and return feedback.

> Rubrics provide guidance for promoting peer feedback. It is also possible for peers to use rubrics to offer feedback. Without rubrics, peer evaluations can be challenging because (a) peers want their colleagues to be successful so may not offer honest feedback, and (b) they often do not recognize which criteria are most salient. Rubrics provide a method for more meaningful peer feedback.

> Rubrics help students learn and improve their efforts. If students can see the expectations and where they fell short or what they did well, they are more likely to be successful in subsequent assignments. In addition, by having a detailed guide of expectations, they have the opportunity to seek clarification before they begin an assignment and as long as they are willing to do the work outlined in the rubric,

should not fail the assignment. In other words, rubrics are criterion-referenced rather than norm-referenced (Hansen, 2011; Oermann & Gaberson, 2021).

➤ Rubrics can promote improvement in developing competency over time through a critical process. For competency development, understanding the rubric's trajectory of development allows students the opportunity to critically self-evaluate their performance against the rubric, noting patterns of improvement and/or recurrent issues. As well, students can use a rubric to self-correct and set goals toward the next level of achievement. Anecdotally, several students at the start of their program expressed relief to me after looking at a developmental rubric and realizing they are exactly where they should be (at the beginning).

➤ Rubrics provide a common language to support student learning. Language is very powerful, and every profession has its own. By using language in rubrics to describe expectations, students begin to learn the language of their profession, and they have the opportunity to better understand and demonstrate the course and/or program outcomes. Additionally, rubrics provide a common language between and among students as well as educators (Kopp & Mayberry, 2021).

➤ Rubrics offer a more equitable approach to assessment. Speaking of language, rubrics can level the playing field by adopting a common language, whether a student speaks another language as primary or is from a different English-speaking country where words or phrases may have different meanings. If the criteria for grading and expectations for student performance are transparent (Jonsson, 2014), subjectivity is minimized, and the educator is more likely to grade equitably and reliably. Enhancement of feedback has been noted as a benefit of rubric use; in other words, feedback can be more useful and targeted with rubrics (Cockett & Jackson, 2018). Rubrics can also provide a more reliable approach to assessment when multiple educators are grading (Minnich et al., 2018).

➤ Rubrics can help educators become better educators. Patterns identified by using common criteria in a rubric allow the educator to recognize teaching strengths, weaknesses, or blind spots. For example, if many students are having difficulties with a particular concept or writing process as evidenced by the rubric for an assignment, that may bring attention that more teaching is needed in that area. (Adapted from Stevens & Levi, 2013, pp. 17–28.)

While one integrative review uncovered that the majority of students found rubrics useful, some students believed that rubrics restricted creativity, added pressure, or were not used in a consistent fashion (Cockett & Jackson, 2018). The following sections address these issues.

GETTING STARTED

Before creating a rubric, there are several critical preliminary considerations. Skipping these may lead to a less-than-successful product, not to mention unnecessary work. Contemplate these:

➤ Know your learners' educational path, where they have come from, and where they are going next in the program. What concepts and skills did they learn in the course before the one in which they are currently enrolled? What level of mastery were the expected to achieve? What are they supposed to learn or experience in the current course? Without the answers to these questions, the bar may be set too high or too low. Positioning it just right in a rubric prevents unnecessary discouragement and also motivates students to stretch their abilities.

> Link the assignment and/or skill to course or program outcomes, considering the importance or weight of outcomes. It is critical and fair that whatever grading scheme you use should reflect the course or program outcomes. This promotes the concepts of curricular alignment discussed in Chapter 7 (Hansen, 2011; Oermann & Gaberson, 2021; Wiggins & McTighe, 2005).

> Assess honestly; if this is an assignment or skill you have evaluated before, reflect on how well your previous assessment strategy worked or did not and why. Identifying these can help to guide your efforts to create a meaningful rubric.

> Carefully read and review a rubric you may have inherited from the course or from a previous educator. Is it usable for you to work with or would it need extensive revision? If the latter, it is probably best to start fresh (Stevens & Levi, 2013).

> Check online for an available rubric that may be suitable for your purposes or easily modifiable (Stevens & Levi, 2013). If published, you may not need to ask permission to use it. Regardless, attribution of the rubric should be a part of your practice; if you intend to modify or adapt the rubric, you should reach out to the creator to let them know your intentions and to ask for permission or suggestions.

As you can see, beginning this way requires some time and reflection so it is best not to wait until the last minute to begin creating or adapting a rubric. Once these steps are complete, it is time to start constructing the rubric; knowing the components is a critical next step.

UNPACKING THE RUBRIC

Whether the rubric is used for a point-in-time assignment, such as a written nursing care plan or project, or for a skill that develops over time, such as therapeutic communication, the components of a rubric are essentially the same. The first step is to identify the skill or concept to be evaluated. In the left-hand column of the grid, the crucial dimensions of the competency or task are listed. The columns to the right are labeled with the levels, for example, Excellent, Satisfactory, and Not Satisfactory. Once the elements of the competency and the levels of achievement are identified, the cells are completed with the details or descriptors for each level for a specific dimension (see Table 16.1). Each of these four components will be discussed in more detail in the following paragraphs.

Task or Title

The competency, assignment, or skill becomes the title of the rubric or at least is identified at the top of the grid. For example, it could be a rubric for a specific

TABLE 16.1

Basic Rubric Grid

		Competency or Task	
Dimensions	**Levels**	——————————————▶	
	Level Descriptors	——————————————▶	
	Level Descriptors	——————————————▶	
	Level Descriptors	——————————————▶	
▼	Level Descriptors	——————————————▶	

assignment, such as a persuasive letter to a stakeholder, advocating for a social change impacting a population (see Table 16.2), or it could be a skill to be developed the length of the program, such as clinical judgment, where everyone starts as a beginner (see Table 16.3).

Dimensions of the Task/Skill

This part of the rubric may require the most work, but it is pre-work that will pay off during the process of grading. It also communicates to students what is most salient for them to demonstrate or learn. Begin by reflecting on the skill or assignment to uncover the critical elements.

A variety of approaches can be used. A very utilitarian approach is to break down a psychomotor skill by steps whereas a non-psychomotor skill may require more nuanced dimensions, reflecting a theoretical or conceptual understanding or approach. Remember, it is important that the dimensions be measurable or observable in some way to provide fair assessment for all learners. Hansen (2011) suggested another strategy: gather a group of representative past assignments and sort them into three or four piles, based on the quality of the content. At that point, it will be easier to determine the important dimensions of the skill/assignment and begin to consider levels of performance.

Levels of Performance

One can label levels, using the university or college's grading system, such as 70–79 percent (C), 80–89 percent (B), and 90–100 percent (A). However, in certain circumstances, it may be more appropriate to use language that describes performance, such as Excellent, Satisfactory, or Unsatisfactory. Another strategy is to use points that imply a range of potential; that is, 1, 3, and 5 with 5 as the highest achievable

TABLE 16.2

Rubric for Written Assignment with Weighting

PERSUASIVE WRITING ASSIGNMENT

CONTENT (130 total pts, must have a minimum of 91 pts in this section to receive a passing grade)

Dimensions	A/A− Level (90–100%)	B/B− Level (80–89%)	C/C− Level (70–79%)	Not Passing Level (<70%)	Points Earned
Identifies SPECIFIC audience (individual or agency that influence) (30 pts)	Audience is specifically identified by individual or group name and has potential or real influence on the issue (24–30)		Audience is alluded to (21–23)	Audience is generic or disorganized, e.g., "all nurses," or reader cannot identify the intended audience (<21)	
Tailors an appropriate message and request to motivate the audience to take a specific action (40 pts)	The message is clear and the request achievable for the audience and is stated near the beginning of the text (unless using option 4) so that the reader knows the specific request or issue (36–40)	The message is mostly clear with few statements that do not seem to apply. The request may appear a bit too much after a bit too much introduction (32–35)	The message and request for action are specified but very late in the text OR there is not a good relationship identified for the audience (28–34)	It is unclear what action the reader should take or how the message relates to the specified action (<28)	
Focuses on one health care issue related to clinical population of focus with broad-reaching implications (30 pts)	The health care issue is clearly identified, and it relates to the writer's clinical population (27–30)	The health care issue is clear but relates to individuals primarily or is distracted from by other minor issues (24–26)	The primary health care issue is present but difficult to identify because of equally presented issues or it is too specific to have a far-reaching effect (21–23)	There is no health care issue identified, or the reader cannot identify the issue in one sentence or less (<21)	

	Current and/or expected burden is clearly expressed with citations to validate (13.5–15)	Current and/or expected burden is cited, but its connection to the issue may not be clear (12–13)	Current and/or expected burden is alluded to in the text but is not clearly stated or cited (10.5–12)	No reference is made to the impact of the issue (<10.5)
Includes a description of the burden or impact of this issue on individuals, families, communities, and/or society in general (15 pts)				
Includes compelling comparison data to support the issue being presented (15 pts)	Data clearly connect to the identified health care issue; comparison data of any type is presented with a citation and numeric values, e.g., percentages/rates (13.5–15)	Data are present and somewhat connects to the identified health care issue; comparison data are presented with citations (12–13)	Comparison data are alluded to or is presented without a citation or numeric values (10.5–12)	No data or comparison data (<10.5)

REFERENCES (30 total pts, must have a minimum of 21 pts in this section to receive a passing grade)

Dimensions	A/A– Level (90–100%)	B/B– Level (80–89%)	C/C– Level (70–79%)	Not Passing Level (<70%)	Points Earned
Content is supported by a minimum of 10 references (at least one government statistical citation, at least one professional association citation, 4–8 peer-reviewed journal articles, 0–4 well-referenced website documents (reviewed by a panel of experts and containing at least 10 high-quality references) (30 pts)	All requirements for references are met as stated; for each inaccurate reference or reference that does not meet the requirement, there is a 3-point deduction (27–30)	Two references do not meet the criteria (24)	Three references do not meet the criteria (21)	Four or more references do not meet the criteria (<21)	

(continued)

TABLE 16.2

Rubric for Written Assignment with Weighting *(Continued)*

FORMAT/TECHNICAL (40 total pts, must have a minimum of 21 pts in this section to receive a passing grade)

Dimensions	A/A– Level (90–100%)	B/B– Level (80–89%)	C/C– Level (70–79%)	Not Passing Level (<70%)	Points Earned
Adheres to APA format expectations as described in Sakai toolbar; summary is written concisely (total length does not exceed 1–2 pages double-spaced, not including reference list or title page) (20 pts)	Each type of APA mistake is worth a 2 pt. deduction; e.g., if there are 1 or there are 3 direct quotes without page numbers, 2 pt. are deducted; no format mistakes or omissions found or only a small error in format (18–20)	Two types of APA and/or format mistakes and/or omissions are present (16–17)	Three types of APA and/or format mistakes and/or omissions are present (14–15)	More than 3 types of APA and/or format mistakes and/or omissions are present (<14)	
Demonstrates excellent sentence structure and use of language and any minor errors do not interfere with understanding the intended meaning (20 pts)	Each sentence has a subject and verb, language use is clear as to meaning and contextually accurate. Spelling and punctuation are mostly accurate. Meaning of each sentence or thought is clear despite small errors (18–20)	Sentences overall are complete; spelling and punctuation are mostly accurate. Some words may lack clarity or statements may lack a bit of context. Overarching meaning of whole text is mostly clear despite a few small errors (16–17)	One or two incomplete sentences are present or punctuation is consistently inadequate; context for statements may be questionable. Overarching meaning of whole text is present despite many small errors (14–15)	Many errors in sentence structure and language use are present. The persuasiveness or cogency of the text is lost because of the number or severity of errors (<14)	
TOTAL POINTS					

Additional comments:

Evaluated by

TABLE 16.3

Lasater Clinical Judgment Rubric

Effective NOTICING involves:	Exemplary	Accomplished	Developing	Beginning
Focused observation	Focuses observation appropriately; regularly observes and monitors a wide variety of objective and subjective data to uncover any useful information	Regularly observes/monitors a variety of data, including both subjective and objective; most useful information is noticed, may miss the most subtle signs	Attempts to monitor a variety of subjective and objective data, but is overwhelmed by the array of data; focuses on the most obvious data, missing some important information	Confused by the clinical situation and the amount/type of data; observation is not organized and important data are missed, and/or assessment errors are made
Recognizing deviations from expected patterns	Recognizes subtle patterns and deviations from expected patterns in data and uses these to guide the assessment	Recognizes most obvious patterns and deviations in data and uses these to continually assess	Identifies obvious patterns and deviations, missing some important information; unsure how to continue the assessment	Focuses on one thing at a time and misses most patterns/deviations from expectations; misses opportunities to refine the assessment
Information seeking	Assertively seeks information to plan intervention: carefully collects useful subjective data from observing the client and from interacting with the client and family	Actively seeks subjective information about the client's situation from the client and family to support planning interventions; occasionally does not pursue important leads	Makes limited efforts to seek additional information from the client/family; often seems not to know what information to seek and/or pursues unrelated information	Is ineffective in seeking information; relies mostly on objective data; has difficulty interacting with the client and family and fails to collect important subjective data

Effective INTERPRETING involves:	Exemplary	Accomplished	Developing	Beginning
Prioritizing data	Focuses on the most relevant and important data useful for explaining the client's condition	Generally focuses on the most important data and seeks further relevant information, but also may try to attend to less pertinent data	Makes an effort to prioritize data and focus on the most important, but also attends to less relevant/useful data	Has difficulty focusing and appears not to know which data are most important to the diagnosis; attempts to attend to all available data

(continued)

TABLE 16.3

Lasater Clinical Judgment Rubric (Continued)

Effective INTERPRETING involves:	Exemplary	Accomplished	Developing	Beginning
Making sense of data	Even when facing complex, conflicting, or confusing data, is able to (1) note and make sense of patterns in the client's data, (2) compare these with known patterns from the nursing knowledge base, research, personal experience, and intuition), and (3) develop plans for interventions that can be justified in terms of their likelihood of success	In most situations, interprets the client's data patterns and compares them with known patterns to develop an intervention plan and accompanying rationale; the exceptions are rare or complicated cases where it is appropriate to seek the guidance of a specialist or more experienced nurse	In simple or common/familiar situations, is able to compare the client's data patterns with those known and to develop/explain intervention plans; has difficulty, however, with even moderately difficult data/situations that are within the expectations for students, inappropriately requires advice or assistance	Even in simple familiar/common situations, has difficulty interpreting or making sense of data; has trouble distinguishing among competing explanations and appropriate interventions, requiring assistance both in diagnosing the problem and in developing an intervention

Effective RESPONDING involves:	Exemplary	Accomplished	Developing	Beginning
Calm, confident manner	Assumes responsibility: delegates team assignments, assesses the client, and reassures them and their families	Generally displays leadership and confidence, and is able to control/calm most situations; may show stress in particularly difficult or complex situations	Is tentative in the leader's role; reassures clients/families in routine and relatively simple situations, but becomes stressed and disorganized easily	Except in simple and routine situations, is stressed and disorganized, lacks control, making clients and families anxious/less able to cooperate
Clear communication	Communicates effectively; explains interventions; calms/reassures clients and families; directs and involves team members, explaining and giving directions; checks for	Generally communicates well; explains carefully to clients; gives clear directions to team; could be more effective in establishing rapport	Shows some communication ability (e.g., giving directions); communication with clients/families/team members is only partly successful; displays caring but not competence	Has difficulty communicating; explanations are confusing, directions are unclear or contradictory, and clients/families are made confused/anxious, not reassured

	Exemplary	Accomplished	Developing	Beginning
Well-planned intervention/ flexibility	Interventions are tailored for the individual client; monitors client progress closely and is able to adjust treatment as indicated by the client response	Develops interventions based on relevant patient data; monitors progress regularly but does not expect to have to change treatments	Develops interventions based on the most obvious data; monitors progress, but is unable to make adjustments based on the patient response	Focuses on developing a single intervention addressing a likely solution, but it may be vague, confusing, and/or incomplete; some monitoring may occur
Being skillful	Shows mastery of necessary nursing skills	Displays proficiency in the use of most nursing skills; could improve speed or accuracy	Is hesitant or ineffective in utilizing nursing skills	Is unable to select and/or perform the nursing skills
Effective REFLECTING involves:	**Exemplary**	**Accomplished**	**Developing**	**Beginning**
Evaluation/self-analysis	Independently evaluates/ analyzes personal clinical performance, noting decision points, elaborating alternatives, and accurately evaluating choices against alternatives	Evaluates/analyzes personal clinical performance with minimal prompting, primarily major events/decisions; key decision points are identified and alternatives are considered	Even when prompted, briefly verbalizes the most obvious evaluations; has difficulty imagining alternative choices; is self-protective in evaluating personal choices	Even prompted evaluations are brief, cursory, and not used to improve performance; justifies personal decisions/choices without evaluating them
Commitment to improvement	Demonstrates commitment to ongoing improvement: reflects on and critically evaluates nursing experiences; accurately identifies strengths/weaknesses and develops specific plans to eliminate weaknesses	Demonstrates a desire to improve nursing performance: reflects on and evaluates experiences/ identifies strengths/ weaknesses; could be more systematic in evaluating weaknesses	Demonstrates awareness of the need for ongoing improvement and makes some effort to learn from experience and improve performance but tends to state the obvious, and needs external evaluation	Appears uninterested in improving performance or unable to do so; rarely reflects; is uncritical of himself/herself, or overly critical (given level of development); is unable to see flaws or need for improvement

TABLE 16.4

Rubric with Scoring Flexibility

FORUM DISCUSSION ASSESSMENT

Points	5 Points (per cell)	3 Points (per cell)	1 Point (per cell)	0 Points
Quality of post	Appropriate comments: thoughtful, reflective, and respectful of others' postings	Appropriate comments responding respectfully to others' postings	Responds, but with minimum effort. (e.g., "I agree with Bill")	No posting
Relevance of post	Posts topics related to discussion and prompts further discussion	Posts topics that are related to discussion	Posts topics that do not relate to the discussion; makes short or irrelevant remarks	No posting
Contribution to the learning community	Aware of needs of the community; attempts to further the group discussion; presents creative approaches to topic	Attempts to direct the discussion and occasionally present relevant viewpoints for consideration by group	Does not make effort to participate in learning community as it develops	No feedback to fellow students
Initial post	Initial post is on time (according to the due dates)	Initial post is 2 days late (according to the due dates)	Initial post is 4 days late (according to the due dates)	Initial post is 5 or more days late or never done (according to the due dates)
Responses to classmates	Meaningful responses to at least 3 peers	Meaningful responses to 2 peers	A meaningful response is made to 1 peer only.	No meaningful responses to peers

score (see Table 16.4). Language to describe levels is an important communicator. For instance, using the term *Unsatisfactory* may seem too negative, especially in the case of a competency rubric designed to describe progress over the length of the program. *Developing*, *Beginning*, or *Needs Improvement* may be more palatable or encouraging descriptors; however, if the educator is trying to convey that the student really must improve, *Unsatisfactory* may communicate the importance of meeting expected standards most effectively. I recommend never using the term, *Fail*, which undermines student potential.

Inevitably, the question of weighting must be considered. If each dimension is equally salient, there is nothing extra to be done. However, in the case of grading an assignment that includes criteria for punctuation and grammar, for example, criteria related to content are likely more important, thus a scheme for weighting is required (see Table 16.2). The determination of the importance of the dimensions should be considered from the outset of rubric construction.

The question often arises regarding how many levels a rubric should have, and the quick (but not so easy) answer is, "As many as are needed!" But what is meant by this? A good rule of thumb is to start with three to keep it simple and begin to describe the levels of performance. If it becomes difficult to describe the levels, it may be that additional levels are necessary; Stevens and Levi (2013) recommend no more than five. However, if the evaluator finds it challenging to distinguish between two levels and keeps wishing there was a level in between, it may well be that another level will be useful. If it is problematic to distinguish between the levels, fewer may be better. However, the real test comes when you begin using the rubric, and the level descriptors are the key.

Level Descriptors

The level descriptors of performance are the meat of the rubric. The labels create a starting place, but we all interpret labels differently. Through the use of well-worded level descriptors, students and educators become familiar with objective actions that are expected. For that reason, it is critical to consider how the terminology aligns with the course or program outcomes the rubric is addressing.

An empty grid can be daunting, but with some reflection, the educator can start by describing what is acceptable or satisfactory, then complete the highest and lowest levels of performance. In other words, what would you expect to see in an assignment at the *Excellent* level vs. *Satisfactory*? Or perhaps it is easier to start with descriptors that outline the very highest level or the unacceptable level. There is no one right way to do this; rather, it is up to the rubric creator to determine how to start describing the levels. No matter where the educator begins, the process will inevitably be iterative and require going back and forth between levels to hone the descriptions.

Creating a rubric is not an occasion for creative writing or choosing a variety of synonyms. Rather, consistent language is critical for clarity; therefore, choose words wisely. Avoid the passive voice when possible; use action verbs where appropriate, such as *describe, define, state,* or *choose.* Alignment of language between the cells, particularly verbs, is also a key to understanding what is meant by the level descriptors. The rubric can help shape program language or vice versa so that educators and students use a similar vocabulary when discussing the assignment or a program's competency. If a common language already exists, it will be important to use it in rubrics.

For certain dimensions, it is easy to quantify the descriptors. For example, the rubric might be an assessment tool for a paper in which including 10 peer-reviewed references is required. The level descriptors may read: Cites 1–4 peer-reviewed references (Unsatisfactory); Cites 5–8 peer-reviewed references (Satisfactory); Cites 9–10 peer-reviewed references (Excellent).

For the educator, the descriptors, accurately written in consistent, understandable language with enough detail, minimize subjectivity. For the student, the descriptors offer a clear guide for completing the assignment and/or elucidating the next steps in competency development. Again, there will be a need during the development process to go back and forth between levels to ensure consistent language and that distinguishing between the levels is possible or to return to the outcomes the assignment or competency is addressing to be sure they clearly connect (Oermann Gaberson, 2021).

Parenthetically, you will notice in the rubrics provided as examples, the levels an level descriptors tend to move from right to left, that is, from lowest to highest in different direction from how we read in English. This appears to be the conventiona approach for no reason I have discovered. However, it is logical for me to think abou a trajectory moving in the direction of the specific targeted dimensions in the left-han column.

TYPES OF RUBRICS AND SOME EXAMPLES FOR DIFFERENT USES

There have already been references to different types of rubrics, but in this section descriptions of three different types will be explained and illustrated with exam ples: (a) holistic rubrics, where one score covers multiple aspects of the assignment (b) point-in-time or analytic rubrics, e.g., written assignments, skill demonstrations posters, presentations; and (c) developmental rubrics used to assess a skill or com petency that develops over time (e.g., length of course or program). As an aside, there is evidence that co-constructed rubrics (between students and educators) may have positive benefit on learning, learning self-regulation, and student satisfaction with feed back (Cockett & Jackson, 2018; Fraile et al., 2017; Kiss et al., 2017).

Holistic Rubrics

Oermann and Gaberson (2021) state that using a holistic rubric for scoring "yields one overall score that considers the entire response to the item rather than scoring its com ponent parts separately" (p. 114). This type of rubric is very effective when assessing student contributions to weekly assignments, such as online discussion forums or a low-scoring part of the overall course grade. An otherwise arduous grading process can become one that takes just a few minutes and offers timely feedback. Table 16.5 is an example of this type of rubric.

Point-in-Time or Analytic Rubrics

Consider using this type of rubric for written assignments or presentations, particularly when they account for a significant part of the students' grades or are complex assign ments. Because the content I teach is not wholly fact-driven and I want to know how students apply their learning, I prefer to require a writing assignment that is an opportu nity for students to synthesize and apply their learning in a real-world way rather than a final examination. Table 16.2 is an example of a rather complex point-in-time rubric that includes an example of the weighting of sections for a final paper. The rubric is complex because it represents a summation of the students' work for the course. The trick with point-in-time rubrics is not to spell out so much detail to limit students' creativity but rather to offer guidelines for the successful completion of the assignment (more generic vs. specific; Hansen, 2011). Table 16.4 also offers an example of scoring flexibility by having dimensions for 5 points, 3, points, 1, and 0 points.

TABLE 16.5

Holistic Rubric

FORUM DISCUSSION WITH PEERS
(30 percent of course grade)

Score	Description
4	Comments reveal the ability to make subtle connections between own and others' work with regard to the assignments. Arguments are well-supported by evidence from the literature and critically consider the plausibility of other perspectives. Aware of own limitations in understanding. Meaningfully responds to at least 3 peers.
3	Comments reveal the ability to make subtle connections in own work with regard to the assignments. Theory supporting arguments is clearly articulated, but evidence from the literature may be missing. Other perspectives are considered in relation to one's own. Generally aware of what is and is not understood. Responds in some measure of depth to at least two peers.
2	Comments are descriptive rather than analytic or evaluative with regard to the assignments. Theory is used exclusively to support arguments and assertions. Generally aware of what is and is not understood. Responds to peers in occasionally meaningful ways and/or limits responses to one peer.
1	Comments are descriptive of reading/topic and demonstrate little or no understanding. Relevancy of comments to readings or topic not clear. No theories or concepts were used to analyze or support statements. Not clear about what is and is not understood. Does not respond to classmates' statements relevantly or does not respond at all.

For interest, contrast two rubrics, Table 16.4 (point-in-time, analytic) with Table 16.5 (holistic). Both evaluate students' participation in online forums but in different ways. Which do you find more satisfying or easier to work with? Which balances feedback with the educator's time for grading? Which type of rubric will best provide feedback to facilitate learning and help students to meet expected standards?

Developmental Rubrics

This type of rubric focuses on a competency or skill where the student begins as a novice; hence, the use of this type of rubric is more about formative than summative assessment. Table 16.3 is such a rubric where a trajectory of development of clinical judgment is laid out from Beginning to Exemplary for 11 dimensions over the length of a program (Lasater, 2007). By having a visible trajectory, students and educators can use it for learning about clinical judgment, goal-setting, and formative assessment. This particular rubric was developed with the intention that prelicensure graduates would achieve the Accomplished level by the end of their programs; however, the Exemplary level was included to (a) give students a vision for the next steps beyond graduation, and (b) account for transferrable skills students may bring to nursing in keeping with a developmental process.

Rubrics are a highly adaptable method for learning and assessment. But with validation, developmental rubrics can also be used as tools for research. For example for data collection purposes, one can assign a number value to the levels, such as 4 = Exemplary, 3 = Accomplished, 2 = Developing, 1 = Beginning in the case of Table 16.3.

How Will the Rubric Be Used?

As part of the planning process, it is a good idea to consider how to use the rubric most effectively. For a course assignment, consider the inclusion of the rubric in the course materials or syllabus. In this way, students can begin to see how their assignment aligns with the course outcomes (Oermann & Gaberson, 2021), and when they can see the link, they are less likely to consider the assignment "busy work." At the very least, students should have access to a grading rubric before they undertake an assignment. If the rubric assesses a skill, such as clinical judgment, having the rubric available helps students begin to understand how such a concept fits into what they are learning about nursing and to visualize a trajectory of development over the specified period of time.

How to use the rubric for actual evaluation? There are many choices here. First of all, determine if the rubric will be available digitally or in hard copy. Depending on the assignment or skill as well as when and where the assessment will take place, consider the idea of an online template so that feedback can be returned digitally to the student for placement in an e-portfolio or be easily filed in the educator's digital gradebook. Either way, a checkbox can be inserted into each cell so the evaluator can simply check the appropriate box, or the language in the cell can be circled or highlighted. In fact, students can engage in self- and/or peer-evaluation by simply marking the appropriate words or phrases with a highlighter (Lasater, 2011). It is always wise to leave a little space at the end of the rubric or perhaps for each dimension for a few brief comments; however, it should not be necessary to write a lot if the rubric spells out what is most important.

When Is It Done?

This is a little like a child asking a parent, "Are we there yet?" on a road trip. Like an artist, it is sometimes challenging to know when the product or work of art is finished. If the steps outlined above have been completed and the cells are full of descriptors, it is now time to test the rubric. If it is based on an assignment/competency within a course, it would be an excellent idea to share it with the course leader or a trusted colleague who is familiar with the course well before the course launches. If the rubric is based on a theory or model created by someone else, it is recommended to check in with that person for some assurance that your use of the rubric is consistent with the intended purpose (Lasater, 2007). Prior to the course beginning, or at least before an assignment is announced, the students should have access to the rubric so the expectations are transparent, and they can see where the bolus of points is for the assignment. If you use an online learning management system, such as Blackboard, Moodle, or Sakai, the course materials section is a logical place to post the rubric.

TESTING THE RUBRIC

They say the proof is in the pudding! So, it is now time to try out the rubric. Start with the recognition that there will likely need to be minor adjustments that the first experience of using will bring to light.

You will undoubtedly find that pure objectivity is nearly impossible (Kopp & Mayberry, 2021), but hopefully, you will discover that the process of grading is much more enjoyable, more reliable, and less tiring than before. As you work through the stack of assignments, you may find a pattern that indicates the wording between levels is not clear enough to distinguish between them, or the emphasis or weight is not exactly where it needs to be. Jot down these notes so you can address them the next time you have completed the grading process.

Once you've worked through the stack, go back to the rubric to make the changes or adjustments that need to be made for the next time. I recommend this be done after each use of the rubric; in other words, use the evidence from one use to inform future use.

USING RUBRICS FOR CLINICAL EXPERIENCE/SIMULATION

Rubrics, particularly developmental rubrics, can be useful tools in clinical settings, including simulation. Beyond focusing on skills, they can be advantageous in other ways in these settings. Consider these uses:

▸ Students, preceptors, and educators can use them for formative assessment of a particular skill at a point in time, such as midterm;

▸ Educators can use them as guides to formulate deeper-level questions about a concept or skill or to facilitate a debriefing;

▸ If a rubric focuses on a psychomotor skill, the completed rubric becomes evidence of growth toward mastery; and

▸ Students can track their own progress for specific skills and use the rubric to set goals for next steps in their development of the skill. (Adapted from Lasater, 2011.)

CHAPTER SUMMARY

Creating rubrics is an art based on good pedagogical practice and evidence; there is no one right way to create an excellent rubric, and all rubrics require ongoing fine-tuning. However, rubrics hold great potential to save time and effort in grading for the educator and promote student learning. Through trial and error, educators can use rubrics to convey clear expectations, link the rubric's dimensions to course and/or program outcomes, offer a common language, and encourage self-evaluation.

References

Black, P., & Wiliam, D. (1998). Assessment and classroom learning. *Assessment in Education: Principles, Policy & Practice, 5*(1), 7–74. https://doi.org/10.1080/0969595980050102

Cheng, M. W., & Chan, C. K. (2019). An experimental test: Using rubrics for reflective writing to develop reflection. *Studies in Educational Evaluation, 62,* 176–182. https://doi.org/10.1016/j.stueduc.2019.04.001

Cockett, A., & Jackson, C. (2018). The use of assessment rubrics to enhance feedback in higher education: An integrative literature review. *Nurse Education Today, 69,* 8–13. https://doi.org/10.1016/j.nedt.2018.06.022

Fink, L. D. (2013). *Creating significant learning experiences: An integrated approach to designing college courses.* Jossey-Bass.

Fraile, J., Panadero, E., & Pardo, R. (2017). Co-creating rubrics: The effects on self-regulated learning, self-efficacy and performance of establishing assessment criteria with students. *Studies in Educational Evaluation*, *53*, 69–76. https://doi.org/10.1016/j.stueduc.2017.03.003

Hansen, E. J. (2011). *Idea-Based Learning: A Course Design Process to Promote Conceptual Understanding*. Stylus Publishing.

Howell, R. J. (2014). Grading rubrics: Hoopla or help? *Innovations in Teaching and Education International*, *51*(4), 400–410. https://doi.org/10.1080/14703297.2013.785252

Jonsson, A. (2014). Rubrics as a way of providing transparency in assessment. *Assessment & Evaluation in Higher Education*, *39*, 840–852. https://doi.org/10.1080/02602938.2013.875117

Kiss, A., Steiner, C., Grossman, P., Langewitz, W., Tschudi, P., & Kiessling, C. (2017). Students' satisfaction with general practitioners' feedback to their reflective writing: A randomized trial. *Canadian Medical Education Journal, 8*(4), e54–e59. https://doi.org/10.36834/cmej.36929

Kopp, M. L., & Mayberry, A. L. M. (2021). An end-of-life communication performance rubric. *Journal of Hospice & Palliative Nursing*, *23*(5), 429–434. https://doi.org/10.1097/NJH.0000000000000772

Lasater, K. (2007). Clinical judgment development: Using simulation to create an assessment rubric. *Journal of Nursing Education*, *46*, 496–503. https://doi.org/10.3928/01484834-20071101-04

Lasater, K. (2011). Clinical judgment: The last frontier for evaluation. *Nurse Education in Practice*, *11*(2), 86–92. https://doi.org/10.1016/j.nepr.2010.11.013

Lasater, K., Holloway, K., Lapkin, S., Kelly, M., McGrath, B., Nielsen, A., Stoyles, S., Dieckmann, N. F., & Campbell, M. (2019). Do preregistration nursing students' backgrounds impact what they notice and interpret about patients? *Nurse Education Today*, *78*, 37–43. https://doi.org/10.1016/j.nedt.2019.03.013

Minnich, M., Kirkpatrick, A. J., Goodman, J. T. Whittaker, A., Chappell, H. S., Schoening, A. M., & Khanna, M. M. (2018). Writing across the curriculum: Reliability testing of a standardized rubric. *Journal of Nursing Education*, *57*(6), 366–370. https://doi.org/10.3928/01484834-20180522-08

Oermann, M. H., & Gaberson, K. B. (2021). *Evaluation and Testing in Nursing Education* (6th ed.). Springer Publishing.

Rucker, M. L., & Thomson, S. (2003). Assessing student learning outcomes: An investigation of the relationship among feedback measures. *College Student Journal*, *37*(3), 400–405. https://doi.org/10.1177/2158244015615921

Stevens, D. D., & Levi, A. J. (2013). *Introduction to Rubrics: An Assessment Tool to Save Grading Time, Convey Effective Feedback, and Promote Student Learning* (2nd ed.). Stylus Publishing.

Wiggins, G., & McTighe, J. (2005) *Understanding by Design* (2nd ed.). Pearson Education.

17

Assessment of Clinical Judgment

Christine Tanner, PhD, RN (ret), FAAN, ANEF
Paula Gubrud, EdD, RN, CHSE, FAAN, ANEF

CHAPTER OVERVIEW

This chapter focuses on Tanner's model of clinical judgment as a framework for teaching and assessing clinical judgment. We provide an overview of Tanner's model and include recent updates. We recommend assessment approaches that emphasize performance in addressing authentic clinical situations; to that end, we will focus on performance assessment through observation and discussion of actual or simulated clinical situations, as these approaches hold great face validity for evaluating clinical reasoning and are particularly important in formative assessment. We discuss several clinical performance measures and offer guidelines for using these instruments for summative evaluation. We explore the use of Entrustable Professional Activities (EPAs) developed in schools of medicine over the last decade as an important tool for communicating individual learners' level of competencies related to typical workplace activities.

BACKGROUND

Nursing curricula are designed to prepare students to practice safely in rapidly changing and complex health care environments. Curricula in nursing education and other health care professions are transitioning to competency-based frameworks to facilitate this preparation (Giddens et al., 2022; Lucey, 2018; National League for Nursing [NLN], 2023). Nursing as the health care profession with the largest number of clinicians must prepare students with a complex range of competencies for current and continuous change in the health care system. Benner et al. (2010) following their study of nursing education called for radical reform, particularly in using teaching and assessment methods that will promote learners' ability to make sound clinical judgments. In response to these calls, the National Council of State Boards of Nursing (NCSBN) developed a framework for defining and assessing clinical judgment called the NCSBN-Clinical Judgment Measurement Model (CJMM) indicating the model is intended for high-stakes evaluation of clinical judgment competency (Dickison et al., 2019). NCSBN-CJMM was developed to guide the development of Next Gen NCLEX and is not recommended as a guide to develop teaching or formative assessment strategies (Dickison et al., 2019). The NCSBN-CJMM integrates Tanner's Clinical Judgment Model and incorporates two other models and multiple factors identified as influencing clinical judgment (Dickison et al., 2019).

Findings from a recent nationally distributed survey of nursing program deans and directors confirm nursing programs should adopt a model of clinical judgment to fully support teaching and assessment practices (Nielsen et al., 2023). Using a consistent framework throughout a curriculum creates a common language for faculty to discuss clinical judgments, supports intentional scaffolding of concepts and constructs, and can guide the design of assessments used to evaluate the development of clinical judgment as students' progress through the program (Tyo & McCurry, 2019; Nielsen et al., 2023). Tanner's Clinical Judgment Model (Tanner, 2006) is widely used as a model to facilitate teaching, learning, and assessment of the clinical reasoning approaches (Gonzalez, 2018; Gonzalez et al., 2021; Jessee, 2021; Jessee & Tanner, 2016; Jessee et al., 2023; Tyo & McCurry, 2019). Other models have been used as guides for structuring scenarios and debriefing simulations (Dreifuerst, 2012).

TANNER'S CLINICAL JUDGMENT MODEL

The original model, developed over 15 years ago, was based on a review of nearly 200 studies exploring how nurses make clinical judgments, describing the complex reasoning processes needed to make sound judgments. In 2022, we updated the model with more recent research, drawing linkages between clinical reasoning and evidence-based practice (Tanner, 2006; Tanner et al., 2022). We encourage the reader to review the original work, as it has been widely cited in the nursing education literature as a framework for instruction and for commonly used assessment approaches. Here we will review specific areas of the model which were clarified, amplified, or modified as a result of the 2022 literature review. We will also highlight aspects of the model particularly relevant for application to formative and summative assessment.

Tanner (2006) and Tanner et al. (2022) describe clinical reasoning as the processes nurses and other clinicians use to make judgments. Clinical reasoning includes the deliberate process of identifying alternatives, intentional consideration of the evidence to use for rationale, and choosing the most appropriate option. Clinical reasoning also includes using patterns of thought characterized as engaged, practical reasoning (e.g., recognizing a pattern, an intuitive clinical grasp, or a response without deliberate forethought). A clinical judgment is the result of clinical reasoning leading to "…an interpretation or conclusion about a patient's needs, concerns, or health problems, and/or the decision to take action (or not), use or modify standard approaches, or improvise new ones as deemed appropriate by the patient's response" (Tanner, 2006, p. 204).

Briefly, as shown in Figure 17.1, the model has two major components: factors influencing clinical judgment and clinical reasoning processes across five phases: noticing, interpreting, responding, reflecting *in* practice, and reflecting *on* practice. These phases are not linear but rather are iterative. The model also includes a description of three broad reasoning patterns: (1) intuition operating as a function of experience; (2) analytic, viewed as the more rational, conscious reasoning process; and (3) narrative, which is engaged while listening to patient accounts of their illness experiences.

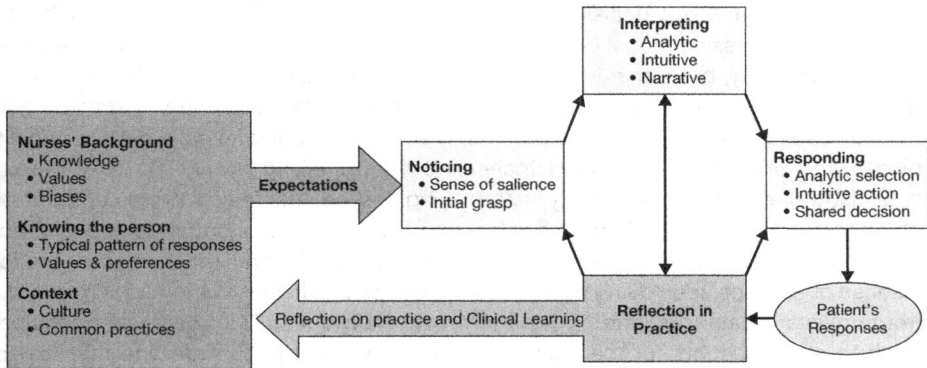

FIGURE 17.1 Tanner Model of Clinical Judgment. (Reprinted with permission from Tanner, C., Messecar, D., & Delawska-Elliott, B. (2022). Chapter 13, evidence based practice. In L. Joel (Ed.), *Advanced practice nursing: Essentials for role development* [5th ed.]. F.A. Davis.)

Most of the studies supporting the original model were based on nursing practice in acute care and hence were concerned with the nurses' focus on supporting their patients' recovery from illness and preventing and/or quickly responding to complications. Clinical reasoning thus originates with noticing, e.g., that there has been a change in the patient's condition, a troublesome pattern appears, or there is a gap between what the nurse expects to observe and what is evident in the situation. Noticing depends on what the nurse brings to the situation; theoretical and practical knowledge, experience with similar patients or situations, the nurse's relationship with this particular patient, understanding what is important to them, and knowing their typical pattern of responses. Noticing also depends on the clinical context; for example, complaints of low back pain on a maternity unit are expected while on a general medical unit with older adults, this might signal that something is awry. The culture of the unit also affects what nurses generally pay attention to; for example, a unit that has focused quality improvement on pain management is likely to show that their clinicians are more attuned to evidence of a patient's pain.

Both intuitive and analytic decision-making have received greatly increased attention in the health professions literature over the last decade, fueled, in part, by the best-selling book, *Thinking, Fast and Slow,* authored by behavioral economist and Nobel Laureate, Daniel Kahneman (2011). The book draws on decades of research on decision-making, exploring heuristics (short-cut rules) and cognitive biases. Kahneman's theory divides the mind's thinking processes into two distinct systems with each pathway characterized by its own important attributes:

Type 1 is a fast, intuitive, pattern recognition-driven method of problem solving, which places a low cognitive burden on the user, and allows one ideally to make rapid and accurate decisions. Other mental activities become fast and automatic through prolonged practice. Type 2 is the mind's slower, analytical mode, where reason dominates. It places a higher cognitive burden on the user but allows them to appraise data more critically, look beyond patterns, and may be more suitable for more complex problems.

As applied to medical decision-making, Kahneman's model is commonly referred t as the dual processing model (Norman et al., 2017). The two types of thinking do not oper ate independently, but rather in tandem. It has become a dominant model in researc on diagnostic reasoning because of recent attention to diagnostic error and the cogni tive biases that may lead to it; it is commonly thought that diagnostic error and implici biases are more likely to result from unchecked type 1 thinking (Norman et al., 2017; Lawsor 2018). However, both type 1 and type 2 thinking can be affected by biases and unreli able shortcuts (heuristics). Current opinion among psychologists is that we spend abou 95% of our time in Type 1 thinking. For the experienced clinician, intuition accounts fo a sense of salience, identifying plausible diagnostic hypotheses, distinguishing relevan from irrelevant data, recognizing a pattern over individual bits of data, and noticing Intuition also accounts for the early warning of imminent patient decline that exper nurses often describe (Benner et al., 2009), and has been reported as a more reliable indi cator than objective early warning scores (Lavoie et al., 2020).

Reflection in and on practice are critical phases of clinical reasoning. Experienced nurse: continuously observe the patient's responses to their actions, modifying their actions a: necessary. For example, nurses question impacts such as: how do positional change: together with analgesic medication and reassurance influence the level of pain in this situa tion? Nurses experiencing an early warning will engage in deliberative rationality, collectinç specific data to confirm or disconfirm their sense of potential deterioration of patient statu: before calling the rapid response team. Reflection is essential for learners to identify subtle influences on their reasoning, realizing gaps in knowledge needed for a particular situation biases introduced by recent experiences, or the effect of having just studied some topic ir theory class. Reflection on clinical experience is critical for clinical learning.

Two areas that have gained increasing emphasis since the original model was pub lished were reviewed for relevant research and incorporated into the revision: (1) the potential impact of implicit bias on clinical reasoning; and (2) involvement of the patien and family in clinical decision-making.

Implicit Bias Impact on Clinical Reasoning

The role of implicit bias in health care has been extensively studied since the publica- tion of Unequal Treatment: Confronting Racial and Ethnic Disparities in Health Care (Institute of Medicine, 2003). Implicit bias includes not only racial bias, but many other biases against groups judged negatively by one or more characteristics, such as low socia economic status (SES), sexual orientation, and weight (Costa et al., 2016; Robstad et al., 2019 Schaa et al., 2015). Implicit bias can occur in several ways: prejudice (negative attitudes toward a group); stereotypes (overgeneralization of positive or negative characteristics of a group); and, discrimination (behavior which reveals to the patient the prejudice anc negative stereotypes held by the provider through their interactions, their interest ir hearing the patient's story, and their engagement of the patient in health care decision- making). Health care provider implicit bias contributes to health disparities by eroding the patient's trust and confidence in the provider's health counseling (Schultz & Baker, 2017, and by making poor clinical judgments based on biased interpretations of the patient's concerns. Implicit bias training may be helpful but not sufficient to fully address health disparities (Ochs, 2023).

Patient- and Family-Centered Care

Shared decision-making between the clinician and patient/family has been viewed as essential for patient-centered quality of care (Institute of Medicine, 2001). This is especially important in treatment decision-making, when there are several treatment options, each with varying degrees of effectiveness and potential side effects, and the patient's choice among these options is essential (Milky & Thomas, 2020). The clinician is likely to use an analytic process to derive appropriate treatment options, considering what they understand of patient preferences, and their experience with the use of one or more of the treatments. In shared decision-making with an engaged patient, the clinician explains the clinical problem and identifies possible actions, and describes what factors need to be considered to make a good decision, i.e., what are the potential side effects, what is the likelihood that these would occur, what is the likelihood of the patient's preferred outcome?

Some General Guidelines

Tanner's model of clinical reasoning captures the processes that experienced nurses use as they go about making judgments. It was developed to create a vision of the kind of clinical judgment that we aspire for our learners; with some experience, our learners may occasionally reach the level described. The practice of learners in pre-licensure programs is characteristically described as novice practice. As Benner (2001) showed clearly in her landmark study of the development of expertise, elaborated in a subsequent study of critical care nurses' development (Benner et al., 2010), there are stages to development in practice disciplines just as there are instructional approaches that are more or less suited for the stage of development. Benner and co-authors (2010) in their study of nursing education, highlighted both clinical and classroom teaching approaches that were characterized by engaging students in real clinical situations, coaching them, pointing out salient features of clinical situations, and situating content in clinical cases. These approaches help learners begin to develop a sense of salience, recognize the need for informed judgment, and begin moving beyond rule-based approaches. Approaches to help students develop clinical judgment are informed by these assumptions:

Clinical reasoning and judgment are contextually bound. How the student's clinical reasoning unfolds is influenced by the characteristics of the situation and what the clinician brings to the situation.

Because of the situational nature of clinical reasoning, the assessment approach with the highest face validity will be the assessment of performance in actual patient situations, with high-fidelity simulation running a close second. This also suggests that there may be variability in students' performance from one situation to another simply because there is variability in relevant aspects of the situation, in knowledge the student brings to the situation, as well as in other factors that influence clinical reasoning. This also suggests that the instructor should search for multiple situations in which the student engages in clinical reasoning, observing for patterns in performance—e.g., failure to notice relevant data, jumping to conclusions about required action, and failure to consider alternative interpretations. Summative evaluation should never rest on a single performance but rather on the patterns shown over several situations.

For the clinical coach, understanding a student's reasoning processes, including what knowledge they bring to the situation and how they interpreted their observations requires that the student be able to verbalize their thinking (Jessee & Tanner, 2016). This requires tactful, respectful questioning by the coach, showing curiosity about how the student thought through the situation.

For a student to engage in clinical reasoning, they need to be presented with a clinical situation that requires judgment on their part. The situation may be in the simulation environment in which scenarios are developed which portray a problematic situation and presented to the student or team of students as if the student were responsible for the care of that simulated patient. It may also be a situation presenting itself during the student's actual clinical experience. Neophyte students may need help in recognizing a decision to be made or a situation calling for a judgment.

ASSESSING COMPETENCY-GENERAL GUIDELINES

There have been a number of approaches purporting to assess learners' clinical judgment or decision-making in the health professions literature. Daniel et al. (2019) describe several approaches using paper-and-pencil or computer-based exams, many of which are in widespread use in schools of nursing for summative evaluation of learners. Multiple-choice exams and short-answer and essay exams are typically tests of knowledge or factual recall. Some written tests have been developed to assess varying components of clinical reasoning. For example, the patient-management problem (PMP) presents a realistic written clinical scenario, providing specific resources to collect additional assessment data or take specific actions. The examinee chooses from among these, then receives the assessment data or the patient's response to the action. In a linear-branching format, the examinee proceeds through the problem seeking additional data information; their path through the problem is determined by what resources they select in each section.

Multiple studies and nursing education experts identify the need for the development of methods and instruments to assess clinical judgment and other core competencies new graduates need to provide safe quality patient care (Lewallen & Van Horn, 2019; Nielsen et al., 2023; Wilson et al., 2021). Comprehensive guidelines identified through a scoping review completed by Daniel et al. (2019) can be used to develop systematic approaches used to assessing clinical judgment. The systematic plan must balance assessment used for supporting learning (formative assessment) and evaluation of student performance designed to determine competency (summative assessment). Table 17.1 identifies guidelines to apply when developing a comprehensive and systematic plan for assessing clinical judgment competency.

Formative Assessments Used to Assess Students Learning About Clinical Judgment

Helping students verbalize their thinking. Formative assessments serve multiple purposes. Formative assessment can be designed to illustrate the learner's thinking, provide opportunity to demonstrate a skill, and can make professional attitudes and

TABLE 17.1

Guidelines for Assessing Clinical Judgment Competency

Guideline	Rationale	Reference
Adopt a clinical judgment model	Nursing programs should adopt a clinical judgment model to integrate throughout the entire curriculum. This creates shared language needed to teach and assess competency.	Nielsen et al., 2023 Tyo & McCurry, 2019
Use multiple assessment methods	Use multiple assessment methods including performance observations in patient care and simulation. Verbal reflections in response to coaching and feedback and in debriefing provide assessment data. Non-observable measures such as reflective journaling, concept maps, case studies with unfolding diagnostic information, and screen-based simulations.	Daniel et al., 2019 Nielsen, et al., 2023 Tyo & McCurry, 2019
Observe performance in multiple clinical situations	Clinical reasoning is contextually bound and knowledge dependent. Errors in reasoning are to be expected in new learners. To reach a summative judgment, observe for patterns of behavior that occur over several situations.	Norman, 2017 Tanner, 2006
Provide faculty development—include adjuncts	Clinical judgment is a clinical competency. Coaching and providing feedback in the clinical learning environment should incorporate language from the agreed-upon model. Faculty should become experts in the model to effectively support student development in clinical judgment.	Nielsen et al., 2023 Jesse, 2018
Design an intentional longitudinal plan to assure progress in developing clinical judgment competency	To ensure clinical judgment competency, use a variety of assessments, administered longitudinally (throughout a program of study), covering a variety of problems, in a variety of settings to accommodate content and context specificity.	Daniel et al., 2019 Watling & Ginsburg, 2019
Scaffold the complexity of patient situations	Clinical judgment is a process used when the situation is ambiguous and/or ill-defined. Make sure the problem at hand is within the student's capability to address. Simple problems with minimal data to discern are appropriate for beginning students. As students progress, the complexity of the ill-defined problem can be increased.	Tanner, 2006 McGaghie et al., 2020 Watling & Ginsburg, 2019
Use formative assessment as the primary approach to evaluating clinical judgment competency	Formative assessments serve a dual purpose as a process used to evaluate students' developing clinical judgment competency and teaching clinical judgment. Assess for patterns of evidence the student is progressing in their clinical judgments. Assess the student's response to feedback to assure they are applying new learning and corrections in new situations.	Daniel et al., 2019 McGaghie et al., 2020 Watling & Ginsburg, 2019

(continued)

TABLE 17.1

Guidelines for Assessing Clinical Judgment Competency *(Continued)*

Guideline	Rationale	Reference
Assure integrity of assessment methods and instruments	Assess methods and instruments (i.e., rubrics) used for validity, feasibility, defensibility, and fit (i.e., alignment with course and/or program outcomes). Consider ease of use.	Daniel et al., 2019
Use high-stakes summative assessment sparingly and with caution	The defensibility of using observed clinical performance assessments for summative decisions can be questionable because, from a generalizability theory perspective, several measurements in several clinical contexts are needed to reach acceptable reliability for judgments regarding student performance. Ensuring evaluation by multiple raters trained to use tools and standardized processes over time is also essential for observed high-stakes clinical performance assessment.	Watling & Ginsburg, 2019

values visible. Formative assessment can identify gaps between expectations and student proficiency related to the knowledge, thinking, skilled know-how, and attitudes needed to provide safe, quality patient-centered care. The data obtained from formative assessment is used to deepen learning, improve skill performance, and address gaps in knowledge and/or errors in application to clinical situations. Formative assessment is often described as a process used as a catalyst for learning, as compared with summative assessment, which is typically an evaluation of learning. Providing feedback to learners regarding their clinical judgment competency should be planned and intentional and also take advantage of unplanned teachable moments. Curricular adaptation of a model or framework of clinical judgment creates shared language critical to engaging the students in feedback designed to either acknowledge sound thinking and actions or guide the learner to reframe the mental model used when making a clinical judgment or reconsider actions taken when there is a gap. Using consistent language and an agreed-upon clinical judgment model facilitates progression from one course to the next and helps identify if the student has a pattern of a clinical reasoning error.

Giving feedback to students about their clinical judgment requires a combination of instructor values, attitudes, and skills. Two interrelated learner-centered assumptions are embedded in the *Debriefing with Good Judgment* method of debriefing using questioning and feedback (Fey et al., 2022): (1) hold learners to high standards; and (2) hold learners in high regard (Fey et al., 2022). These two assumptions convey to the student an appreciation for them as learners, who you expect to meet high standards. When a student makes an error in clinical judgment, the teacher must consider the root cause of the gap in clinical reasoning. Instructional and learner gaps are outlined and questions for consideration are presented in Table 17.2. First, the teacher should consider the possible instructional gaps. Questions for consideration include:

TABLE 17.2

Questions for Assessing Gaps in Clinical Reasoning

Gap	Questions
Instructional	➤ Is the problem encountered aligned with the student's level of experience and expected performance? ➤ Have clear expectations regarding roles and responsibilities to make clinical judgments been established? ➤ Does the student have the background knowledge needed to make a sound clinical judgment? ➤ Did the learner have an opportunity to prepare for the situation at hand? ➤ Is there an undue influence related to the culture of the environment creating a gap in clinical judgment?
Learner	➤ Is there a gap in knowledge? ➤ Is there a bias that got in the way of making a sound clinical judgment? ➤ Did the learner fail to notice the significance of salient data? ➤ Is there a gap in the interpretation phase of clinical judgment? ➤ Did the learner notice what was salient and interpreted the data correctly but was unable to respond appropriately?

Exploring the gap with the learner requires transparent and respectful dialogue embedded in the assumptions of the *Debriefing with Good Judgment* method (Fey et al., 2022). Instruction and learner gaps may have both contributed to the error. Once the root cause(s) of the lapse in clinical judgment has been identified the teacher should provide feedback that articulates the desired standard of care to be met, with high regard for the learner. The teacher should dialogue with the learners as "...intelligent, capable individuals who are sincerely trying to do their best and want to get better" (Fey et al., 2022, p. 3). McAllister and co-authors (2007, p. 304) describe feedback that aims to correct misunderstandings or expand the student's thinking as "gentle interruptions." They posit creating a transformative teaching environment in the clinical setting requires the instructor to assess students' thinking and to provide feedback as an essential and frequent teaching-learning activity that is designed to keep students and patients safe and facilitate continuous improvement and growth (McAllister et al., 2007). In summary, verbal interaction and feedback between the learner and teacher is a primary means of formative assessment.

The faculty can use a pre-encounter dialogue before the student enters a patient situation to uncover what the student expects to see and use the conversation to probe the learner's thinking, suggest important assessment data the student didn't identify, and correct any misunderstandings. The clinical teacher should affirm sound thinking and provide a rationale for why the student's thinking is appropriate for the apparent situation at hand. Simply stating "good thinking" is not enough. Using language from Tanner's model provides a shared mental framework to ground the pre-encounter conversation. See Table 17.3 for sample pre-encounter questions.

TABLE 17.3

Pre-Encounter Clinical Judgment Coaching Questions

Tanner's Clinical Judgment Model	Questions
Uncovering student's background	▸ Tell me what you know about this patient and is there anything you are curious about?
Identifying expectations	▸ Describe what you expect to find when you meet the patient.
Describing past experiences that may influence noticing	▸ Have you ever cared for a similar patient? ▸ What do you think you will see and do based on that previous experience?
Uncovering conscious or unconscious bias	▸ Can you identify any bias (positive or challenging) you may have related to this patient?
Exploring background knowledge	▸ Is there anything about the care the patient has been receiving that makes you curious?
Uncovering anticipated concerns	▸ What concerns do you have about this patient?
Coaching the student to consider areas of focused assessment	▸ Describe what your focused assessment will look like.

Once the encounter is complete, the faculty can continue to perform formative assessments through a post-encounter debriefing. The conversation can be facilitated to assess the *noticing and interpretation phases* of Tanner's model by asking what was unexpected and if their observations and interaction mirror what they anticipated. The teacher should probe to uncover the learner's interpretation of their findings, their reflection on their interpretation, and if they need additional data to bolster their interpretations. The teacher should also probe what actions might be warranted and how they will know if they are working. The conversation can include the student's reflection on the *responding phase* of Tanner's model and conclude with questions that encourage the learner to consider how what they have learned can be applied to future patient encounters. If the student has cared for similar patients in the past, ask questions to help the student identify possible patterns. For example, when caring for a post-operative patient, talking with the student about the usual trajectory of pain control used can help the student develop pattern recognition. See Table 17.4 for sample questions to use for assessing students' application of Tanner's clinical judgment model during the post-encounter.

Using the language of Tanner's Clinical Judgment model, while articulating desired standards to be met and holding the student in high regard will serve the dual purposes of formative assessment: to evaluate students' clinical reasoning and to facilitate learning. Non-judgmental questioning techniques help students frame their thinking that ground their clinical judgments. Providing non-judgmental feedback supports learning and facilitates development of sound clinical judgment.

In addition to one-to-one conversations with the student that may be planned, or quite possibly unplanned, two formative assessment techniques stand out as effective

TABLE 17.4

Post-Encounter Clinical Judgment Coach Questions

Tanners Clinical Judgment Model	Question
Noticing	➤ What did you notice when you walked into the patient's room?
Noticing and interpretation	➤ Tell me about the expected findings and any unexpected findings you found.
Interpretation	➤ I am curious about your interpretation of those findings. Tell me about the patient's condition and situation.
Responding	➤ What actions did you take in response to that thinking?
Interpretation	➤ Tell me about the patient's response to your actions.
Reflection on practice	➤ Do you have any unanswered questions or lingering concerns about this patient?

means to use in a plan to assess a student's clinical judgment: (1) SBAR [Situation, Background, Assessment, Recommendation] (Coolen et al., 2020; Parry & Selvaraj, 2023; Scolari et al., 2022) handoff reports; and (2) concept mapping. Incorporating an SBAR report or summary into a dialogue or as a post-clinical written assignment helps the student organize their thinking with the various phases of Tanner's model. Using SBAR guides the student in providing a glimpse into their thinking about a particular situation and is an opportunity to correct misunderstandings or expand understanding. Describing the *Situation* at hand using the SBAR format requires the learner to identify what is salient. Presenting the *Background* also prompts the student to discern what is important for another provider to know about the problem requiring a clinical judgment. The learner must organize the data encountered and consider the connections between the situation and the background to provide a cogent report. The *Assessment* aspect of the SBAR requires the student to articulate a conclusion about what they think is going on. Articulating or describing the situation, background, and assessment of a patient's problem corresponds to the noticing and interpreting phases of Tanner's model. The *Recommendation* aspect of an SBAR prompts the learner to articulate what should be done (or a conscious decision to do nothing) to address the patient's problem. The recommendation aspect of SBAR aligns with the responding phase of Tanner's model as the student describes a plan or actual patient intervention provided in response to the situation, background, and assessment. In addition to the SBAR report, the teacher can include verbal or written questions that prompt the student to reflect on the situation, their own thinking, and the responses or interventions provided to care for the patient. A question asking the student to forecast how they can apply what was learned to future practice situations promotes the reflection-on-action phase of Tanner's model that is critical to building a progressive repertoire of knowledge, skills, and attitudes used when making clinical judgments. In addition to helping the student reflect on their clinical reasoning, repetitive practice with SBAR may help improve handover reports as they begin their clinical practice (Scolari et al., 2022).

Concept mapping is an established educational strategy used in nursing over th past two decades and has been used to replace traditional care plans (Daley et al., 201 Eisenmann, 2021). Concept maps allow learners to show their knowledge and understand ing of connections between health and illness problems or concepts, and prescribe treatments, including medications and nursing interventions. The traditional concep map can be constructed freehand by the student, or a computer template can be pro vided. The purpose of a concept map is to create an illustration that represents studer knowledge and understanding of connections between concepts. The students ma the patient problems illustrating connections between disease process and assessmen findings to include physical assessment data, lab and other diagnostic reports, medica tions, and other treatments (Daley et al., 2016).

The key to effective concept mapping is creating guidelines that help the studen see connections between concepts used to provide care. Concept mapping can b challenging for beginning students as the process represents movement away fron memorization and fact description. Facilitating concept mapping in a group settin with novice students can provide modeling and guidance using a coaching approach Creating guidelines for developing the concept maps with an example will help th learners develop the thinking skills focused on making connections embedded ir patient care situations. Using the language of Tanner's model in the guidelines anc exemplars will facilitate the student's ability to complete the assignment which car be used as a formative assessment. See Box 17.1 for an example of a concept map assignment.

Formative Classroom Assessments

Classroom activities can be designed to facilitate the development of clinical judg ment (Gonzalez, 2018; Gonzalez et al., 2021; Nielsen et al., 2023; Sommer et al., 2021). Classroom Assessment Techniques (CATs) (Angelo & Cross, 1993; Barkley & Major, 2016) can be used as formative assessments providing data to the teacher about student learning about the effectiveness of the classroom teaching approaches and facilitating the learner's antici patory thinking, a process used in sound clinical reasoning. For example, the *Background Knowledge Probe CAT* (Angelo & Cross, 1993) is essentially a short quiz designed to identify what students know and understand about a particular topic. The short quiz is adminis tered before the class begins. Consider a class focused on a patient with diabetes and COPD. The quiz asks five to six questions about the pathophysiology, symptoms, and common medications used for this type of patient. The quiz is completed anonymously which confirms the formative nature of the assessment and the results are used to assess the group's collective background knowledge of the patient's problems. Results are used to guide the design and implementation of learning activities. The answers are reviewed, and misunderstandings are corrected. Often the students share their knowledge with each other, and the teacher coaches and guides them to create a shared and accurate frame of reference needed to address the problems presented in the case study focusing on the important cues to facilitate the noticing aspect of clinical judgment. This activity prompts the anticipatory thinking described as the foundation for what a nurse is likely to notice. Another CAT is a modified Johari window (South, 2007) (Box 17.2). Students

BOX 17.1

Concept Mapping Assignment

Tanner's Clinical Judgment Model/Gidden's Concepts of Nursing Practice Mapping Assignment

Used by permission of Carol Thorn, MSN, RN

Objectives:

➤ Identify relevant priorities of care at various stages of information gathering.

➤ Determine significant data to be interpreted to guide priority/care delivered.

➤ Appropriately interpret salient data in the prioritization/delivery of patient care.

➤ Apply relevant response(s) to pertinent/identified concepts of nursing practice.

Answer the following questions in the space/pages provided for you.

1. You will receive a report on a patient. In your group, complete the following:

   ➤ As you are reading the report, please highlight information that you 'noticed' or that caused questions or concerns (related to patient, family, nurse, etc.). Limit highlighting to the top 8 things that you noticed that may be of concern while caring for this patient.

   ➤ In the rectangle space in the top center of the concept map (last page of assignment), group members need to identify the top 5 pieces of information (from the information that was highlighted) that will cause the nurse the most concern and/or harm to the patient.

      ➤ In other words, what are the top 5 things that you 'noticed' in the report that brought up potential concerns/problems related to this patient that you will/may have to consider as you plan their care?

   ➤ In the boxes surrounding the rectangle, identify **a minimum of 8** nursing concepts/problems you will/may be worried about or need to monitor throughout your shift.

      ➤ There should be at least 1 psych-social concern addressed during your shift.

      ➤ You do not need to provide a rationale if your concern is self-evident (e.g., someone is on a vent and you are concerned about airway management).

         ➤ However, if you think there may be some difficulty understanding why you listed a psych-social issue in place of ABCs, please provide rationale for your decision.

   ➤ Prioritize these problems/concerns as "High, Medium, or Low" as related to your overall concern. Be prepared to alter your prioritization as needed as more information about the patient is interpreted.

2. As a group, choose five concepts from your list and complete the following:

   ➤ Under each concept chosen, identify data that would need to be interpreted to provide safe, efficient care to this patient.

      ➤ Such as, if your patient has an oxygenation issue you may want to know their oxygen saturation, respiratory rate, hemoglobin level, lung assessment findings, etc.

   ➤ List corresponding data that you would like for each concept, even if it is already listed under a different concept. This will help you determine the importance/relevance of the data (i.e., if respiratory rate trending is identified as data to be reviewed in 4 out of the 5 problems, it would increase the importance of knowing this information to safely care for the patient).

3. Based on the information provided in the report and related to the above 5 identified concepts/problems, list at least 2 complications that this patient is at risk of developing.

(continued)

BOX 17.1

Concept Mapping Assignment *(Continued)*

Does the data identified under each concept capture the ability to notice any abnormalities if the complication were to develop? If not, list additional information/data points needed under the concept but in a different color ink/pencil.

4. Related to the above complications, fill in the spaces below by answering the questions posed.

List 2 things the nurse can do to help prevent the complication from developing.	Complication # 1	List at least 2 signs and/or symptoms that would be found on assessment if this particular complication were to develop.

Based on the group's identification of data needed for interpretation, the group is provided additional information/patient data at this time.
- First-year students may be provided additional information that is salient to the patient's condition that they did not recognize as important.
- Second-year students are only provided the information that was deemed relevant based on the concept map assignment.

5. After having the opportunity to interpret the additional information provided for this patient (lab values, vital signs, etc.), is there a need for additional information that was not previously identified? If so, list additional needed data for interpretation below:

List 2 things the nurse can do to help prevent the complication from developing	Complication # 2	List at least 2 signs and/or symptoms that would be found on assessment if this particular complication were to develop.

6. After having the opportunity to interpret the additional information provided for this patient (lab values, vital signs, etc.), does the group want to alter the prioritization of the nursing concept/problems? If so, how would the prioritization change and why?
7. Develop a plan of care for this patient based on the current prioritization of the top 5 problems/concepts. Identify how the nurse should respond to the data provided and what actions should be taken at this time/during the first few hours of the shift. This does not need to be in NANDA language.

BOX 17.1

Concept Mapping Assignment *(Continued)*

	Top information from report	
Fluid Balance Priority:		Hemodynamics/Perfusion Priority:
Mood/Affect Priority:		Glycemic Control Priority:
Electrolyte Balance Priority:		Safety Priority:

Bowel/Urinary Elimination Priority:	Oxygenation Priority:	Acid/Base Balance Priority:	Activity Tolerance Priority:
Support System Priority:	Infection Priority:	Mental Status Priority:	Nutrition Priority:
Stress Priority:	Priority:	Priority:	Coping Strategies Priority:
Knowledge Priority:	Priority:	Priority:	Skin Integrity Priority:

BOX 17.2

Formative Assessment Exemplar: Johari Window

Please enter your responses to the top 2 window panes before coming to class. Bring your Johari window to class.

We will be completing a case study on Mr. C. He has been admitted to the hospital with acute respiratory distress and has a diagnosis of COPD.

At the end of class, we will complete the bottom 2 window panes. You will be asked to submit the Johari window. You are not required to include your name in your submission.

What I know about COPD and acute respiratory distress	What I don't know about COPD and acute respiratory distress
What I learned about COPD and acute respiratory distress	What I need to learn more about COPD and respiratory distress

complete the top two panes of the window before the class begins and complete the bottom panes of the window when the class is complete. The instructor has clear evidence of what knowledge and understanding the students are bringing to the case study and what the students learned. A completed Johari window identifies what remaining questions, concepts, and content should be addressed after the class session is completed. Gaps in knowledge needed to make sound clinical judgments are identified. Students identify what they need to learn more about.

Several established formative assessment techniques can be used to help the teacher understand the learners' development of sound clinical judgment. Table 17.5 provides a list and short descriptions of intentional formative assessments that correspond with the various phases of Tanner's Clinical Judgment Model.

Summative Assessments

Competency-based education has created pressure on educators to assess students' clinical judgment and determine when students are ready to practice independently (Giddens et al., 2022; NLN, 2023). Clinical judgment competency is the bedrock of safe patient-centered care in a highly complex and dynamic health care delivery system (Kavanagh & Sharpnack, 2021) and nurse educators must make summative evaluations regarding students' clinical judgment competency before they graduate. Summative assessments are referred to as making *assessments of learning* and often require the learner to demonstrate observable competency in simulation or in the clinical environment. Summative assessments may include exams using multiple-choice questions. The Next Gen NCLEX is an example of a summative high-stakes exam that has recently been developed to provide questions that require the participant to make a clinical judgment (Dickison et al., 2019).

Challenges with a point in time, high-stakes summative assessments are consistently called into question (NLN, 2020; Watling & Gingsberg, 2019). As health professions education adopt competency-based curriculum frameworks, guidelines, and criteria for using high-stakes summative assessments are emerging. NLN (2020, 2023) has created vision statements educators can use to create assessment policies. Watling & Gingsberg (2019) posit that sound summative competency assessment aspires to both facilitate learning and evaluate the learner's ability to safely practice independently. This requires a systematic approach focused on multiple and ongoing formative assessments, which evaluate the students' growing competency as they progress through the program. Because nurse educators must assess clinical judgment and other critical competencies, the challenges and best practices in developing summative competency assessment are complex. Recent literature reviews identify and describe instruments and methods used to evaluate clinical reasoning and judgment that can be used to develop a systematic plan to make summative assessments of students' competency (Brentnall et al., 2022; Clemett & Raleigh, 2021; Daniel et al., 2019).

Instruments

Some instruments are designed to measure more than one competency and clinical judgment is embedded as one component (Brentnall et al., 2022; Clemett & Raleigh, 2021;

TABLE 17.5

Formative Assessment Techniques to Assess Clinical Judgment

Clinical Judgment Phase	Formative Assessment Methods	Description
Uncovering expectations	Pre-conference discussion	Individual and small group discussion with questions about what students know about their patients and what they expect to see when they walk into the room
	Clinical preparation	Students complete preparation worksheets to guide their assessments and prepare for any procedures they may complete. Content includes: ▸ Brief summary of relevant Pathophysiology ▸ Expected signs and symptoms ▸ Possible complications ▸ List of medications with purpose statements (let them use their drug manuals for details!)
	Bias check	Ask students if they recognize any conscious or should consider unconscious bias that may be influencing their pre-encounter mental models about the patient
Noticing and Interpretation	Student rounds and huddles	Individual meetings with students before and after they encounter the patient
	SBAR reports	Oral or written SBAR report to summarize the thinking
	Think aloud	Ask the student to verbally share their thinking as they assess the patient—Instructor shares their thinking as well as a direct observer
	Concept Maps	Students use a visual illustration to draw connections between patient condition, assessment findings, and treatments/interventions
Responding	SBAR	Focused questions on the Recommendations of the SBAR report
	Coaching and feedback	Instructor provides feedback and coaching as student interacts with the patient. The coaching and feedback may occur after the encounter as faculty helps students with what went well or what could be enhanced or done differently (Plus/Delta)
Reflection in action	Think aloud	Student verbally shares thinking while responding
Reflection on action	Post-clinical conferences	Students describe patients, and care provided. Faculty helps students see similarities and differences between patients with comparable conditions to help recognize patterns (e.g., what do post-op patients have in common regarding pain control, what variables create differences)
	Guided reflective journaling	Students complete guided reflective journaling post-clinical experience. Guidelines should specify page limits and ask students to address salient questions related to clinical judgment. Assignments can be organized using language from the phases of the clinical judgment model

Daniel et al., 2019). An example is the widely used Creighton Competency Evaluatio Instrument (CCEI) (Hayden et al., 2014; Manz et al., 2022). The CCEI is designed to meas ure multiple competencies and includes eight subscales used to measure students clinical judgment. The subscale items do not align with a clinical judgment model o framework. The Lasater Clinical Judgment Rubric (LCJR) (Lasater, 2007) was develope to assess the use of Tanner's Clinical Judgement Model (Tanner, 2006) and is identi fied in published systematic reviews as the dominant instrument used in prelicen sure nursing education to assess clinical judgment (Brentnall et al., 2022; Clemett & Raleigh 2021; Daniel et al., 2019). The LCJR has been used extensively in nursing programs an research projects as it has established reliability (Adamson et al., 2012). See Chapter 16 *Rubric Development*, for an in-depth description of the LCJR. See Table 17.6 for : selected list of instruments used in clinical education and simulation to assess clinica judgment competency.

TABLE 17.6

Selected Instruments that Assess Clinical Judgment

Author	Instrument	Comments
Hayden et al., 2014 Manz et al., 2022	Creighton Competency Evaluation Instrument	Developed for the National Council State Boards of Nursing simulation to evaluate clinical competency in simulation and patient care environments. Is not organized by a clinical judgment framework or model. There are 4 categories of clinical competency assessed. Each category has subscales. The clinical judgment category has 8 subscales. The tool uses a dichotomous scale to evaluate student performance making the instrument essentially a competency checklist. Several studies have established reliability and validity.
Lasater, 2007	Lasater Clinical Judgment Rubric (LCJR)	A rubric developed to assess Tanner's Clinical Judgment Model in both clinical patient care settings and simulation environments. Extensive global use with several studies establishing reliability. Has not been modified to reflect changes to Tanner's model.
Prion et al., 2017	Quint Leveled Clinical Competency Tool	A rubric designed to assess student progress over time in simulation and patient care clinical environments. Aspects of Tanner's Clinical Judgment Model are evident in the tool which also integrates the nursing process.
Sweeney et al., 2020	Sweeney-Clark Simulation Evaluation Rubric	Described as a rubric overlaying Benner's novice-to-expert framework and Bloom's taxonomy. Is not organized by a clinical judgment framework or model. Clinical judgment is one of 8 performance categories assessed. Some reliability and validity established.

Objective Structured Clinical Examinations

Objective Structured Clinical Examinations (OSCEs) have been used extensively in medical education to evaluate clinical competencies (Holmboe et al., 2018). OSCEs typically use mini-clinical scenarios with standardized patients who are actors trained to portray a patient presentation. The actors are trained to respond to the clinician in a prescribed way. The patient scenario is designed to focus on select clinical competencies and scoring instruments are developed by the program faculty to score the student performance. The students are directly observed as they interact with the standardized patient. Sometimes both the actor and the faculty evaluate the learner's demonstrated behaviors using a scoring rubric or checklist. Often several stations are developed, and the students have multiple encounters with various clinical scenarios during an evaluation session. OSCEs can be designed so the student must confront an ill-defined problem and make a clinical judgment and OSCEs are used for formative and summative assessment. When OSCEs are used for summative assessment, the evaluation is completed by more than one trained rater, and the instruments used to guide the ratings are carefully constructed with a focus on reliability (Holmboe et al., 2018). See Chapter 12, *Best Practices in Simulation Learning* for further discussion of OSCEs.

While the practice of assessing clinical judgment competency is in the nascent stage of practice in nursing education, general assessment principles and emerging best practices can be used to develop a systematic approach to summative assessment of clinical judgment. See Chapter 7, *Backward Design: Aligning Outcomes, Assessments, and Activities* and Chapter 14, *Equitable Assessment Practices* for important background related to general assessment principles used in instructional design and equitable grading practices.

Entrustable Professional Activities

Nearly 20 years ago, ten Cate (2005) introduced the concept of entrustable professional activities to be associated with the competencies medical students must demonstrate before they advance to residency. "Entrustable" designates the extent to which the learner is 'trusted' to perform the activity with what degree of supervision. Wagner and colleagues were able to demonstrate the applicability of EPAs in the evaluation of competencies in quality and safety in advanced practice nursing (Wagner et al., 2018). Other investigators have explored their usefulness in undergraduate education (Lau et al., 2020a; 2020b) and in transitioning nurse practitioner students to practice (Hodges et al., 2019). The nearly 15 years of research and application in graduate and undergraduate medical education provide excellent groundwork for other health disciplines, including nursing, to explore this promising approach to the challenges of authentic clinical performance assessment in competency-based education (ten Cate et al., 2020; ten Cate & Chen, 2020; ten Cate & Taylor, 2021). See Box 17.3 for an example of an EPA designed to address the application of clinical judgment in safe medication administration.

The NLN's vision statement addressing competency-based education cites EPAs as an essential component in competency-based education and assessment (NLN, 2023). The NLN indicates they are building a toolkit of resources for faculty to develop curriculum in competency-based programs of study. EPAs will be included in the toolkit (NLN, 2023).

BOX 17.3

Entrustable Professional Activity Template and Exemplar

Preamble

Wagner et al. (2018) indicate EPAs are defined as "tasks or responsibilities that faculty entrust to a trainee to execute unsupervised, once they have obtained adequate competence" (p. 238). EPAs were originally developed in medicine and are described as tasks or responsibilities that faculty entrust to a learner to perform unsupervised once they have demonstrated adequate competence (ten Cate & Taylor, 2021). The goal of entrustment is to allow the learner to perform the activities without direct supervision in the next stage of clinical training. The template below synthesizes recommendations for designing EPAs (Holmboe et al., 2018; ten Cate & Taylor, 2021; Wagner et al., 2018).

Entrustable Professional Activity	
1. Title	Short title describing the EPA
2. Description (include specification/limitations)	Describe the "what and when" with specifications/limitations
3. Align with a competency framework	List competency domains used by program/school (i.e., QSEN, AACN, or program-specific)
4. Required experience and knowledge, skills and attitudes (competencies)	List knowledge, skills, attitudes addressed in this EPA
5. Assessment methods to assess progress and summative decision	List assessment methods, both progressive and summative, evaluation allowing students to perform the EPA independently
6. When is unsupervised practice expected?	Identify at what point in the curriculum student is expected to become independent
7. When and context of formal evaluation	When and in what context(s) does formal entrustment occur?

EPA Tracking

EPA				
EPA title	1 Observe/Lab Practice	2 Direct Supervision	3 Indirect Supervision	4 Oversight

Levels of Supervision

1. Observation/lab/practice—The skill or task is introduced and the learner practices the skill in a lab or simulation. Active coaching is provided using a deliberate practice approach (see Chapter 10, *Current Concepts in Clinical Education*)
2. Direct supervision—The student performs the skill in an authentic patient care environment. Supervising faculty or designated staff nurse is in the patient's room and provides direct supervision while the task is performed.

BOX 17.3

Entrustable Professional Activity Template and Exemplar *(Continued)*

3. Indirect supervision—The student performs the skill in the authentic patient care environment The supervising faculty or designated staff nurse helps the student prepare for the task but is not present during the patient encounter. The supervising faculty/designated staff nurse is readily available to help during the student/patient encounter.
4. Oversight—The student performs the skill in an authentic patient care environment. The supervising faculty is available for assistance but may be in a different patient care area or off-site and can be contacted by phone.

EPA Example

Background

Medication administration errors account for 1.5 million preventable adverse reactions to drugs annually in the United States (Lee & Wessol, 2021). The ability to safely administer medications in a variety of settings is a ubiquitous nursing function in a variety of patient care environments. Administering medications safely is a nursing skill new graduates are expected to perform independently once they begin practicing.

Lee & Wessol (2021) found a positive correlation when students applied Tanner's model of clinical judgment to safe medication administration practices. This Entrustable Professional Activity (EPA) is designed to assure students have a progressive opportunity to apply clinical judgment to safe medication practices with the aim of preparing them to perform this skill independently as they enter their final capstone clinical practicum.

Entrustable Professional Activity—Competencies and Milestones	
1. Title	Safe oral medication administration
2. Description (include specification/limitations)	Uses sound clinical reasoning, evidence-based practice standards, and patient-centered care to administer oral medications in a variety of settings. Learners should demonstrate progressive competency culminating in the ability to independently administer oral medications to a group of patients (3 or more) by the end of the advanced medical/surgical course.
3. Align with a competency framework	Clinical reasoning/judgment Evidence-based practices Patient-centered care
4. Required experience and knowledge, skills and attitudes (competencies)	Pathophysiology, pharmacology (purpose, side effects, drug interactions, normal dose); connects pathophysiology to prescribed medication, assesses patient responses and outcomes r/t medication, uses safe medication standards of practice (adheres to the *rights* of medication administration), individualizes administration to patient situation, demonstrates commitment to patient safety.
5. Assessment methods to assess progress and summative decision	Dosage calculation test, multiple patient medication mastery demonstration in skill lab, mastery of safe medication administration in simulation, demonstrates minimum of 6 accurate medication administrations in patient care environment.

(continued)

BOX 17.3

Entrustable Professional Activity Template and Exemplar *(Continued)*

6. When is unsupervised practice expected?	Week 10 advanced med/surg course
7. When does formal entrustment occur?	Formative ▸ Lab demonstration end of fundamental course ▸ Simulation ▸ Med/Surg 1 course Summative ▸ Clinical demonstration by week 10 of advanced Med/Surg Course ▸ May include demonstration in long-term care

EPA Tracking

EPA Safe Medication Administration	1 Observe/Lab Practice	2 Direct Supervision	3 Indirect Supervision	4 Oversight
Safe oral medication administration— 1–2 patients	11/11/24	4/3/25 4/4/25 4/10/25 4/11/25 4/18/25 4/29/25	5/5/25 5/6/25 5/12/25 5/13/25 5/15/25 5/16/2	6/10/25
Safe oral medication administration—4 or more patients	8/20/25	9/3/25 9/4/25 9/10/25 9/11/25 9/18/25 9/29/25	10/5/25 10/6/25 10/12/25 10/13/25 10/15/25 10/16/2	11/3/25

Adapted from Holmboe et al., 2018; ten Cate & Taylor, 2021; Wagner et al., 2018.

CHAPTER SUMMARY

The ability to make sound clinical judgments is the cornerstone of providing safe, quality, and patient-centered care. Consistent use of an established and evidence-based clinical judgment model or framework is essential to facilitating teaching and learning practices that promote the progressive development of clinical judgment in nursing students. Tanner's model of clinical judgment has been used and researched extensively; recent updates address the influence implicit bias may have in making sound clinical judgments and emphasize the transition to patient-centered health care that includes the patient and family perspective and participation in clinical decision-making. Formative assessment using a variety of methods facilitates the learners' development. Providing feedback that embeds high regard and high standards for the student promotes learning through formative assessment. Creating a variety of methods and opportunities using formative assessment strategies assures students have ample opportunity to demonstrate evolving clinical judgment competency. Single high-stakes evaluation to assess students' clinical judgment competency should be avoided. Faculty evaluation of students' clinical judgment should include a variety of methods and be based on a pattern of performance. Entrustable Professional Activities (EPAs) are a method developed in medical education to evaluate a student's trusted competence as an independent clinician. As nursing education transforms to a competency-based model, EPAs may be used as one method used to assess workplace activities associated with clinical judgment competency.

References

Adamson, K., Gubrud, P., Sideras, S., & Lasater, K. (2012). Assessing the reliability, validity, and use of the Lasater Clinical Judgment Rubric: Three approaches. *Journal of Nursing Education*, *51*(2), 66–73.

Angelo, T. A., & Cross, K. P. (1993). *Classroom assessment techniques*. Jossey-Bass.

Barkley, E. F., & Major, C. H. (2016). *Learning assessment techniques*. Jossey-Bass.

Benner, P. (2001). *From novice to expert: Excellence and power in clinical nursing practice*. Prentice-Hall.

Benner, P., Sutphen, M., Leonard, V., & Day, L. (2010). *Educating nurses: A call for radical transformation*. Jossey-Bass.

Benner, P., Tanner, C. A., & Chesla, C. A. (2009). *Expertise in nursing practice: Caring, clinical judgment, and ethics* (2nd ed.). Springer.

Brentnall, J., Thackery, D., & Judd, B. (2022). Evaluating the clinical reasoning of student health professionals in placement and simulation settings: A systematic review. *International Journal of Environmental Research and Public*, *19*, 936. https://doi.org/10.3390/ijerph19020936

Clemett, V. J., & Raleigh, M. (2021). The validity and reliability of clinical judgment and decision-making skills assessment in nursing: A systematic literature review. *Nurse Education Today*, *102*, 104885. https://doi.org/10.1016/j.nedt.2021.104885

Coolen, E., Engbers, R., Draaisma, J., Heinen, M., & Fluit, C. (2020) The use of SBAR as a structured communication tool in the pediatric non-acute care setting: bridge or barrier for interprofessional collaboration?, *Journal of Interprofessional Care*, 1–10. https://doi.org/10.1080/13561820.2020.1816936

Costa, A. B., Pas, P. F., de Camargo, E. S., Guaranha, C., Caetano, A. H., Kveller, D., da Rosa Filho, H. T., Catelan, R. F., Koller, S. H., & Nardi, H. C. (2016). Effectiveness of a multidimensional web-based intervention program to change Brazilian health practitioners: attitudes toward lesbian, gay, bisexual and transgender population. *Journal of Health Psychology*, *20*, 2138–2144.

Daley, B. J., Morgan, S., & Black, S. B. (2016). Concept maps in nursing education: A historical literature review and research directions. *Journal of Nursing Education*, *55*(11), 631–639. https://doi.org/10.3928/01484834-20161011-05

Daniel, M., Rencic, J., Durning, S. J., Holmboe, E., Santen, S. A., Lang V., Ratcliffe, T., Gordon, D., Heist, B., Lubarsky, S., Estrada, C. A., Ballard, T., Artino, A. R., Jr., Sergio Da Silva, A., Cleary, T., Stojan, J., & Gruppen, L. D. (2019). Clinical reasoning assessment methods: A scoping review and practical guidance. *Academic Medicine*, *94*(6), 902–912. https://doi.org/10.1097/ACM0000000000002618

Dickison, P., Haerling, K. A., & Lasater, K. (2019). NCSBN Clinical Judgment Measurement Model clarification. *Journal of Nursing Education*, *59*(7), 365. https://doi.org/10.3928/01484834-20200617-02

Dreifuerst, K. T. (2012). Using debriefing for meaningful learning to foster development of clinical reasoning in simulation. *Journal of Nursing Education*, *51*(6), 326–333. https://doi.org/10.3928/01484834-20120409-02

Eisenmann, N. (2021). An innovative clinical concept map to promote clinical judgment in nursing students. *Journal of Nursing Education*, *60*(3), 143–148. https://doi.org/10.3928/01484834-20210222-04

Fey, M. K., Roussin, C. J., Rudolph, J. W., Morse, K. J., Palaganas, J. C., & Szyld, D. (2022). Teaching, coaching or debriefing "With Good Judgment" across the simzones. *Advances in Simulation*, *7*, 39. https://doi.org/10.1186/s41077-022-00235-y

Giddens, J., Douglas, J. P., & Conroy, S. (2022). The revised AACN Essentials: Implications for nursing regulation. *Journal of Nursing Regulation*, *12*(4), 16–22.

Gonzalez, L. (2018). Teaching clinical reasoning piece by piece: A clinical reasoning concept-based learning method. *Journal of Nursing Education*, *57*(12) 727–735. https://doi.org/10.3928/01484834-20181119-05

Gonzalez, L., Nielsen, A., & Lasater, K. (2021). Developing students' clinical reasoning skills: A faculty guide. *Journal of Nursing Education*, *6*(9), 485–493. https://doi.org/10.3928/014834-20210708-01

Hayden, J., Keegan, M., Kardong-Edgren, S., & Smiley, R. A. (2014). Reliability and validity testing of the Creighton Competency Evaluation Instrument for use in the NCSBN Simulation Study. *Nursing Education Perspectives*, *35*(4), 244–252. https://doi.org/10.58480/13-1130.1

Hodges, A. L., Konicki, A. J., Talley, M. H., Bordelon, C. J., Holland, A. C., & Galin, F. S. (2019). Competency-based education in transitioning nurse practitioner students from education into practice. *Journal of the American Association of Nurse Practitioners*, *31*, 675–682. https://doi.org/10.1097/JXX.0000000000000327

Holmboe, E. S., During, S. J., & Hawkins, R. E. (2018). *Evaluation of clinical competence* (2nd ed.). Elsevier.

Institute of Medicine. (2001). *Crossing the quality chasm: A new health system for the 21st century*. Committee on Quality of Health Care in America, National Academies Press

Institute of Medicine. (2003). *Unequal treatment: Confronting racial and ethnic disparities in health care*. The National Academies Press. https://doi.org/10.17226/12875

Jessee, M. A. (2018). Pursuing improvement in clinical reasoning: An integrated clinical education theory. *Journal of Nursing Education*, *57*(1), 7–13. https://doi.org/10.3928/01484834-20180102-03

Jessee, M. A. (2021). An update on clinical judgment in nursing and implications for education, practice and regulation. *Journal of Nursing Regulation*, *12*(3), 50–57.

Jessee, M. A., Nielsen, A., Monagle, J., Lasater, K., & Dickison, P. (2023). A national report on clinical judgment model use in prelicensure curricula. *Nursing Education Perspectives*, *44*(1), 4–10. https://doi.org/10.1097/01.NEP.0000000000001062

Jessee, M. A., & Tanner, C. A. (2016). Pursuing improvement in clinical reasoning: Development of the clinical coaching interactions inventory. *Journal of Nursing Education*, *55*(9), 495–504. https://doi.org/10.3928/01484834-20160816-03

Kahneman, D. (2011). *Thinking fast and slow*. Macmillan.

Kavanagh, J. M., & Sharpnack, P. A. (2021). Crisis in competency: A defining moment in nursing education. *Online Journal of Issues in Nursing*, *26*(1), Article 2. https://doi.org/10.3912/OJIN.Vol26No01Man02

Lasater, K. (2007). Clinical judgment development: Using simulation to create an assessment rubric. *Journal of Nursing Education*, *46*(11), 496–503.

Lau, S. T., Ang, E., Samarasekera, D. D., & Shorey, S. (2020a). Development of undergraduate nursing entrustable professional activities to enhance clinical care and practice. *Nurse Education Today*, *87*, 104347. https://doi.org/10.1016/j.nedt.2020.104347

Lau, S. T., Ang, E., Samarasekera, D. D., & Shorey, S. (2020b). Evaluation of an undergraduate nursing entrustable professional activities framework: An exploratory qualitative research. *Nurse Education Today*, *87*, 104343. https://doi.org/10.1016/j.nedt.2020.104343

Lavoie, P., Clarke, S. P., Clausen, C., Purden, M., Emed, J., Mailhot, T., Fontaine, G., & Frunchak, V. (2020). Nurses' judgment of patient risk of deterioration at change-of-shift handoff: Agreement between nurses and comparison with early warning scores. *Heart & Lung, 49*(4), 420–425.

Lawson, T. N. (2018). Diagnostic reasoning and cognitive biases of nurse practitioners. *Journal of Nursing Education, 57*, 203–208. https://doi.org/10.3928/01484834-20180322-03

Lee, K. C., & Wessol, J. L. (2021). Clinical reasoning, judgment and safe medication administration practices in senior nursing students. *Nurse Educator, 47*(1), 51–55. https://doi.org/10.1097/NNE.0000000000001059

Lewallen, L. P., & Van Horn, E. R. (2019). The state of the science on clinical evaluation in nursing education. *Nursing Education Perspectives, 40*(1), 4–10. https://doi.org/10/1097/01.NEP.0000000000000376

Lucey, C. R. (2018). Achieving competency-based, time-variable health professions education. Proceedings of a conference sponsored by Josiah Macy Jr. Foundation in June 2017; New York, NY: Josiah Macy Jr. Foundation.

Manz, J. A., Tracy, M., Hercinger, M., Todd, M., & Hawkins, K. (2022). Assessing competency: An Integrative Review of The Creighton Simulation Evaluation Instrument (C-SEI) and Creighton Competency Evaluation Instrument (C-CEI). *Clinical Simulation in Nursing, 66*, 66–75. https://doi.org/10.1016/j.ecns.2022.02.003

McAllister, M., Tower, M., & Walker, R. (2007). Gentle interruptions: Transformative approaches to clinical teaching. *Journal of Nursing Education, 45*(6), 304–312.

McGaghie, W. C. (2020). Mastery learning: Origins, features and evidence from the health professions. In W. C. McGaghie, J. H. Barsuk & D. B. Wayne (Eds.), *Comprehensive healthcare simulation: Mastery learning in the health professions*. Springer.

Milky, G., & Thomas, J., 3rd. (2020). Shared decision making, satisfaction with care and adherence among patients with diabetes. *Patient Education & Counseling, 103*, 661–669. https://doi.org/10.106/j.pec.2019.10.008

National League for Nursing (NLN). (2023). *NLN Vision Series: Integrating Competency-Based Education in the Nursing Curriculum*. https://www.nln.org/detail-pages/news/2023/02/09/nln-publishes-new-vision-statement-integrating-competency-based-education-in-the-nursing-curriculum accessed 2-13-23.

Nielsen, A., Gonzalez, L., Jessee, M. A., Monagle, J., Dickison, P., & Lasater, K. (2023). Current practices of teaching clinical judgment. *Nurse Educator, 48*(1), 7–12. https://doi.org/10.1097/NNE.0000000000001268

NLN. (2020). *NLN Vision Series: The Fair Testing Imperative in Nursing Education*. https://www.nln.org/docs/default-source/uploaded-files/advocacy-public-policy/nln-fair-testing-vision-series.pdf accessed 2-13-23.

Norman, G. R., Monteiro, S. D., Sherbino, J., Ilgen, J. S., Schmidt, H. G., & Mamede, S. (2017). The causes of errors in clinical reasoning: Cognitive biases, knowledge deficits, and dual process thinking. *Academic Medicine, 92*(1), 23–30. https://doi.org/10.1097/ACM.0000000000001421

Ochs, J. H. (2023). Addressing health disparities by addressing structural racism and implicit bias in nursing education. *Nurse Education Today, 121*, 105670. https://doi.org/10.1016/j.nedt.2022.105670

Parry, A., & Selvaraj, N. (2023). Effective handovers on escalation of care for the deteriorating patient. *Nursing Standard, 38*(3), 77–81. https://doi.org/10.7748/ns.2023.e12078

Prion, S. K., Gilbert, G. E., Adamson, K. A., Kardong-Edgren, S., & Quint, S. (2017). Development and testing of the Quint Leveled Clinical Competency Tool. *Clinical Simulation in Nursing, 13*(3), 106–115. https://doi.org/10.1016/j.ecns.2016.10.008

Robstad, N., Westergren, T., Siebler, F., Söderhamn, Y., & Fegran, L. (2019). Intensive care nurses' implicit and explicit attitudes and their behavioral intentions towards obese intensive care patients. *Journal of Advanced Nursing, 75*, 3621–3642.

Schaa, K. L., Roter, D. L., Biesecker, B. B., Cooper, L. A., & Erby, L. H. (2015). Genetic counselors' implicit racial attitudes and their relationship to communication. *Health Psychology, 34*(2), 111–119. https://doi.org/10.1037/hea0000155

Schultz, P. L., & Baker, J. (2017). Teaching strategies to increase nursing student acceptance and management of unconscious bias. *Journal of Nursing Education, 56*(11), 692–696. https://doi.org/10.3928/01484834-20171020-11

Scolari, E., Soncini, L., Ramelet, A. S., & Schneider, A. G. (2022). Quality of the situation-background-assessment recommendation tool during nurse-physician calls in the ICU: An observational study. *Nursing in Critical Care, 27*(6), 796–803. https://doi.org/10.1111/nicc.12743

Sommer, S. K., Johnson, J. D., Clark, C. M., & Mills, C. M. (2021). Assisting learners to understand and incorporate functions of clinical judgment into nursing practice. *Nurse Educator, 46*(6), 372–375. https://doi.org/10.1097/NNE.0000000000001020

South, B. (2007). Combining mandala and the Jahari Window: An exercise in self-awareness. *Teaching and Learning in Nursing, 2*, 8–11. https://doi.org/10.1016/j.teln.2006.10.001

Sweeney, N., Rollins, M. C., Gantt, L., Swanson, M., & Ravitz, J. (2020). Development and reliability testing of the Sweeney-Clark simulation evaluation rubric. *Clinical Simulation in Nursing, 41*, 22–32. https://doi.org/10.1016/j.ecns.2019.04.002

Tanner, C. A. (2006). Thinking like a nurse: A research-based model of clinical judgment in nursing. *Journal of Nursing Education, 45*(6), 204–211. https://doi.org/10.3928/01484834-20060601-04

Tanner, C., Messecar, D., & Delawska-Elliott, B. (2022). Chapter 13, evidence based practice. In L. Joel (Ed.), *Advanced practice nursing: Essentials for role development* (5th ed.). F.A. Davis.

ten Cate, O. (2005). Entrustability of professional activities and competency-based training. *Medical Education, 39*, 1176–1177. https://doi.org/10.1111/j.1365-2929.2005.02341x

ten Cate, O., & Chen, C. H. (2020). The ingredients of a rich entrustment decision. *Medical Teacher, 42*(12), 1413–1420. https://doi.org/10.1080/0142159X.2020.1817348

ten Cate, O., & Taylor, D. R. (2021). The recommended description of an entrustable professional activity: AMEE Guide No. 140. *Medical Teacher, 43*(10), 1106–1114. https://doi.org/10.1080/0142159X.2020.1838465

Tyo, B. M., & McCurry, M. K. (2019). An integrative review of clinical reasoning teaching strategies and outcome evaluation in nursing education. *Nursing Education Perspectives, 40*(1), 11–17. https://doi.org/10.1097/01.NEP.0000000000000375

Wagner, L. M., Dolansky, M. A., & Englander, R. (2018). Entrustable professional activities for quality and patient safety. *Nursing Outlook, 66*, 237–243.

Watling, C. J., & Gingsberg, S. (2019). Assessment, feedback and alchemy of learning. *Medical Education, 53*, 76–85. https://doi.org/10.1111/medu.13645

Wilson, R. D., Wilson, B. L., & Madden, C. (2021). Creating a national standard for prelicensure clinical evaluation in nursing. *Journal of Nursing Education, 60*(12), 686–689. https://doi.org/10.3928/01484834-20211004-0

18

Ethical and Legal Considerations in Assessment

Paula Gubrud, EdD, RN, CHSE, FAAN, ANEF

CHAPTER OVERVIEW

Ethical and legal considerations for providing a safe and fair assessment of learners are reviewed in this chapter. Topics include methods to reduce bias and misconduct in the learning environment and concepts of just culture for the academic nursing learning environment and provision of reasonable accommodations to support effective learning environments. An introduction to using program evaluation standards for continuous quality improvement is presented.

INTRODUCTION

The nurse educator's role in evaluating student competency involves the dual responsibility of facilitating learning and evaluating competency performance to assure students are fit for practice as new graduates. This complex obligation requires ethical comportment that embodies high standards as an educator and as a nurse. The nurse educator must incorporate standards and expected practices embedded in higher education with the ethics of the nursing profession which includes protecting the public and promoting health and safety for patients as a licensed professional nurse. The nurse educator must use best practices in assessment and integrate moral and legal obligations to provide and contribute to safe and effective patient care. Adhering to standards of assessment with professional ethical obligations related to patient safety can require the nurse educator to reconcile competing values and expectations. As a licensed professional, the nurse educator must utilize academic policies generated from the broader institution and within the nursing program. Familiarity with the regulatory rules that govern nursing education programs can inform the legal obligations the nurse educator is required to fulfill.

QUALITY AND SAFETY EDUCATION FOR NURSES (QSEN) AND JUST CULTURE

Background

Nursing education has considered patient safety a crucial construct used to organize curriculum, evaluate student performance in skills and clinical activities, and guide supervisory practices when students are engaged in patient care experiences. In 199 the Institute of Medicine (IOM) landmark publication reported an alarming rate of preventable errors in health care citing medical errors as the third leading cause of death in the United States (IOM, 1999). In a follow-up to this report, the IOM (2003) published *Health Professions Education: A Bridge to Quality.* This publication presented cor competencies with recommendations for all health profession education programs to integrate these core competencies into curriculum framework and learning activities The Robert Wood Foundation continued supporting a focus on safety and quality and funded a national initiative called the Quality and Safety Education for Nurses (QSEN to define competencies that should be integrated into prelicensure nursing education (QSEN Institute, n.d.). See Table 18.1 for the IOM Health Professions Core Competencie and QSEN Competencies.

QSEN Safety Competency

Concerns for patient safety have been a long-standing concern in nursing education It's common to hear a faculty voice concerns about unsafe behaviors when considering whether to allow a student to progress in the program or graduate. Concerns regarding safety are well founded as despite the emphasis on safety in health care, errors continue to occur at an alarming rate. A 2022 report from the Office of the Inspector General indicates 25% of hospitalized patients experienced harm in October of 2018 (U.S Department of Office of Health & Human Services, Inspector General, 2022). The National Council of State Boards of Nursing (NCSBN) collects data on nursing student errors and near

---

TABLE 18.1

Institute of Medicine (2003) Health Professions Core Competencies and QSEN Competencies

IOM Core Competencies	QSEN Competencies for Nurses
Provide patient-centered care	Patient-centered care
Work in interdisciplinary teams	Teamwork and collaboration
Employ evidence-based practice	Evidence-based practice
Apply quality improvement	Quality improvement
Use informatics	Safety
	Informatics

Source: Cronenwett et al., 2007; QSEN Institute, n.d.

misses from prelicensure programs in 43 states. Analysis of data from 204 programs over a three-year period indicated that the majority of errors that occurred in a patient care clinical setting were related to medications. The top five occurrences were medication errors, deviation in protocol, inadequate clinical preparation, needlesticks, and ineffective preparation. Even more significantly, 10.8 percent of these errors resulted in harm, either to the patient or to the student. The authors concluded that these errors and near misses were related to the following patient safety issues: lack of adherence to protocols related to checking patient identification and allergy status and following the five rights of medication administration (Silvestre & Spector, 2023).

The QSEN competencies emphasize the importance of developing a curriculum that includes knowledge, skills, and attitudes that prepare students to function in a complex and constantly evolving health care system. The QSEN safety competency reframes perceptions of patient safety away from sole individual accountability for patient safety to an awareness that the health care system must be designed to help nurses keep patients safe (Armstrong, 2019). The QSEN competencies are each described in terms of knowledge, skills, and attitudes (KSAs) required to develop proficient behaviors (Armstrong, 2019). The KSAs for patient safety include attributes of just culture and an appreciation for the role complex systems play in the provision of safe nursing care.

Unfortunately, nursing education programs have a history of responding with a punitive response when a student makes a safety error when engaged in clinical learning in the patient care environment (Disch et al., 2017). A large study completed by Disch et al. (2017) found errors occurring in the clinical environment frequently result in disciplinary action from verbal warning to dismissal from the program. The survey found significant numbers of students reported that when an error occurs, the focus of documentation is on the person, not the problem, and that mistakes were held against them (Disch et al., 2017). The result of using a disciplinary response to students' clinical errors, or near misses results in creating a culture of secrecy, shame and blame, and a belief that the student clinician could have prevented the error through personal diligence and attention to detail (Barnsteiner et al., 2023).

Just Culture

In addition to the IOM's (1999) recommendations to address the need for improvements in patient safety, the report also emphasized the importance of transforming culture to a non-punitive stance that recognizes the role of systems as a contributing cause of error in most situations (Barkell & Synder, 2021). In nursing education programs, it is imperative to embrace the understanding that according to safety science, the results of harsh discipline are contrary to mitigating future errors, solving system problems, and improving practice (Barnsteiner et al., 2023). Transitioning to a system of just culture focuses on learning from errors by reducing the focus on "blame and retrain," to a holistic approach that seeks to understand the root cause of errors. Research in health care organizations has consistently found that implementing and supporting just culture increases reports of errors and near misses which reduces error through learning by using root cause analysis and addressing weaknesses in the system that contribute to mistakes (Barkell & Snyder, 2021; Marx, 2019).

What Is Just Culture?

Just culture balances the standard of individual accountability with system accountability when an error or near miss occurs (Walker et al., 2020). It's important to acknowledge just culture is not punitive, nor is it blame-free (Armstrong, 2019). It's a system based on trust that encourages people and systems to identify the sources of errors and engage in forward-thinking problem-solving to prevent reoccurrence (Barnsteiner et al., 2023). Just culture is described as an environment that supports learning from errors and assigning accountability for individual behaviors that contribute to or cause errors (Walker, 2019). Petschonek et al. (2013) identified six core dimensions and definitions to use when developing, assessing, and improving just culture within a health care organization. The six core dimensions are 1) balance, 2) trust, 3) openness of communication, 4) quality of the event-reporting process, 5) feedback and communication about the events, and 6) overall goal of continuous improvement. Table 18.2 provides a description of each dimension adapted for academic nursing organizations.

Experts in just culture cite multiple assumptions that can be used to develop and enhance a just culture within an organization (Armstrong, 2019; Barnsteiner, 2023; Barnsteiner & Disch, 2017; Walker, 2019). Common core assumptions are:

> Health care is provided by humans and humans make mistakes.
> Just culture embraces an atmosphere of trust, rewarding people for identifying sources of error and engaging in problem-solving to prevent reoccurrence.

TABLE 18.2

Assessing and Improving Just Culture

Dimension	Definitions
Balance	One's perceptions of fair treatment within the organization as it is related to error, error reporting, and the organization system's approach to a safety error.
Trust	The extent to which individual trusts the organization, their supervisors, and their peers.
Openness of communication	The willingness of individuals to communicate information upward to clinical faculty, supervisors, and the clinical facility supervisors and administrators. Examples include: willingness to share events information and suggestions for making improvements or preventing a reoccurrence.
Quality of the event-reporting process	Perceived quality of the event reporting system. Whether the individual is given time and assistance to complete a report and to what extent the student believes the reporting system is monitored and maintained
Feedback and communication	Belief regarding whether the school and clinical organization effectively shares information about the events and outcome(s) of evaluating the event
Overall goal of continuous improvement	Belief the organizations (school and clinical learning organization) demonstrates a goal of continuous improvement, characterized by a willingness to learn from events and make improvements to the school and clinical learning environment systems

Adapted from Petschonek et al., 2013.

> Medical errors and near misses are usually multifactorial and involve individual and system accountability.

> Just culture does not eliminate the possibility that some events require sole individual accountability.

> Just culture uses a systematic process focused on root cause analysis to fully understand the antecedents contributing to the error. Root cause analysis is necessary for determining accountability, transparency, reliance on evidence that lends to the individual learning from the mistake, and revising system issues that contribute to or create the likelihood of an error.

Understanding the error. Determining the root cause or causes of an error begins with the embodiment of the same values used to debrief and coach students as described in Chapter 17, *Assessment of Clinical Judgment*. The process should hold the learners in high regard and hold them to high standards (Fey et al., 2022). In the case of an error, patient safety standards provide the benchmark used to frame the concern and process of understanding what happened. The NCSBN (2012) provides a helpful step-by-step process for conducting a root cause analysis. Barnsteiner et al. (2023) suggest the inquiry begin by answering five questions.

1. What happened?
2. Has it happened before?
3. Could it happen again?
4. What caused it to happen?
5. Who should be told?

Errors are often multifactorial and can involve more than one level of systems failure, and there may be acceptable behavior and potentially unacceptable behavior on the part of the student that may be involved in the error (Barnsteiner et al., 2023). In just culture, errors are described in terms of three possible levels: human errors, at-risk behaviors, and reckless behavior (Barnsteiner et al., 2023; Marx, 2019).

> Human errors are considered level-one errors. Human errors are unintended mistakes occurring because of a gap in knowledge or skill or practicing above what should be expected of the level of the learner. Human factors, including fatigue, an overwhelming cognitive load, such as caring for multiple complex patients in a chaotic situation, creates opportunity for human error.

> At-risk behaviors are the second level of error and involve the individual doing something inappropriate but with the genuine belief the action will not result in untoward consequences, or the risk is inconsequential. Workarounds to a procedure are sometimes considered at-risk behavior. Failing to conduct two-person identification with a patient the nurse has already had encounters with is an example of at-risk behavior.

> Reckless behavior, the third level of error, occurs when individuals make mistakes "…with impunity or reckless behavior" (Barnsteiner et al., 2023, p. 140). These kinds of errors occur when an individual has a disregard for policies and procedures or devise their own rules. In extreme situations the individual intentionally causes harm.

Response to the error. The actions and reactions to an error should be determined b the level and sometimes the frequency of errors. A pattern of human error should rais concern and a plan for improvement should be considered. Punitive corrective actio for unintentional human errors or system failures reduces the reporting of errors, n the occurrence of errors (Barnsteiner et al., 2023; Walker et al., 2023). Marx (2019) suggest creating psychological safety in just culture involves assuring the response to the err is appropriate for the level of the mistake. When the root cause of a mistake is du to human error and/or system failure, the approach is to accept the error. This doe not mean the error is ignored but is used as a learning opportunity to improve prac tice and/or initiate system change. Root cause analysis will unpack the circumstanc es and causes of the error and inform steps to prevent future similar mistakes. Th North Carolina Board of Nursing (2022) has developed a Student Event Practice Even Evaluation Tool (SPEET) for the analysis of an error in Nursing Education program (see Chapter 2, *Teaching in a Practice-Based Profession* for further description of th SPEET). The NCSBN (n.d.) provides a debriefing template developed by Dr. Gerry Alt miller that faculty can use to guide the student through learning about patient safet and taking action to improve practice behaviors. Reckless errors require a differer response. The individual needs to be coached, and reconciliation regarding the risk behavior and a commitment to improvement is required (Marx, 2017). Closer supervisio when the student is engaged in patient care may be necessary to assure patient safet and the individual may need to demonstrate re-mastery of a skill or a knowledge ga may need to be addressed and remedied. When the root cause of an error is due t reckless behavior the individuals must be held accountable through a disciplinary pro cess described in the policy. According to Barnsteiner et al. (2023), these types of error are very infrequent. When errors occur because of reckless behavior serious discipline is likely an appropriate response. Discipline for a reckless error or established pat tern of errors resulting from at-risk behaviors may include dismissal from the program (Barnsteiner et al., 2023).

Policy

Nursing education programs need policies in place to promote a just culture. Nursing programs should have tools and processes in place to track errors and near misses Reporting tools should use clear, non-judgmental language. Tracking data should be de-identified and reviewed according to a regular schedule so trends and patterns o common errors can be identified, and program improvements can be made. For exam- ple, if there are numerous medication errors or near misses occurring in a particula course by multiple students, faculty may need to revise or add learning activities related to safe medication administration in skills lab and simulation.

Nursing education programs should develop policies that clearly describe reckless, unacceptable behavior and potential actions and consequences (Barnsteiner et al., 2023). Due process policies must be in place to assure students' legal rights are upheld dur- ing disciplinary processes. Faculty have a responsibility to understand and adhere to due process procedures (Walker, 2019; Walker, 2021), which should be approved by college or university student services. When a student is disciplined, college and university policies must align with program policy to avoid conflict of interest. Academic nurse leaders may need to educate college administration on the importance of using safe standards in patient care and provide information and research on the impact of human errors in health care so non-nurse academic administrators understand the facets of just culture.

Walker (2019) states ongoing defensible clinical evaluation is also a component of due process. Clinical evaluations should be conducted according to school policy and course requirements. Clinical faculty have a responsibility to inform students when they are not meeting standards of practice. Conversely, opportunities must be provided to facilitate student achievement of learning outcomes. Concerns should be documented, and the student should have an opportunity to respond in writing to the matters described by the faculty. Both the faculty and student should sign the document so it's clear the student was informed of the concerns, acknowledges the steps they should take to improve, and describes desired outcomes that must demonstrate. Documentation should be filed and available for review so concerns and evidence of improvement can be monitored as students progress through clinical courses. Consistent documentation also records trends or patterns of unsafe behavior. The NCSBN has developed resources to assist with tracking and analysis of student errors and near misses (NCSBN, 2021). Safe Student Reports and a national data repository allow nursing education programs to benchmark their data with national data.

Curriculum

Developing a just culture requires intentional curricular actions to assure faculty and students have the requisite knowledge, skills, and attitudes needed to embrace a just culture. Barnsteiner and Disch (2017) call for a shared accountability model that includes students, faculty, and organizational leaders. They purport all stakeholders need the opportunity to discuss issues that arise, mechanisms for decision-making, and support for discerning new ideas. They identify faculty development as an important aspect of implementing a just culture (Barnsteiner & Disch, 2017). Faculty may not have been exposed to safety science in formal or continuing education and related topics such as high-reliability organizations, human factors, system complexity, and quality improvement may need to be included in new faculty orientation. Clinical faculty need to be oriented to policies and resources that support just culture.

Walker et al. (2023) provide descriptions of several just culture learning activities that can be integrated throughout the curriculum. They advocate for assuring safety science and improvement is integrated into clinical, including simulation-based learning experiences, and laboratory courses, not just in theory as lecture content. Some examples are 1) including questions and observations regarding safe behavior in simulation scenarios, 2) addressing safety issues including observed near misses in clinical post-conferences, and 3) reflective journaling assignments can also address students' observations and analysis of safety issues and experiences encountered when involved in patient care. Several schools have adopted programs that reward students for catching and reflecting on near misses and have demonstrated these interventions increase error reporting and create a culture that is safety conscious and values continuous improvement (Tanz, 2018; Walker et al., 2023).

Evaluating Just Culture

Multiple experts in just culture suggest the adaptation of just culture begins wit assessing related organizational values and attributes (Armstrong, 2019; Barnsteiner et a 2023; Barnsteiner & Disch, 2017; Hays & Kruse, 2022; Walker, 2019; Walker et al., 2023). Walker (2019 developed an assessment tool that aims to describe the current culture and can b used at specific time intervals so the current state can be recognized, successful inter ventions are identified and enhanced, and the effectiveness of actions taken can b monitored. The *Just Culture Assessment Tool* originally created for the practice envi ronment (Petschonek et al., 2013) was adapted for academia (Walker, 2019). The revised too is called the *Just Culture Assessment Tool for Nursing Education* (JCAT-NE) and ha established reliability and validity (Walker, 2019). 6 items were added to the original tool t address issues specific to assessing just culture in nursing academia. Understandin current culture within a program can provide the motivation for change and ongoin administration and analysis of the JCAT-NE can provide benchmarks for programs, indi vidual faculty, and students (Walker, 2019).

DISABILITY INCLUSION IN NURSING EDUCATION

Background

Nursing education and practice have embraced values of diversity, inclusivity, anc belonging as essential for a workforce situated to promote health equity and miti gation of health disparities in the United States (Hassmiller & Wakefield, 2022; Sumpte et al., 2022). Unfortunately, the lack of diversity in nursing education, which ha downstream consequences for developing a diverse nursing workforce is widel acknowledged (Gonzalez & Hasiao, 2020). Nursing education and health professior programs, in general, have historically limited access for people with disabilities (Gonzales & Hasiao, 2020) as disability is often viewed through the medical model lens (Marks & McCulloh, 2016; Marks & Sisirak, 2022). Students with disabilities (SWD) are ofter excluded from nursing education programs because of outdated perceptions sug gesting a disability creates risk and liability for unsafe practice situations (Marks & MCCulloh, 2016). As discussed previously in this chapter most health care errors are largely due to system processes and environmental conditions, not individual mis takes. Furthermore, there is no documented evidence demonstrating a causal rela tionship between health care workers with disabilities and increased patient safety risk and error (Englund & Lancaster, 2022; Gonzales & Hasiao, 2020; Marks & McCulloh, 2016). People with disabilities often recognize their limitations and find work that allows them to utilize their strengths. With the call for expanding nurses in primary care, and other community-based settings, the opportunity for nurses to practice in non acute settings will be expanding (Hassmiller & Wakefield, 2022). Expanding access to nursing education for SWD is one step toward meeting the nursing workforce rec ommendations and goals described in the *Future of Nursing 2020–2030* report. As with other marginalized groups, developing a workforce that includes clinicians with disabilities improves the care for patients with disabilities (Gonzales & Hasieo, 2020; Marks & Sisirak, 2022).

Historical nursing education policies and practices have excluded pre-nursing SWD from even applying to nursing school (Epstein et al., 2021; Gonzales & Hasiao, 2020; Matt et al., 2015). Specifically, these policies and practices include the ubiquitous use of Core Performance Standards or Essential Functions (Englund & Lancaster, 2022; Gonzales & Hasiao, 2020; Matt et al., 2015). Core Performance Standards or Essential Functions frequently focus on the perceived physical requirements for bedside nurses practicing in acute care settings and fail to acknowledge: potential accommodations that can be implemented in the hospital environment, or explore utilizing non-acute clinical practice environments available to SWD after graduation (Epstein et al., 2021; Elting et al., 2021; Gonzales & Hasiao, 2020). Neal-Boylan and Miller (2020, p. 239) recommend "Avoiding confusing essential functions of the nursing role with academic requirements to succeed in nursing school and practice as a safe novice nurse."

Americans with Disabilities Act (ADA)

The passage of the ADA of 1990 transformed the quality of life and opportunity for people with disabilities. However, health care professions have been slow to improve accommodations that support workers and SWD (Marks & Sisirak, 2022). After the ADA Amendments Act (ADAAA) of 2008, access to professions for people with physical disability improved (Elting et al., 2021). Marks and McCulloh (2016) conclude the ADAAA of 2008 "…served to rekindle the spirit, intent, and protections of the ADA of 1990" (p. 10). Developing accommodations to eliminate discrimination against SWD should incorporate the spirit and the letter of both the original ADA and the ADAA (Englund & Lancaster, 2022; Epstein et al., 2021; Marks & McCulloh, 2016).

Accommodations

In post-secondary education, accommodations refer to "the process of making adjustments or alternative arrangements in the educational environment to ensure a discriminatory effect does not occur because of the student's disability" (May, 2014, p. 241). A student's request for reasonable accommodation is a legal right protected under the ADA and the ADAAA. The request for reasonable accommodation must be initiated by the student using the university or college process and policy through the institution's disability services. Reasonable accommodations are described as interventions that do not create an undue burden on the program and do not require faculty to transform the curriculum to implement an assigned accommodation (Horkey, 2019). A reasonable accommodation should be designed to mitigate the potentially discriminatory effect of the disability, providing equal opportunity to successfully meet course and program outcomes when compared with non-disabled students (Horkey, 2019). To receive accommodations, the disability must be diagnosed by a qualified clinician. Accommodations are then identified and assigned by the institution's disability services and the faculty may not be aware of the diagnosed disability. Legally, the student is not required to disclose their disability to faculty and should never be pressured to do so (May, 2014). Faculty's legal responsibility involves the effective implementation of the assigned accommodation (Horkey, 2019; May, 2014). Studies show faculty are more effective when they receive

training on the effective implementation of accommodations (Horkey, 2019) and shoul
not hesitate to collaborate with the institution's disability services to fully understand th
obvious and nuanced aspects of implementing the assigned accommodations. Estab
lishing a collaborative partnership with disability services using a shared framewor
committed to both promoting inclusivity and upholding standards of care will facilitat
student and program success. It is especially important to keep up-to-date on bes
practices in supporting students with accommodations as the landscape of disabilit
support for nursing students continues to evolve. The American Association of Co
leges of Nursing (AACN) (n.d.) has developed a comprehensive and helpful tool kit o
resources that can assist nurse educators with providing and advocating for accom
modating students with disabilities.

Classroom accommodations. Classroom accommodations are becoming more com
mon with the increase in SWD seeking higher education and improved adaptatio
of the ADA and ADAAA (Neal-Boylan & Miller, 2017). Classroom accommodations ca
address both physical and cognitive disabilities. Students with sight or hearin
disability may need to be seated in an optimum place in the classroom and hav
access to audio textbooks, or large print. When using a slide deck, the faculty ma
be asked to provide a copy to the student in advance or provide access to large
print. Accommodations for students with disabilities such as dyslexia and atten
tion deficit disorder may also include allowing students to record lectures and ac
cess visual and auditory learning materials. A common accommodation involves
providing a longer time for test taking in a quiet space. Students with chronic ill
nesses may receive accommodations for alterations in attendance, assignment
and assessment due dates. The faculty's responsibility is to provide the assigned
accommodations provided by disability services. Offering solutions to enhance the
accommodations is allowable when a collaborative partnership with disability ser
vices is established and when all stakeholders involved in promoting the student's
success will be realized.

Clinical accommodations. Clinical accommodations are more complicated to develop
and identify. Expanding the collaborative partnership that includes the clinica
organization will enhance the probability of avoiding discriminatory behavior and
actions toward the student. Multiple studies found students were more likely to
"mask" their disability due to fear of discrimination in the clinical environment (Elting
et al., 2021; Englund & Lancaster, 2022; Epstein et al., 2021; Gonzales & Hsiao, 2020). Unfortunately
SWD consistently reports faculty, staff, and peer attitudes toward disability create
more significant barriers than the disability itself (Englund & Lancaster, 2022; Epstein et al.
2021). In a scoping review, Epstein et al. (2021) found students feel labeled and are
sometimes excluded from clinical experiences, and therefore mask their disability
and forego accommodations, and suggest policies need to embrace their strengths
and contributions rather than their disability. Englund & Lancaster (2022) suggest
discriminatory attitudes are rooted in concerns for patient safety and the reliance on
medical-surgical clinical experiences and the persistent focus on psychomotor tasks
and skills as the driver of nursing work. There is no evidence that a nursing student's
disability compromises patient safety. Research findings indicate the opposite is true

as students with disabilities find safe ways to compensate for limitations (Gonzales & Hsiao, 2020).

As noted previously, the faculty's legal responsibility involves implementing the assigned accommodations provided by disability services which can include creative problem-solving. The disability services officer may need help understanding the nature of the work and learning the student will undertake in the clinical learning environment. Horkey (2019) indicates flexibility is key to successfully accommodating students in the clinical environment. They also suggest accommodations may need to be redesigned with each new clinical environment as procedures may be variable based on the characteristics of the physical environment. Additionally, accommodations may change as the student progresses in the program as the student may not have enough clinical experience to anticipate what is needed as the level of care provided becomes more complex and advances. Horkey (2019) also suggests faculty collaborate with the clinical environment to develop strategies needed to provide reasonable accommodations. Whenever, possible accommodations should be tested in a safe environment, such as the lab and simulation environment, before being implemented in the clinical setting (Hokey, 2019).

Universal Design for Learning

Universal design instruction (UDI) aims to enhance educational opportunities for all learners by meeting the needs of diverse learners and providing learning activities addressing multiple senses (auditory, visual, and kinesthetic) as students engage in developing nursing knowledge and skilled know-how (Coffman & Draper, 2022). Chapters 5 and 6 in this text provide a foundational discussion of universal design for learning and how its incorporation as a framework in a nursing education program can promote an inclusive learning environment for all students including students with disabilities.

PROGRAM REGULATION AND ACCREDITATION
Background

Nursing education requires investment from multiple stakeholders. Schools and universities invest significant resources to provide quality curricula and instruction provided by nursing faculty, dedicated to the dual responsibility of educating students, who design inclusive quality learning experiences and assure students practice safely with high-quality nursing care in a variety of settings. Clinical partners contribute to nursing education programs through the provision of learning environments that allow students to practice and learn in a psychologically safe setting, and they facilitate time and resources for staff to contribute to the students' clinical learning. Finally, and perhaps most importantly, students and their families dedicate time, financial resources, and extraordinary personal commitment to a program of study designed to prepare learners competent to practice as a professional registered nurse. Regulatory bodies in each state and accreditation organizations provide the standards to which nursing education programs must incorporate with the aim to provide a quality education that adheres to nursing practice standards.

Systematic Plan for Evaluation

In Chapter 2 we describe regulatory and accreditation agencies that address nursing education. Developing and implementing a systematic plan for evaluation is a standard that must be addressed for regulatory approval and to attain accreditation (Oermann 2023). The purpose of developing and implementing a systematic plan for evaluation is to engage the faculty and university in a continuous cycle of improvement. Oermann (2023) explains:

> Program evaluation is a systematic process of collecting data for making decisions about a nursing program and judging its value . . . With evaluation that is done continuously, faculty, administrators, and other stakeholders learn what is working well in their nursing program and where changes are needed to improve quality and outcomes. (p. 1)

Schools are required to develop a self-study every 8 to 10 years that is submitted to regulatory and accrediting organizations. The regulatory and accreditation process should not begin with writing a self-study that addresses how standards are met and end with the follow-up peer site visit. The process requires programs to develop and maintain a systematic plan for evaluation to assure program challenges and problems are identified early, and strengths can be enhanced. Meeting the accreditation standards for program evaluation includes demonstrating and documenting how data was to make program improvements. In summary, the accrediting process and standards are designed to promote an evidence-based cycle of using data to make quality improvements. Table 18.3 lists the areas of assessments that are addressed in regulatory and accreditation self-studies (Oermann, 2023).

TABLE 18.3

Assessment Areas for Accreditation

USDE Educational Standards	Examples of Evidence
Student achievement	NCLEX pass rate, clinical evaluation, employment rates, program completion rates
Curricula	Curriculum documents demonstrating alignment, course syllabus, evaluation methods
Faculty	Evidence of faculty qualification (e.g., RN, license, academic transcripts) Faculty satisfaction surveys
Facilities equipment and supplies	Description of classroom, lab, and clinical facilities. Annual equipment and supply budgets and record of purchases.
Fiscal and administrative capacity	Organizational chart, annual budget documents
Student support services	Description of available student support services, awarded financial aid, student satisfaction surveys
Policies about advertising and publications	Catalog and websites. Marketing materials used to recruit
Records of student complaints	Documentation of student complaints, including responses

Program outcome assessment and assessment of end-of-program student learning outcomes or terminal competencies are critical components of a systematic plan of evaluation (Al-Alawi & Alexander, 2020; Beasley et al., 2018). Program outcome data points include but are not limited to NCLEX pass rates, program completion rates, and post-graduation employment rates (Nunn-Ellison et al., 2018). The data required for each accreditation agency varies and programs also may include program satisfaction surveys completed by students at the end of the program and employer satisfaction with new graduates.

Assessing how students demonstrate they have met the end of the program student learning outcomes (EPSLOs), often referred to as terminal competencies is complex and uses multiple sources of data. NCLEX pass rates are used to measure some EPSLOs. Aggregate data mined from final clinical evaluations and capstone projects are also common measures and each program can identify what measures they want to use (Al-Alawi & Alexander, 2020; Beasley et al., 2018). The classroom nurse educator may not be directly involved in developing, implementing, and reporting on the systematic plan for evaluation. However, faculty and students contribute to the collection of data used in the plan for evaluation. Faculty are expected to understand the plan, contribute data, and use the results toward improvement. When clinical evaluations and capstone projects are used for learning outcome, evaluation using best practices in grading and learning assessment is critical to assuring the systematic plan for evaluation is a quality process and yields results that can be used for program improvement. We encourage faculty to become familiar with their program's systematic program assessment, and participate and use the data collected and analyzed to improve their practice as a nurse educator.

CHAPTER SUMMARY

Nurse educators fulfill a complex role that must balance the goals of facilitating inclusive quality learning experiences that address the unique instructional needs of each student with assuring graduates have the competencies needed to provide safe, quality care. The QSEN competencies provide a framework for assessing the facets of quality and safe nursing care. Just culture assures students have the opportunity to develop competency without fear of reprisal for the inevitability of being involved in human and/or system errors. The dual application of QSEN competencies and just culture will promote a safe, productive learning environment that prepares high-quality graduates.

As the nursing profession strives to become a more inclusive, diverse workforce, SWD needs improved access to nursing education. Historically this population has been excluded from nursing education due to concerns about safety. There is no evidence that disabled students have safety violations more than other students. However, there is evidence outcomes for patients who are disabled improves when cared for by clinicians with disabilities. Nurse educators must work with the degree-granting institution's disability services and clinical partners to facilitate meaningful learning for SWD and to provide and facilitate assigned accommodations that will contribute to student success.

Regulatory and accreditation agencies provide standards that nursing education programs are required to meet. Programs are required to create systematic plans for evaluation of standards and results should be used to assure there is a continuous cycle of assessment and improvement. Nursing faculty contribute to collecting and analyzing data and use results to improve their practice as educators.

References

Al-Alawi, R., & Alexander, G. L. (2020). Systematic review of program evaluation in baccalaureate nursing programs. *Journal of Professional Nursing, 36*(4), 236–244. https://doi.org/j.profnurs/2019.003

American Association of Colleges of Nursing. (n.d.). *Accommodating Students with Disabilities*. https://www.aacnnursing.org/Education-Resources/Tool-Kits/Accommodating-Students-with-Disabilities

Armstrong, G. (2019). QSEN safety competency: The key ingredient is just culture. *The Journal of Continuing Education in Nursing, 50*(10), 445–447. https://doi.org/10.3928/00220124-20190917-05

Barkell, N. P., & Snyder, S. S. (2021). Just culture in healthcare: An integrative review. *Nursing Forum, 56*(1), 103–111. https://doi.org/10.1111/nuf.12525

Barnsteiner, G., Disch, J., Johnson, M., & Spector, N. (2023). Applying principles of a fair and just culture to a student scenario. *Journal of Nursing Education, 62*(3), 139–145. https://doi.org/10.3928/01484834-20230109-03

Barnsteiner, J., & Disch, J. (2017). Creating a fair and just culture in schools of nursing. *The American Journal of Nursing, 117*(11), 42–48. https://doi.org/10.1097/01.NAJ.0000526747.84173.97

Beasley, S. F., Farmer, S., Ard, N., & Nunn-Ellison, K. (2018). Systematic plan of evaluation Part I: Assessment of end-of-program student learning outcomes. *Teaching and Learning in Nursing, 13*, 3–8. https://doi.org/1016/jteln.2017.09.003

Coffman, S., & Draper, C. (2022). Universal design for learning in higher education. *Teaching and Learning in Nursing, 17*, 36–41. https://doi.org/1016/j.teln.2021.07.009

Cronenwett, L., Sherwood, G., Barnsteiner, J., Disch, J., Johnson, J., Mitchell, P., Sullivan, D. T., & Warren, J. (2007). Quality and Safety Education for Nurses. *Nursing Outlook, 55*(3), 122–131. https://doi.org/10.1016/j.outlook.2007.02.006

Disch, J., Barnsteiner, J., Connor, S., & Brogren, F. (2017). Exploring how schools of nursing handle student errors and near misses. *American Journal of Nursing, 117*(10), 24–31.

Elting, J. K., Avit, E., & Gordon, R. (2021). Nursing faculty perceptions regarding students with physical disabilities. *Nurse Educator, 46*(4), 225–229. https://doi.org/10.1097/NNE.0000000000000940

Englund, H. M., & Lancaster, R. J. (2022). Difference in Marginality between nursing students with and without disabilities. *Journal of Nursing Education, 6*(8), 429–437. https://doi.org/10.3928/01484834-20220602-03

Epstein, I., Khanlou, N., Ermel, R. E., Sherk, M., Simmonds, K. K., Balaquiao, L., & Chang, K. Y. (2021). Students who identify with a disability and instructors' experiences in nursing practice: A scoping review. *International Journal of Mental Health and Addiction, 19*, 91–118. https://doi.org/10.1007/s11469-019-00129-7

Fey, M. K., Roussin, C. J., Rudolph J. W., Morse, K. J., Palaganas, J. C., & Szyld, D. (2022). Teaching, coaching or debriefing "With Good Judgment" across the simzones. *Advances in Simulation, 7*, 39. https://doi.org/10.1186/s41077-022-00235-y

Gonzalez, H. C., & Hasiao, E. L. (2020). Disability inclusion in nursing education. *Teaching and Learning in Nursing, 15*, 53–56. https://doi.org/1016/j.teln.2019.08.012

Hassmiller, S. B., & Wakefield, M. (2022). The future of nursing 2020–2030: Charting a path to achieve health equity. *Nursing*

Outlook, *70*, S1–S9. https://doi.org/
10.1066/j.outlook.2022.05.013

Horkey, E. (2019). Reasonable accommodation
implementation in clinical nursing education:
A scoping review. *Nursing Education Perspectives*, *40*(4), 205–209. https://doi.org/
10.1097/01.NEP.0000000000000469

Institute of Medicine. (1999). *To err is human:
Building a safer health care system. Execu-
tive summary*. The National Academies
Press.

Institute of Medicine. (2003). *Health profession
education: A bridge to quality*. The National
Academies Press.

Marks, B., & McCulloh, K. (2016). Success for
students and nurses with disabilities: A call
to action for nurse educators. *Nurse Educator*, *41*(1), 9–12. https://doi.org/10.1097/
NNE.0000000000000212

Marks, B., & Sisirak, J. (2022). Nurses with
Disability: Transforming Healthcare for All.
Online Journal of Issues in Nursing, *27*(3),
1–16.

Marx, D. (2019). Patient safety and the just
culture. *Obstetrics and Gynecology Clinics
of North America*, *46*, 239–245.

May, K. A. (2014). Nursing faculty knowledge
of the Americans With Disabilities Act.
Nurse Educator, *39*(5), 241–245. https://doi.
org/10.1097/NNE.0000000000000058

NCSBN. (n.d.). *Template for Debriefing Following a Student Error using Reflection
and Quality and Safety Competencies*.
Retrieved from https://www.ncsbn.org/
public-files/Student_Error_Debriefing_
Template.pdf

NCSBN. (2012). *Root cause analysis steps*.
Retrieved from https://www.ncsbn.org/
public-files/Root_Cause_Analysis_Steps.pdf

NCSBN. *About U.S. regulatory bodies*.
https://www.ncsbn.org/nursing-regula-
tion/about-nursing-regulatory-bodies.
page

NCSBN. Approval of nursing education
programs. https://www.ncsbn.org/nursing-
regulation/education/approval-of-nursing-
education-programs.page

NCSBN. (2021). *Safe student reports (SSR)
research study*. https://www.ncsbn.org/safe-
student-reports.htm

Neal-Boylan, L., & Miller, M. (2017). Treat
me like everyone else: The experience of
nurses who had a disability while in school.
Nurse Educator, *42*(4), 176–180. https://doi.
org/10.1097/NNE.0000000000000348

Neal-Boylan, L., & Miller, M. (2020). How inclusive are we, really? *Teaching and Learning in
Nursing*, *15*(4), 237–240.

North Carolina Board of Nursing. (2022). Just
Culture/SPEET. Retrieved from https://www.
ncbon.com/education-resources-for-program-
directors-just-culture-information

Nunn-Ellison, K., Ard, N., Beasley, S., &
Farmer, S. (2018). Systematic plan of evaluation Part II: Assessment of end-of-program
student learning outcomes. *Teaching and
Learning in Nursing*, *13*, 113–118.
https://doi.org/1016/jteln.2017.11.001

Oermann, M. (2023). *A systematic approach
to evaluation of nursing programs* (2nd ed.).
United States: National League for Nursing.

Petschonek, D., Burlison, J., Cross, C.,
Martin, K., Laver, J., Landis, R. S., &
Hoffman, J. M. (2013). Development of
the just culture assessment tool (JCAT):
Measuring the perceptions of healthcare
professionals in hospitals. *Journal of
Patient Safety, 9*(4), 190–197.

QSEN Institute. (n.d.). The evolution of the Quality and Safety Education for Nurses (QSEN)
Initiative. Retrieved from https://qsen.org/
about-qsen/project-overview/

Silvestre, J. H., & Spector, N. (2023). Nursing
student errors and near misses: Three
years of data. *The Journal of Nursing Education*, *62*(1), 12–19. https://doi.org/10.3928/
01484834-20221109-05

Sumpter, D., Blodgett, N., Beard, K., & Howard,
V. (2022). Transforming nursing education in
response to the Future of Nursing 2020–2030
report. *Nursing Outlook, 70*, S20–S31.
https://doi.org/10.1016/j.outlook.2022.02.007

Tanz, M. (2018). Improving safety knowledge,
skills, and attitudes with a good catch
program and student-designed simulation. *Journal of Nursing Education*, *57*(6),
379–384. https://doi.org/10.3928/01484834-
20180522-11

U.S. Department of Office of Health & Human
Services, Inspector General. (2022). *Adverse*

events in hospitals: A quarter of Medicare patients experienced harm in October 2018. https://oig.hhs.gov/oei/reports/OEI-06-18-00400.pd

Walker, D., Altmiller, G., Hromadik, L., Barkell, N., Barker, N., Boyd, T., Compton, M., Cook, P., Curia, M., Hays, D., Flexner, R., Jordan, J., Jowell, V., Kaulback, M., Magpantay-Monroe, E., Rudolph, B., Toothaker, R., Vottero, B., & Wallace, S. (2019). Nursing students' perceptions of just culture in nursing programs: A multisite study. *Nurse Educator*, *45*(3), 133–138. https://doi.org/10.1097/NNE.0000000000000739

Walker, D., Barkell, N., & Dodd, C. (2023). Error and near miss reporting in nursing education: The journey of two programs. *Teaching and Learning in Nursing*, *18*, 197–203. https://doi.org/10.1016/j.teln.2022.10.001

Walker, S. Y. (2019). Courage in clinical instruction part II: Protecting patients while assuring due process. *Teaching and Learning in Nursing Education*, *14*, 312–313. https://doi.org/10.1016/j.teln.2019.06.012

Walker, S. Y. (2021). Due process in nursing education: Reprise. *Teaching and Learning in Nursing Education*, *16*, 189–190. https://doi.org/10.1016/j.teln.2021.01.002